GW01145431

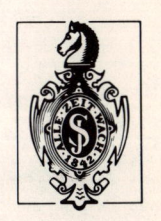

Current Concepts in Critical Care

Already published in the Series:

Shock and the Adult Respiratory Distress Syndrome
Edited by W. Kox and D. Bihari

Imaging and Labelling Techniques in the Critically Ill
Edited by W. Kox, J. Boultbee and R. Donaldson

With the compliments of

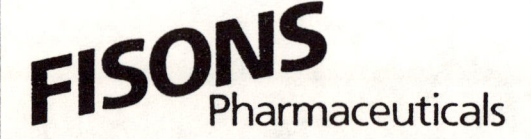

FISONS Pharmaceuticals

David Bihari and Guy Neild (eds.)

Acute Renal Failure in the Intensive Therapy Unit

With 63 Figures

Springer-Verlag
London Berlin Heidelberg New York
Paris Tokyo Hong Kong

David Bihari, MA, MRCP
Director of Intensive Care Services, Department of Intensive Care,
Guy's Hospital, St Thomas St, London SE1 9RT, UK

Guy Neild, MD, FRCP
Senior Lecturer in Nephrology, Department of Renal Medicine,
Institute of Urology, UCMSM, St Philip's Hospital, Sheffield St,
London WC2A 2EX, UK

ISBN 3-540-19588-2 Springer-Verlag Berlin Heidelberg New York
ISBN 0-387-19588-2 Springer-Verlag New York Berlin Heidelberg

British Library Cataloguing in Publication Data
Acute renal failure in the intensive therapy unit.
  1. Man. Kidneys. Acute Failure & Chronic Renal Failure
    I. Bihari, David, *1954–*   II. Neild, Guy, *1948–*   II. Series
616.6'14
ISBN 3-540-19588-2

Library of Congress Cataloging-in-Publication Data
Acute renal failure in the intensive therapy unit/David Bihari and Guy Neild (eds.).
  p. cm. – (Current concepts in critical care)
  Based on workshop held in Avignon, France in Sept., 1988, sponsored by Fisons PLC.
  Includes bibliographical references.
  ISBN 0-387-19588-2
  1. Acute renal failure – Congresses. 2. Critical care medicine – Congresses. I. Bihari, David, 1954– . II. Neild, Guy, 1948–. III. Fisons Limited. IV. Series
[DNLM: 1. Critical Care – methods – congresses. 2. Intensive Care Units – congresses. 3. Kidney Failure, Acute – therapy – congresses. WJ 342 A18955 1988]
RC918.R4A345 1990
616.6'14 – dc20
DNLM/DLC
for Library of Congress   89-21930
                                                                                        CIP

Apart from any fair dealing for the purposes of research or private study, or criticism or review, as permitted under the Copyright, Designs and Patents Act, 1988, this publication may only be reproduced, stored or transmitted, in any form or by any means, with the prior permission in writing of the publishers, or in the case of reprographic reproduction in accordance with the terms of licences issued by the Copyright Licensing Agency. Enquiries concerning reproduction outside those terms should be sent to the publishers.

© Springer-Verlag Berlin Heidelberg 1990
Printed in Great Britain

The use of registered names, trademarks etc. in this publication does not imply, even in the absence of a specific statement, that such names are exempt from the relevant laws and regulations and therefore free for general use.

Product Liability: The publisher can give no guarantee for information about drug dosage and application thereof contained in this book. In every individual case the respective user must check its accuracy by consulting other pharmaceutical literature.

Filmset by Wilmaset, Birkenhead, Wirral
Printed by The Alden Press, Osney Mead, Oxford, UK
2128/3916-593210   Printed on acid-free paper

This book is dedicated to the memory of Dr. Paul Noone – a gifted and valued colleague who is sorely missed

Preface

There is, today, some concern within the medical community that whilst there has been an enormous proliferation of meetings and publications in various fields of clinical investigation, this has not been accompanied to the same extent by any great benefit for patients. Thus, whilst doctors and clinical scientists meet around the world and discuss what they consider to be the important issues, little of this erudition is translated directly into improvements in care, and patients continue to die from their underlying disease. This may sound a little cynical but is particularly true of patients who develop acute renal failure in the Intensive Therapy Unit. It is often said of these patients that rates of survival have not substantially changed over the last 40 years.

Some would say that one of the great achievements of modern-day surgical practice and peri-operative care has been the reduction in prevalence of acute renal failure associated with biliary, aortic and cardiac surgery. Renal "protection" (volume loading, mannitol, low-dose dopamine, loop diuretics) in the Intensive Therapy Unit remains a contentious issue but has obviously contributed in some way to the falling prevalence in these cases. Other than volume loading, it has been difficult to judge the efficacy of the available strategies, particularly in the more complicated patients with sepsis or trauma and other organ failure.

Whilst the incidence of acute renal failure is indeed probably falling, and the spectrum of cases undoubtedly changing from the young and previously healthy to the elderly, infected and chronically diseased, renal replacement therapy is one of the most rapidly evolving aspects of intensive care. Yet, it continues to be fraught with difficulties, not least in the nomenclature and abbreviations (PD, HD, CAVH, CVVH, CAVHD, CVVHD, CUPID) used to describe the techniques available. Physicians who attend in the Intensive Therapy Unit have three specific "gut" feelings about patients who develop renal failure: first, it is a bad thing and is best prevented. Second, it is better to have patients passing some urine than no urine at all since fluid balance is easier and the patient tends not to die from pulmonary oedema nor hyperkalaemia. For this reason, many physicians would attempt to convert oliguric acute renal failure into the polyuric form by the administration of large doses of frusemide together with low-dose dopamine and mannitol. Finally, it would seem that these patients require some sort of aggressive nutritional support and they should receive dialysis (or whatever) so that this can be achieved. Whilst no-one would seriously question the first principle, there are few data to support the second and third suppositions. Yet, their practice remains ubiquitous in the Intensive Care Unit and, as usual in medicine, the development and strength of expression of an opinion concerning the efficacy of a treatment directly reflects the absence of any convincing objective data, one way or another. So often, *ex cathedra* statements are made concerning the importance of mannitol, low-dose dopamine or branched-chain amino acids as if there was a mass of evidence to justify their use routinely.

For these reasons, we were convinced that the subject "Acute Renal Failure in the Intensive Therapy Unit" required an extensive and lengthy airing in the setting of a small closed workshop of invited experts. At the same time, we were somewhat hesitant of convening such a meeting. Again, our concern centred upon the possible conclusions of such a workshop and whether any worthwhile contribution could be made in terms of understanding the pathogenesis of the condition and improving patient care. There are many standard texts available on acute renal failure and there have been a number of excellent editorials published recently in leading journals. There are regular large symposia in North America and Europe at which new data can be presented. We did not want to produce another set of *ex cathedra* statements to confuse busy clinicians. Nevertheless, the quest for some sort of "consensus" amongst nephrologists and specialists in intensive care from around the world was thought to be unusual enough to deserve support. Our hope was that it might lead to some new ideas and a different perspective on pathogenesis, prevention and treatment. Thus, with some trepidation, we convened a workshop in Avignon, France in September 1988, most kindly sponsored by Fisons PLC, UK and organized by Mr Philip White, Fisons PLC.

This book is the direct result of that meeting and contains much of the thought and discussion that went on in Avignon. Original research papers pertinent to the subject are mixed with reviews of specific issues. As usual, a publication of this nature can never hope to be definitive but reflects the interests of the editors and their contributors. Inevitably, there has been some duplication of content but each group of authors contributes their own perspective to a difficult subject. Whilst the reader has to judge for himself, we believe that the group has achieved a clear expression of both the conventional and some novel ideas regarding pathogenesis and management. They have highlighted those areas of which little is known and which require further investigation. What about the patients – will they benefit from this corporate endeavour? Sadly, in the short term, probably not! What is apparent is that there are no magic solutions to the problem of established acute renal failure in the Intensive Therapy Unit. But if we have stimulated the reader to think about the problem and the questions which inevitably arise from that thought, we do the subject a service and sooner or later, the patient will benefit.

London
March 1989

David Bihari
Guy Neild

Contents

List of Contributors xv

SECTION I: Definitions and Epidemiology

1 Acute Renal Failure in the ITU: The Nephrologist's View
  J. S. Cameron 3

2 Epidemiology of Acute Renal Failure in France Today
  D. Kleinknecht 13

3 Acute Renal Failure and Sepsis: A Microbiologist's View
  P. Noone 23

4 Acute Renal Failure at a Crossroads
  K. Solez and L. C. Racusen 35

5 Acute Renal Failure in Old Age
  J. F. Macias 41

SECTION II: Some Aspects of Renal Physiology

6 Cortical and Juxtamedullary Glomerular Blood Flow After Temporary Ischaemia
  M. Steinhausen, M. Fretschner, E. Gulbins and N. Parekh   47

7 Are Atrial Pressures Involved in the Regulation of Sodium and Water Balance? Studies in Conscious Animals
  G. Kaczmarczyk, E. Schmidt, K. Falke and
  H. W. Reinhardt 59

SECTION III: Pathogenesis of Acute Renal Failure in the Intensive Therapy Unit

8 Endothelial and Mesangial Cell Dysfunction in Acute Renal Failure
  G. H. Neild 77

9 Role of the Medulla in Acute Renal Failure
   P. H. Epstein, M. Brezis and S. Rosen 91

10 Ischaemic Acute Renal Failure in an Intact Animal Model
   P. J. Ratcliffe, Z. H. Endre, J. D. Tange and
   J. G. G. Ledingham 103

11 Eicosanoids and Acute Renal Failure
   A. Schieppati and G. Remuzzi 115

12 Disturbances in Renal Function Associated with Hepatic Dysfunction
   J. M. Lopez-Novoa 131

13 A Review of Mediators and the Hepatorenal Syndrome
   K. Moore, V. Parsons, P. Ward and R. Williams 143

14 Drug-Induced Acute Renal Failure
   A. L. Linton 157

15 Nature of Postischaemic Renal Injury Following Aortic or Cardiac Surgery
   B. D. Myers 167

16 Acute Renal Failure in Sepsis
   A. L. Linton 181

SECTION IV: Clinical Features of Acute Renal Failure in the Intensive Therapy Unit

17 Strategies in Management of Acute Renal Failure in the Intensive Therapy Unit
   R. W. Schrier, W. T. Abraham and J. Hensen 193

18 Acute Renal Failure and Crush Injury
   O. S. Better 215

19 Renal Function After Open Heart Surgery
   H. M. Koning and J. A. Leusink 223

20 Acute Renal Failure Following Heart and Heart–Lung Transplantation
   M. E. Rogerson, G. H. Neild and F. D. Thompson 235

21 Bleeding in Acute Renal Failure
   K. Andrassy 243

22 Mechanisms of Uraemic Encephalopathy
   A. I. Arieff and C. L. Fraser 255

23 Measuring Severity of Illness
J. Bion 269

SECTION V: Strategies in Management of Acute Renal Failure

24 Prophylaxis of Acute Renal Failure in the Intensive Care Unit
J. M. Lazarus 279

25 Appropriate Renal Support in the Management of Acute Renal and Respiratory Failure: Does Early Aggressive Treatment Improve the Outcome?
K. Simpson, M. Travers and M. Allison 311

26 The Role of Spontaneous and Pumped Haemofiltration
J. C. Mason 319

27 Renal Replacement Therapy in the ICU: Approaches in Switzerland
P. M. Suter, R. Malacrida, M. Levy and H. Favre 331

28 Anticoagulation and Extracorporeal Circuits: The Role of Prostacyclin
M. J. Weston 337

29 Nutritional Support in Acute Renal Failure in the Critically Ill
R. A. Little, I. T. Campbell, C. J. Green, R. Kishen and S. Waldek... 347

30 The Prevention of Severe Combined Acute Respiratory and Renal Failure in the Intensive Therapy Unit
D. J. Bihari 359

Subject Index 387

Contributors

W. T. Abraham, MD
Department of Medicine, University of Colorado School of Medicine,
Denver, Colorado 80262, USA

Marjorie Allison, MD, FRCP
Renal Unit, Glasgow Royal Infirmary, Glasgow, UK

K. Andrassy, MD
Klinikum der Universität Heidelberg, Sektion Nephrologie,
Bergheimerstrasse 56A, 6900 Heidelberg 1, West Germany

A. I. Arieff, MD, FACP
Geriatrics Section, Veterans Administration Medical Center,
University of California School of Medicine, 4150 Clement St,
San Francisco, California 94121, USA

O. S. Better, MD
Faculty of Medicine, Technicon, Israel Institute of Technology, and
Department of Nephrology, Rambam Hospital, Haifa 35254,
31096 Israel

D. J. Bihari, MA, MRCP
Department of Intensive Care, Guy's Hospital, London SE1 9RT, UK

J. Bion, MBBS, MRCP, FFARCS
Department of Anaesthetics and Intensive Care,
University of Birmingham, and Queen Elizabeth Hospital,
Birmingham B15 2TH, UK

M. Brezis, MD
The Charles A. Dana Research Institute,
Harvard-Thorndike Laboratory of Beth Israel Hospital,
Departments of Medicine and Pathology, Harvard Medical School
and Beth Israel Hospital, Boston, MA 02215, USA

J. S. Cameron, MD, FRCP
Department of Renal Medicine, Clinical Science Laboratories,
Guy's Hospital, London SE1 9RT, UK

I. T. Campbell, MB
University Department of Anaesthesia, Royal Liverpool Hospital,
Liverpool, UK

Z. H. Endre, MD
Nuffield Department of Clinical Medicine, John Radcliffe Hospital,
Oxford OX3 9DU, UK

F. H. Epstein, MD
The Charles A. Dana Research Institute,
Harvard-Thorndike Laboratory of Beth Israel Hospital,
Departments of Medicine and Pathology, Harvard Medical School
and Beth Israel Hospital, Boston, MA 02215, USA

K. Falke, MD
Institute of Anaesthesiology and Operative Intensive Medicine,
Free University of Berlin, Klinikum Rudolf-Virchow,
Standort Charlottenburg, Berlin, West Germany

H. Favre, MD
Divisions des Soins Intensifs de Néphrologie,
Départements d'Anaesthesiologie et de Médicine,
Hôpital Cantonal 1211 Geneva 4, Switzerland

C. L. Fraser, MD
Geriatrics Section, Department of Medicine,
Veterans Administration Medical Center and
University of California School of Medicine, San Francisco,
California 94121, USA

M. Fretschner, MD
Physiologisches Institut der Universität Heidelberg,
Heidelberg, West Germany

C. J. Green, MD
University Department of Anaesthesia, Royal Liverpool Hospital,
Liverpool, UK

E. Gulbins, MD
Physiologisches Institut der Universität Heidelberg,
Heidelberg, West Germany

J. Hensen, MD
Department of Medicine, University of Colorado School of Medicine,
Denver, Colorado 80262, USA

G. Kaczmarczyk, MD
Institute of Anaesthesiology and Operative Intensive Medicine,
Free University of Berlin, Klinikum Rudolf-Virchow,
Standort Charlottenburg, Berlin, West Germany

R. Kishen, MB
North Western Injury Research Centre, Intensive Therapy Unit,
Hope Hospital, Salford, UK

D. Kleinknecht, MD
Service de Néphrologie et de Reanimation Polyvalente,
Centre Hospitalier, 56 Boulevard de la Boissiere, 93105 Montreuil,
France

H. M. Koning, MD
Medisch Centrum Department Anaesthesiology, Leeuwarden,
The Netherlands

J. M. Lazarus, MD
End-Stage Renal Disease Program, Brigham and Women's Hospital,
Harvard Medical School and Harvard Center for the Study of
Kidney Diseases, Boston, MA 02215, USA

J. G. G. Ledingham, DM, FRCP
Nuffield Department of Clinical Medicine, John Radcliffe Hospital,
Oxford OX3 9DU, UK

J. A. Leusink, MD
St Antonius Ziekenhuis,
Department of Anaesthesiology and Intensive Care,
Nieuwegein/Utrecht, The Netherlands

M. Levy, MD
Divisions des Soins Intensifs de Néphrologie,
Départements d'Anaesthesiologie et de Médicine, Hôpital Cantonal,
1211 Geneva 4, Switzerland

A. L. Linton, MB, FRCP, FRCPC
Department of Medicine, Victoria Hospital, 375 South St, London,
Ontario N6A 4GS, Canada

R. A. Little, PhD, MRCPath
North Western Injury Research Centre, University of Manchester,
Hope Hospital, Salford M6 8HD, UK

J. M. Lopez-Novoa, MD
Consejo Superior de Investigaciones Cientificas,
Renal Physiopathology Laboratory, Medical Research Institute,
Fundacion Jiminez Diaz, Avenida Reyes Catolicos 2, 28040 Madrid,
Spain

J. F. Macias, MD, PhD
Ministerio de Sanidad y Consumo, Instituto Nacional de la Salud,
Hospital Clinico Universitario, 37007-Salamanca, Spain

R. Malacrida, MD
Divisions des Soins Intensifs de Chirurgie,
Départements d'Anaesthesiologie et de Médicine, Hôpital Cantonal,
1211 Geneva 4, Switzerland

J. C. Mason, MD, MRCP
Wessex Regional Renal Unit, St Mary's Hospital, Milton Road,
Portsmouth PO3 6AD, UK

K. Moore, MRCP
Liver Unit, King's College Hospital School of Medicine and
Dentistry, Denmark Hill, London SE5 9RS, UK

B. D. Myers, MB, MRCP
Division of Nephrology, Stanford University Medical Center,
Stanford, California 94305, USA

G. H. Neild, MD, FRCP
Department of Renal Medicine, Institute of Urology,
St Philip's Hospital, Sheffield St, London WC2A 2EX, UK

P. Noone, MB, FRCPath
Department of Microbiology, Royal Free Hospital,
London NW3 2QG, UK

N. Parekh, MD
Physiologisches Institut der Universität Heidelberg, Heidelberg,
West Germany

V. Parsons, DM, FRCP
Renal Unit, King's College Hospital School of Medicine and
Dentistry, Denmark Hill, London SE5 9RS, UK

L. C. Racusen, MD
Department of Pathology, Johns Hopkins School of Medicine,
Baltimore, MD, USA

P. J. Ratcliffe, MRCP
Nuffield Department of Clinical Medicine, John Radcliffe Hospital,
Oxford OX3 9DU, UK

H. W. Reinhardt, MD
Institute of Anaesthesiology and Operative Intensive Medicine,
Free University of Berlin, Klinikum Rudolf-Virchow,
Standort Charlottenburg, Berlin, West Germany

G. Remuzzi, MD
Division of Nephrology and Dialysis, Ospedali Riunti, Bergamo, and
Mario Negri Institute for Pharmacological Research,
via Gavazzani 11, 24100 Bergamo, Italy

M. E. Rogerson, MB, MRCP
Institute of Urology and St Peter's Hospitals, St Philip's Hospital,
Sheffield St, London WC2A 2EX, UK

S. Rosen, MD
The Charles A. Dana Research Institute,
Harvard-Thorndike Laboratory of Beth Israel Hospital,
Departments of Medicine and Pathology, Harvard Medical School
and Beth Israel Hospital, Boston, MA 02215, USA

A. Schieppati, MD
Division of Nephrology and Dialysis, Ospedali Riunti, Bergamo, and
Mario Negri Institute for Pharmacological Research, Bergamo, Italy

E. Schmidt, MD
Institute of Anaesthesiology and Operative Intensive Medicine,
Free University of Berlin, Klinikum Rudolf-Virchow,
Standort Charlottenburg, Berlin, West Germany

R. W. Schrier, MD
Department of Medicine, University of Colorado Medical Center,
Denver, Colorado 80262, USA

K. Simpson, MD, MRCP
Renal Unit, Glasgow Royal Infirmary, Glasgow, UK

K. Solez, MD
Department of Pathology, University of Alberta,
5B4 02WC Mackenzie Health Sciences Centre, Edmonton, Alberta,
Canada T6G 2R7

M. Steinhausen, MD
Physiologisches Institut der Universität Heidelberg,
Heidelberg D6900, West Germany

P. M. Suter, MD
Divisions des Soins Intensifs de Chirurgie,
Départements d'Anaesthesiologie et de Médicine, Hôpital Cantonal,
Universitaire de Geneve, 1211 Geneva 4, Switzerland

J. D. Tange, MD
Nuffield Department of Clinical Medicine, John Radcliffe Hospital,
Oxford OX3 9DU, UK

F. D. Thompson, MD, FRCP
Institute of Urology and St·Peter's Hospitals, St Philip's Hospital,
Sheffield St, London WC2A 2EX, UK

M. Travers, MB
Renal Unit, Glasgow Royal Infirmary, Glasgow, UK

S. Waldek, MD, FRCP
Department of Renal Medicine, Hope Hospital, Salford, UK

P. Ward, MD
Department of Clinical Pharmacology,
Royal Postgraduate Medical School, Du Cane Road, London, UK

M. J. Weston, MD, FRCP
Broomfield Hospital, Chelmsford, Essex CM1 5ET, UK

R. Williams, MD, FRCP
Liver Unit, King's College Hospital School of Medicine and
Dentistry, Denmark Hill, London SE5 9RS, UK

Section I
Definitions and Epidemiology

Chapter 1

Acute Renal Failure in the ITU: The Nephrologist's View

J. S. Cameron

Little has changed since I reviewed this topic two years ago (Cameron 1986), but it is useful to take the opportunity to expand on a few points of particular interest and importance: patient selection for admission to the ITU and the two types of acute renal failure (ARF) as seen by the nephrologist; the prevention of ARF; sepsis and catabolism in ARF; and how it's necessary to improve our ability to predict the outcome in individual patients with ARF.

Two Different Disorders: ARF, and ARF as Part of Multiple Organ Failure

Most renal units manage patients referred to them with isolated ARF in their own wards, where peritoneal dialysis (becoming less popular) or haemofiltration/CAVHD (becoming more popular) can cope with the problem almost indefinitely. These patients usually have ARF from "medical" causes: nephrotoxins, particularly drugs giving rise to interstitial nephritis (Cameron 1988), such as non-steroidal anti-inflammatory drugs; forms of glomerulonephritis (Cameron 1984), usually with crescent formation, or as a part of Goodpasture's syndrome of anti-GBM nephritis or vasculitis; or a mixed group of patients in whom rhabdomyolysis (Thomas and Ibels 1985) is increasingly recognized, sometimes of obscure origin.

Other groups of patients who usually do not receive treatment in the ITU are those with antibiotic-induced renal failure, particularly aminoglycosides, and ARF arising from gross mismanagement of electrolyte problems in patients, many of whom already have compromised renal function. Finally an increasing number of elderly patients are recognized to have severe nephrosclerosis and renal arterial disease, whose kidneys may fail suddenly because of occlusion of their better (or only) kidney because of atheromatous renal artery stenosis, or because angiotensin-converting enzyme (ACE) inhibitors such as captopril or enalapril have been administered (Silas et al. 1983). Mismatched blood transfusion and abortions have, in North America and Europe, now disappeared as causes of ARF in all but the exceptional case.

The prognosis for all these patients with isolated single organ ARF is good: collected European data suggest that only 8% die (Cameron 1986). Only pancreatitis (which often evolves into complicated renal failure with multi-system involvement) carries a high mortality. In hospitals in most Western countries, the main reason for referral to the ITU is a need for ventilation, which is rarely present in the patients listed above.

In sharp contrast are the patients – now the majority in most renal units – who have ARF as part of multiple organ failure, arising while they are already in hospital, either in medical or (more commonly) surgical wards, or already in the ITU. In these patients the ARF can be regarded in essence as an indicator of the severity of the underlying disease process(es). Here, the mortality remains implacably high around the 75% mark (Cameron 1986), in all units including our own (Table 1.1). Most of these patients develop ARF following complicated surgery. Naturally, treatment of a peripheral facet of the problem – the acute renal failure, uraemia and inability to regulate electrolyte homeostasis – will have little or no impact on the outcome beyond "purchasing" a period of time in which the underlying problems can be identified and corrected. Their severity and multiplicity means that failure remains usual, although one success story has been the virtual elimination of gastrointestinal haemorrhage as a cause of death, probably as much from better control of uraemia and better nutrition as from local strategies such as antacids and H_2 antagonists.

Table 1.1. Acute renal failure after surgery at Guy's Hospital 1964–1986

Analysis by	Period	Length (yr)	Treatment(s)[a]	n	Died	Mortality (%)	Ventilated		
							n	died	mortality (%)
Cameron	1964–67	3	PD/HD	62	40	65			
Stott	1968–73	4	HD/PD	109	67	62			
Brown	1969–73	3	HD/PD	73	45	62	22	20	91
Neild	1977–78	1	HD	28	14	50	21	15	71
Taube	1981–84	3	HD/HF	143[b]	91[b]	64[b]	29[c]	22[c]	76[c]
Smithies	1985–86	1	HD/HF/CAVHD	20	15	75	31	24	77

Notes: these are selected periods only from a total of 820 patients treated in 1964–86, 436 of whom arose following surgery. The series reported by Stott (1971) and Brown (1973) overlap.

[a] HD, haemodialysis; PD, peritoneal dialysis; HF, haemofiltration; CAVHD, continuous arteriovenous haemodialysis.

[b] All cases, including surgical.

[c] Data for 1984 only.

Thus for the nephrologist ARF in the ITU is a gloomy and exacting affair. The presence of only one other organ failed besides the kidney immediately raises the mortality to 75% or higher; as is well known, the presence of a third organ in failure takes mortality to between 90% and 100%, and almost no patients survive failure of four organs. Once ARF is established in a setting of sepsis, the need for ventilation, cardiovascular support, the development of liver failure, or coma or any combination of these, the ARF itself becomes a peripheral problem; even though in many ITU settings the nephrologist will now be in overall charge of the patient. These points are discussed in more detail in the final section. Given these circumstances, what is there to be done?

Prevention of ARF

Obviously the best solution would be to prevent patients ever going into ARF (Lazarus, Chapter 24). It is probable, but difficult to document, that a number of patients who would have gone into acute renal failure 20 years ago now escape this fate because they are better managed in the medical or surgical wards, or in the ITU. In a few areas such as cardiovascular surgery (Hilberman et al. 1979) data show that this is the case. However, no unit reports a decrease in the number of patients with ARF (Table 1.1). This may in turn result in patients now developing ARF who would have been abandoned without surgery a few years ago, particularly the elderly.

The factors which are preventable in the anticipation and early prevention of post-surgical acute renal failure have been discussed elsewhere (Cameron 1986; Smithies and Cameron 1989b). These include anticipation and early correction of electrolyte imbalance, recognition of pre-existing renal impairment, avoidance of nephrotoxic medical agents and drugs such as aminoglycosides, ACE inhibitors and NSAIDs, early restoration of circulating volume and cardiac output, and above all the early diagnosis and vigorous treatment of sepsis.

The role of pharmacological agents such as frusemide, dopamine or mannitol (Lazarus, Chapter 24) and calcium channel blockers (Schrier et al., Chapter 17) remains speculative. Certainly the vigorous and routine use of frusemide and dopamine seems to reverse the implacable advance of oliguria in a few patients; there is dispute as to the value of urinary electrolyte indices in predicting response (Schrier et al., Chapter 17; Espinel and Gregory 1980; Pru and Kjellstrand 1984) and in practice, by the time the nephrologist sees the patient they have almost always already received a diuretic, usually frusemide, so that the value of the urinary Na^+ concentration is vitiated. Also, it is difficult to separate the effects of these agents from those of concomitant volume replacement or other cardiovascular support. This is especially so for mannitol, which expands plasma volume and improves perfusion because it attracts water from the intracellular space into the extracellular space, by establishing an osmotic gradient.

Calcium channel blockers appear very promising, since defects in calcium translocation seem to be an early and central event in ischaemic injury to the renal tubules, focused on the thick ascending limb with its high energy requirement (Epstein 1985 and Chapter 9). The work of Schrier's group suggests that to be effective, verapamil must be infused directly into the kidney, as it is in preparing donor kidneys for transplantation (Shapiro et al. 1985). This involves renal artery catheterization, but this should give rise to no ethical or practical qualms in a condition with an unchecked mortality of 75% or more, if it gives an increased chance of prevention or earlier recovery. In addition, renal arterial and perhaps also renal venous catheterization in man could provide invaluable data on renal bloodflow, and on substrate delivery to and extraction by the kidney – rather than the whole patient (Bihari et al. 1987) which is all that is available at present. This cannot fail to increase our understanding of acute tubular necrosis.

Sepsis and ARF

Probably the most important single factor in patients with ARF, both as a cause and as a complication, is sepsis; yet a major recent nephrological text on acute renal failure (Brenner and Lazarus 1988) includes no chapter on post-surgical ARF, or on sepsis! The effects of sepsis on the kidney are still poorly understood (Wardle 1982; Clowes 1988), but there is little doubt that sepsis can lead directly to ARF. In patients already in established ARF, or in whom ARF is about to develop, blood cultures are often negative even when the patient appears clinically to be septicaemic. Some of this failure to identify pathogens relates to prior treatment with antibiotics, but more often treatment of sepsis is begun blind, without or before culture data, using broad-spectrum cover. Trials of passive immunization using anti-endotoxin antibody have been rather disappointing (Baumgartner et al. 1985), even though it has been suggested that it is just those patients who fail to develop such antibodies in early life who are prone to overwhelming Gram-negative sepsis later.

There is a strong clinical impression that most patients in ARF who develop infection do so from organisms already present in their own bowel, nares or other body crevices. Thus, given our failure to cope with established sepsis, it becomes attractive to try and "sterilize" the patient with a combination of prophylactic systemic broad-spectrum antibiotics, combined with bowel sterilization using non-absorbable antibiotics. This approach was first introduced by the Gronigen group (Stoutenbeek et al. 1984), and recently the trial in Glasgow (Ledingham et al. 1988) – although open to criticism (Editorial 1988; Bunney 1988; Noone 1988; Inglis 1988) – showed some benefit in severely ill patients, which includes all of the patients under discussion here. No doubt this approach will be studied further. Colonization of the upper gastrointestinal tract is facilitated by inhibition or neutralization of acid, and the net benefits of preventing haemorrhage in patients with ARF, and the relative value of sucralfate, have yet to be defined.

The treatment of sepsis in patients with ARF also deserves comment. There is profound immunosuppression in uraemia (Boulton-Jones et al. 1973), almost every phase of the immune response from antigen presentation to phagocytosis of opsonized organisms being deficient. Thus the patient is wide open to spreading or persisting infections of many types. Intra-abdominal sepsis, often following surgery rather than primary from a perforated viscus, has a particularly poor prognosis in a setting of ARF. It is difficult to diagnose, even more difficult to localize, and carries a very high mortality. Frequent exploration of the abdomen may be necessary for proper diagnosis and drainage (Milligan et al. 1978), but there is an increasing use of percutaneous drainage after localization using ultrasound, CAT scanning and labelled white cell scans, all of which have a role in helping to detect hidden sepsis.

Catabolism in ARF

Compared to other ITU patients, even allowing for sepsis and fever, patients in ARF are markedly catabolic. Until the need for intensive intravenous nutrition was recognized, they wasted visibly from day to day, and outcome seemed to be related to the degree of undernutrition (Giordano et al. 1978). What underlies this profound catabolism (Heidland et al. 1988)?

Extra factors present in uraemia are first, losses of amino acids during haemodialysis (6–8 g per dialysis) or haemofiltration; second (and much more important) additional catabolic factors specific to uraemia. These seem to relate principally to proteolytic enzymes circulating in uraemia, even when sepsis – a known cause of profound proteolysis (Clowes 1988) – is absent; catabolism is also related to raised intracellular proteolysis, particularly in muscle. This in turn may depend on prostaglandin release triggered by interleukin-1, on metabolic acidosis, and the action of glucocorticoids.

Measures to combat this state naturally include feeding large amounts of energy and protein/amino acids, and since this must almost always be done intravenously, the high filtration capacity of CAVH or CAVHD is useful in permitting this without problems of positive fluid balance. The better biocompatibility of the polyacrylonitrile or polysulphone membranes used in the newer techniques, compared with the cellulosic membranes used in conventional haemodialysis, may be of value in limiting neutrophil protease release. Bicarbonate to combat the catabolic effect of acidosis is better than acetate, which has its own toxicity and may not be adequately metabolized to bicarbonate in sick patients; the same is probably true for the lactate used in CAVH, as well as the known defect in liver failure. Protease inhibitors (such as leukopeptin or Ep 475) have been used only in experimental animals, but not in man – although of course fresh frozen plasma will augment levels of alpha-1 antitrypsin and alpha-2 macroglobulin. (Fresh frozen plasma also increases diminished concentrations of fibronectin, which may be an important factor in defence against infection, and is low in septic shock).

The Prediction of Outcome in Individual Cases of ARF

This topic, which is growing in importance, has been dealt with elsewhere (Smithies and Cameron 1989a) but the issues require further discussion.

The high cost, both in economic resources for the hospital service, together with the emotional distress and suffering for patients and relatives, makes better prediction of outcome an important priority. Also, if our management is to be ethical, we must not enter the vicious circle of commitment (Jennett 1985), applying yet further therapy simply because the last treatment failed. There is urgent need – which has been obvious for far too long – for methods of clinical scoring which allow accurate reproducible description, so that we can compare patient groups between studies and between centres. One of the main reasons for our failure to demonstrate progress is the failure of studies to provide information in a form which allows meaningful comparison, as Butkus (1983) has pointed out.

This problem has, of course, been studied closely in the field of general intensive care, in a literature which is too little known in nephrological circles. In recent years, clinical severity scoring systems such as the APACHE II system have allowed much improved description and comparison, and can predict outcome accurately in 80% of cases (Le Gall et al. 1984; Knaus et al. 1985; Chang et al. 1988). Studies of very large numbers of cases in intensive care units have resulted in generally applicable scores that, when weighted for previous health status and diagnostic category, do not lose predictive accuracy to any significant extent. In view of the multiplicity and wide range of causes of ARF, these general scores may be of use in the description and classification of patients with ARF, and warrant further study.

Reports of APACHE II scoring in use, however, suggest that its combination with diagnostic categories may not be as important as sequential scoring to document the response (or lack of it) to therapy, even over a short initial period (Chang et al. 1988); our own preliminary data in ARF (Smithies and Cameron, in preparation) support this contention. In general use, the modified APACHE II score has been reported to give a predictive power of 81% for survivors and 75% for non-survivors in assessing response to initial intensive therapy. This is not yet nearly good enough, of course, to permit ethical discontinuation of treatment in those who may die. Also, the APACHE II system is open to the criticism that the individual physiological scores which make it up were assigned on the basis of discussion, review of previous literature and consensus, rather than from the actual probability of survival in a defined series. As a result, other investigators have turned to multiple logistic regression of patient data to derive relative weight for (supposedly) relevant clinical features, to give an overall probability of death or survival (Lemeshow et al. 1985). Recently Liano et al. (1989) published the first such analysis on patients in ARF, using clinical data obtained at referral to the nephrological unit, and verified prospectively.

Of course, there are a number of previous studies of ARF using multivariate analysis to predict outcome (Cioffi et al. 1984; Lien and Chan 1985; Bullock et al. 1985; Rasmussen et al. 1985; Corwin et al. 1987), but not all have looked at status at referral with easily defined clinical factors (Lohr et al. 1988; Liano et al. 1989). As a result, each of these studies finds rather different clinical factors predictive of outcome. These are: previous state of health; age; clinical setting of the ARF; severity of ARF (oliguria vs no oliguria); complications and other organ failure. Subjectively derived scores such as APACHE II contain, of course, a number of these elements. One factor that multiple linear regression analyses revealed as important in prognosis of ARF was oliguria (urine output <500 ml 24 h^{-1}) vs. non-oliguria (urine output >1000 ml 24 h^{-1}), a point which was missed in the general ITU studies, but which had been recorded in previous series of "non-oliguric" ARF (Anderson et al. 1977; Minuth et al. 1976). This emphasizes that ARF may show different degrees of severity, with different outcomes perhaps relating more to the duration of the state of ARF but marked at presentation by urine volume.

The most striking feature, however, as mentioned above, was the importance of other organ system failure, particularly cardiac, respiratory and neurological. These did not contribute uniformly in all these studies, but their regular appearance suggests how important they are in determining prognosis. It underlines yet again that ARF as seen in the ITU is simply one manifestation of an underlying disease state which has led to multiple organ failure.

Therefore, one might suspect that simple univariate analysis of the number of failing organ systems, particularly in relation to duration, would predict outcome in ARF with some accuracy (Baue 1975; Pine et al. 1983; Fry et al. 1983; Knaus et al. 1985). The largest study was that of Knaus et al. (1985) and Knaus and Zimmerman (1988) of 5677 patients in ITU, including 2719 with organ system failure. Stringent criteria were used to define five organ failures: cardiovascular, respiratory, renal, haematological, and CNS – but not hepatic, which has a bad record if associated with ARF in almost all previous series. Two-organ system failure for more than one day increased the death rate to 60%, and three-organ failure for more than 3 days had a mortality of 92%, only two young, previously fit patients surviving in this category. It is important that future studies give clear comparable definitions of organ system failure, that hepatic failure be evaluated similarly, so that a common database can be developed.

The role of sepsis seems to all observers crucial in the outcome of ARF, but because of negative blood cultures it is difficult to assess. Sepsis may thus be "lost" in analyses such as those described above, even if its secondary effects such as cardiovascular collapse or respiratory distress may be present, and noted as such under these two separate headings. The picture is complicated further by the role of gut or hepatic failure in permitting translocation of organisms of endotoxin into the circulation (Wardle 1982; Clowes 1988), which may in turn lead to other organ failure. It is important that in any system to assess prognosis, sepsis is considered carefully at a clinical as well as a bacteriological level, and described such as in the grading system proposed by Elebute and Stoner (1983).

Another problem in assessment is the role of coma in predicting the outcome of ARF. How can this be assessed in the sedated, ventilated patient? In many units it has become a rare event when an ITU nephrology consultation precedes the patient being narcotized and ventilated, and too few doctors are aware that opiates accumulate in ARF (Ball et al. 1985). Obviously it is wise to give the patient the benefit of the doubt in assessing the CNS (Liano et al. 1989), especially if arrest of treatment is under consideration.

Conclusions

ARF provides a continuing challenge, but uraemia itself can already be treated effectively and indefinitely by dialysis, haemofiltration or CAVHD. It is clear that both nephrologists and intensivists must now regard ARF in the intensive care unit as a grave sign indicating – in almost all instances – that something is gravely amiss elsewhere, upon which patient outcome will depend. We should distinguish sharply, in our practice and in our writing and analysis of data, between ARF *per se* and ARF as part of multiple organ failure. The need for more accurate prognostic indices in ARF as seen in the ITU is urgent. Only when we have a proper database and a reliable method of assessment can we see whether or not any change in management is having an effect, and thus do sensible clinical trials.

It is already clear that a simple "one-off" assessment on referral is not accurate enough for clinical decisions (Smithies and Cameron 1989a; Chang et al. 1988; Smithies and Cameron in preparation; Knaus and Zimmerman 1988; Bion, Chapter 23) especially if withdrawal of treatment is to be considered; repeated assessment over as short a period as a few days may be all that is necessary, however, to reach the required level of certainty; at the moment we simply do not have the data to say. We all remember – perhaps too well – our exceptional patient or patients who survived despite the odds. Above all, we need, desperately, a basis on which to judge when treatment is futile, and further efforts will amount only to the bad management of a death.

References

Anderson RJ, Kinas SL, Berns AS et al. (1977) Non-oliguric acute renal failure. N Engl Med J 296: 1134–1138
Ball M, McQuay HJ, Moore RA et al. (1985) Renal failure and the use of morphine in intensive care. Lancet I: 784–786
Baue A (1975) Multiple progressive or systems failure – a syndrome of the 1970s. Arch Surg 110: 779–781
Baumgartner J-D, Glauser MP, McCutchan JA, Ziegler EJ, van Melle G, Klauber MR, Vogt M, Muehlen E, Luethy R, Chiolero R, Geroulanos S (1985) Prevention of gram-negative shock and death in surgical patients by antibody to endotoxin core glycolipid. Lancet II: 59–63
Bihari D, Smithies M, Gimson A, Tinker J (1987) The effects of prostacyclin on oxygen delivery and uptake in critically ill patients. N Engl J Med 317: 397–403
Boulton-Jones JM, Vick R, Cameron JS, Black PJ (1973) Immune responses in uremia. Clin Nephrol 1: 351–360
Brenner BM, Lazarus MG (eds) (1988) Acute renal failure, 2nd edn. Saunders, Philadelphia
Bullock ML, Umen AJ, Finkelstein M, Keane WF (1985) The assessment of risk factors in 462 patients with acute renal failure. Am J Kidney Dis 5: 97–103
Bunney RG (1988) Selective decontamination in intensive therapy units. Lancet I: 1388 (letter)
Butkus DE (1983) Persistent high mortality in acute renal failure. Are we asking the right questions? Arch Intern Med 143: 209–212
Cameron JS (1984) Acute renal failure in glomerulonephritis. In: Andreucci V (ed) Acute renal failure. Martinus Nijhoff, The Hague, pp 271–295
Cameron JS (1986) Acute renal failure in the intensive care unit today. Intensive Care Med 12: 64–70
Cameron JS (1988) Allergic interstitial nephritis: clinical features and pathogenesis. Q J Med 66: 97–115
Chang RWS, Jacobs S, Lee B et al. (1988) Predicting deaths among intensive care unit patients. Crit Care Med 16: 34–42
Cioffi WG, Ashikaga T, Gamelli RL (1984) Probability of surviving post-operative acute renal failure. Development of a prognostic index. Ann Surg 200: 205–211
Clowes GHA (ed) (1988) Trauma, sepsis, shock. The physiological basis for therapy. Marcel Dekker, New York
Corwin HL, Teplick RS, Schreiber MJ et al. (1987) Prediction of outcome in acute renal failure. Am J Nephrol 7: 8–12
Editorial (1988) Microbial selective decontamination in intensive care patients. Lancet I: 804
Elebute EA, Stoner HB (1983) The grading of sepsis. Br J Surg 70: 29–31
Epstein F (1985) Hypoxia of the renal medulla. Q J Med 57: 807–810
Espinel CH, Gregory AW (1980) Differential diagnosis of acute renal failure. Clin Nephrol 13: 73–77
Fry DE, Pearlstein L, Fulton RL, Pohl HC Jr (1983) Multiple system organ failure. The role of uncontrolled infection. Arch Surg 115: 136–140
Giordano C, de Santo N, Senatore R (1978) Effects of catabolic stress in acute and chronic renal failure. Am J Clin Nutr 31: 1561–1571

Heidland A, Schaefer RM, Heidbreder E, Horl WH (1988) Catabolic factors in renal failure: therapeutic approaches. Nephrol Dial Transplant 3: 8–16
Hilberman M, Myers BD, Carrie NJ et al. (1979) Acute renal failure following cardiac surgery. J Thorac Cardiovasc Surg 77: 880–888
Inglis TJJ (1988) Selective decontamination in intensive therapy units. Lancet I: 1389 (letter)
Jennett B (1985) Inappropriate use of intensive care. Br Med J 289: 1709–1711
Knaus WA, Zimmerman JE (1988) Prediction of outcome from critical illness. In: Ledingham I McA (ed) Recent advances in critical care medicine, 3rd edn. Churchill Livingstone, Edinburgh, pp 1–13
Knaus WA, Draper EA, Wagner DP, Zimmerman JE (1985) Prognosis in acute organ – system failure. Ann Surg 202: 685–693
Ledingham I McA, Alcock SR, Eastway AT et al. (1988) Triple regime of selective decontamination of the digestive tract, systemic cefotaxime, and microbiological surveillance of acquired infection in intensive care unit. Lancet I: 785–789
Le Gall JR, Loirat P, Alperovitch A et al. (1984) A simplified acute physiological score for ICU patients. Crit Care Med 12: 975–977
Lemeshow S, Teres D, Pastides H et al. (1985) A method for predicting survival and mortality of ICU patients using objectively derived weights. Crit Care Med 13: 519–525
Liano F, Gracia Martin F, Gallego A, Orte L, Teruel JL, Marcen R, Matesanz R, Ortuno J (1989) Easy and early prognosis in acute tubular necrosis – a prospective analysis of 228 cases. Nephron 51: 307–313
Lien J, Chan V (1985) Risk factors influencing survival in acute renal failure treated by haemodialysis. Arch Intern Med 145: 2067–2069
Lohr JW, McFarlane MJ, Grantham JJ (1988) A clinical index to predict survival in acute renal failure patients requiring dialysis. Am J Kidney Dis 11: 254–259
Milligan SL, Luft FC, McMurray SD, Kleit SA (1978) Intra-abdominal infection in acute renal failure. Arch Surg 113: 467–471
Minuth AN, Tenell JB, Suki W (1976) Acute renal failure: a study of the course and prognosis of 104 patients and the role of furosemide. Am J Med Sci 271: 317–324
Noone P (1988) Selective decontamination in intensive therapy units. Lancet I: 1388 (letter)
Pine RW, Wertz MJ, Lennard ES, Dellinger EP, Carnico CJ, Minshew BH (1983) Determinants of organ malfunction or death in patients with intra-abdominal sepsis. A discriminant analysis. Arch Surg 118: 242–249
Pru C, Kjellstrand CM (1984) The Fe Na^+ test is of no use in acute renal failure. Nephron 36: 20–23
Rasmussen HH, Pitt EA, Ibels LS, McNeil DR (1985) Prediction of outcome in acute renal failure by discriminant analysis of clinical variables. Arch Intern Med 145: 2015–2018
Shapiro JI, Cheung C, Itabashi A, Chan L, Schrier RW (1985) The effect of verapamil on renal function after warm and cold ischemia in the isolated perfused rat kidney. Transplantation 40: 596–600
Silas JH, Klenka Z, Solomon SA, Bone JM (1983) Captopril induced reversible acute renal failure: a marker of renal artery stenosis affecting a solitary kidney. Br Med J 286: 1702–1703
Smithies M, Cameron JS (1989a) Can we predict the outcome in acute renal failure? Nephron 51: 297–300
Smithies M, Cameron JS (1989b) Acute renal failure following reconstructive vascular surgery. In: Bell PRF, Jamieson CW, Ruckley CV (eds) Surgical management of vascular disease. Balliere Tindall, Eastbourne, (in press)
Stoutenbeek CP, van Saene HKF, Miranda DR, Zandstra DF (1984) The effect of selective decontamination of the digestive tract on colonisation and infection rate in multiple trauma patients. Intensive Care Med 10: 185–192
Thomas MAB, Ibels LS (1985) Rhabdomyolysis and acute renal failure. Aust NZ J Med 15: 623–628
Wardle N (1982) Acute renal failure in the 1980s: the importance of septic shock and endotoxemia. Nephron 30: 193–200

Discussion

The discussion following Professor Cameron's presentation centred upon the differences in outcome in patients with acute renal failure alone compared with those in whom the acute renal failure was just one part of a multi-system disturbance associated with severe trauma and sepsis. Dr Linton emphasized the cost of caring for such patients with multi-system involvement since an estimation of "the marginal cost of a life saved" from multiple organ failure in his institution was something in the order of 1.7 million dollars. All participants agreed that in general acute renal failure as a part of a multi-system disturbance was treated aggressively in all countries, despite the poor outcome and the very high cost of care of each survivor generated.

Following on from this, the discussion centred on the various deleterious effects on renal function of the associated therapies used to treat patients with multiple organ failure. In particular the problem of mechanical ventilation was emphasized and Dr Bihari expressed the view that it was much better to have patients breathing spontaneously on CPAP or pressure support with PEEP, or perhaps IMV. He thought these forms of ventilatory support were more likely to maintain the cardiac output at a higher level and cause less of a reduction in splanchnic and renal blood flow. Similarly, the question of giving large nitrogen loads in the form of amino acids in parenteral nutrition was addressed, since all participants agreed that protein restriction seemed to be beneficial in patients with chronic renal failure. Professor Cameron emphasized the difference between a patient with incipient acute renal failure and one in whom the acute renal failure was established. Perhaps the best support for these two groups in terms of nutrition might be somewhat different! Dr Macias emphasized that the introduction of parenteral nutrition as a part of the treatment for acute renal failure in the elderly greatly improved their survival. However, he admitted that he had not assessed parenteral nutrition in any form of a controlled clinical trial. Dr Epstein wondered whether the early introduction of large amounts of parenteral nutrition in a septic, catabolic patient in whom multiple organ failure was developing, was of any use at all. It was generally agreed that it is difficult to reverse the acute phase response which is a part of a catabolic reaction in the immediate post-injury or septic phase. However, participants also agreed that there was considerable evidence to support the use of parenteral nutrition in a later stage of the illness once the underlying problem of injury or sepsis had been addressed. Dr Hawker emphasized the difficulty of monitoring nutritional therapy in the critically ill. She suggested that circulating factors such as somatomedin C or insulin-like growth factor 1 might be a more useful nutritional index in critically ill patients with renal failure.

Chapter 2

Epidemiology of Acute Renal Failure in France Today

D. Kleinknecht

As in other European countries, acute renal failure (ARF) remains a challenge for any French physician involved in the treatment of patients in the Intensive Care Unit (Cameron 1986). Although the mortality has changed little over the past twenty years, there have been some modifications in aetiology, form and outcome of ARF. This review will centre upon my personal experience and that described in the more recent French literature.

Aetiology and Mortality Rate of ARF

Compared to our previous series, published fifteen years ago (Kleinknecht and Ganeval 1973), further French studies have demonstrated a reduction in the incidence of surgical and post-traumatic ARF, whereas the incidence of ARF due to medical diseases has increased (Table 2.1). These differences are best observed in multidisciplinary units, since the number of surgical or traumatized patients referred to nephrology units is now very low, ranging from 0 to 32%, with wide local variations (Degaichia et al. 1981, Benoit et al. 1982, Laville et al. 1985). ARF associated with obstetric problems has almost disappeared in France, and septic abortion is now exceptional (Pertuiset et al. 1984).

Most patients with ARF have acute tubular necrosis, the incidence of which varies from one-third to two-thirds of cases, whether or not the reports include prerenal failure (Table 2.2). Between 2% and 8% of patients have acute interstitial nephritis and a similar proportion have acute or rapidly progressive glomerulonephritis. The incidence of vascular nephropathy does not exceed 5% of patients. The importance of nephrotoxic substances has been growing over the

Table 2.1. The changing patterns of acute renal failure in France

	Kleinknecht and Ganeval (1973)[a]	Chapman (1978)[b]	Personal series[c]	Personal series[c]
Period	1966–1972	1974–1977	1977–1980	1981–1986
Number of cases	760	3373	263	493
Oliguric	78.8%	62.3%	52.0%	45.6%
Non-oliguric	21.2%	37.7%	48.0%	54.4%
Surgical	38.9%	34.4%	27.4%	24.3%
Post-traumatic	6.7%	7.3%	3.0%	3.3%
Medical	30.2%	53.7%	66.6%	70.2%
Obstetrical	24.2%	4.6%	3.0%	2.1%
Mortality	36.1%	59.5%	51.7%	44.0%
Surgical	50.0%	64.2%	54.2%	49.2%
Post-traumatic	43.0%	68.6%	50.0%	37.5%
Medical	36.0%	58.1%	52.0%	43.4%
Obstetrical	11.0%	23.1%	25.0%	18.2%

[a] Nephrology Unit; [b] Multidisciplinary Units; [c] Nephrology + multidisciplinary ICU.

Table 2.2. Causes of acute renal failure

Causes	Degaichia et al. (1981)[a]	Benoit et al. (1982)[a]	Glaser et al. (1981)[b]	Personal series (1986)[c]
	(Percentage of cases)			
Acute tubular necrosis				
Ischaemic	21.8	39.1	61.1	33.5
Nephrotoxic	21.1	20.0	6.4	
Pigment-induced	0.8	6.1	16.7	
Acute interstitial nephritis	3.5	7.8	–	5.7
Acute or rapidly progressive glomerulonephritis	2.8	3.5	–	7.1
Vascular nephropathy	0.8	2.6	–	5.5
Obstructive nephropathy	11.3	17.4	8.4	2.6
Prerenal failure	19.7	–	7.1	26.2
Others or undetermined	16.2	3.5	0.3	19.4
No. of cases	142	115	311	493

[a] Nephrology Unit; [b] Surgical ICU; [c] Nephrology + multidisciplinary ICU.

years, involving about 20% of patients with ARF hospitalized in nephrology units. This particular aspect will be discussed below.

The majority of patients have a non-oliguric course (Table 2.1), presumably because the incidence of nephrotoxic ARF has increased, and perhaps also as a result of the liberal use of diuretics and dopamine.

Overall mortality may be as low as 16.9% in non-surgical units (Degaichia et al. 1981), but more usually, it ranges from 44% to 66% (Benoit et al. 1982; Brivet et al. 1983; Laville et al. 1985), reaching 75% in surgical intensive care units (ICUs) (Glaser et al. 1981) (Table 2.3). Similar mortality rates are now observed in surgical and medical patients, but are much lower in postpartum ARF (Table 2.1).

Main causes of death are sepsis and respiratory failure, including acute pneumonitis and the adult respiratory distress syndrome (Table 2.3). Bleeding disorders, especially gastrointestinal haemorrhage, are much less frequently

Table 2.3. Causes of death in acute renal failure

Causes of death	Degaichia et al. (1981)[a]	Benoit et al. (1982)[a]	Glaser et al. (1981)[b]	Personal series (1986)[c]
		(Percentage of cases)		
Septicaemia	12.5	14.5	33.9	35.2
Respiratory failure	4.2	14.5	17.1	19.3
Cardiac failure	16.7	7.3	–	13.3
Pre-existing diseases	45.8	16.4	–	10.7
Bleeding disorders	12.5	3.7	12.3	8.1
Coma	–	–	19.9	1.3
Others	8.3	43.6	16.8[d]	11.5
Total	24/142 (16.9%)	55/115 (47.8%)	233/311 (74.9%)	217/493 (44%)

[a] Nephrology Unit; [b] Surgical ICU; [c] Nephrology + multidisciplinary ICU.
[d] Including a surgical complication in 11.2% of total deaths.

involved. In our experience, deaths due to gastrointestinal haemorrhage have decreased from 25% (Kleinknecht and Ganeval 1973) to 3% in the recent years. This decrease has been obtained despite a high incidence of deaths due to septicaemia, which is often associated, on its own, with haemorrhage of the upper gastrointestinal tract (Le Gall et al. 1976). Many patients do not die from renal insufficiency *per se*, but from pre-existing diseases, which are prominent factors in most series (Table 2.3). The high number of deaths due to central nervous disorders or to surgical complications reported by Glaser et al. (1981) is relevant to the surgical orientation of the unit, connected in this case with a neurosurgical service.

In our hands, a better prognosis is observed in cases with glomerulonephritis, interstitial nephritis and prerenal failure, than in cases with acute tubular necrosis and vascular nephropathy (Table 2.4). The worst outcome has occurred in patients with an undefined type of ARF (19.4% of cases) who often die from, or with, one or several coexistent or complicating illnesses.

Table 2.4. Mortality according to the cause of ARF.
Personal series, 1981–1986[a]

Causes of ARF	n	%
Acute tubular necrosis	89/165	53.9
Acute interstitial nephritis	6/28	21.4
Acute glomerulonephritis	2/35	5.7
Vascular nephropathy	15/27	55.6
Obstructive nephropathy	3/13	23.1
Prerenal failure	40/129	31.0
Others or undetermined	63/96[b]	65.6
Total	217/493	44.0

[a] Acute-on-chronic renal failure excluded.
[b] Most cases with multiple organ failure.

The influence of age is a matter of debate. Some authors have found that mortality increases significantly with age (Glaser et al. 1981; Benoit et al. 1982), but others have failed to detect this difference (Brivet et al. 1973; Laville et al.

1985). These discrepancies have been noted in other European studies, with age affecting (Kindler et al. 1985) or not affecting adversely the prognosis (Llano 1984; McInnes et al. 1987; Lameire et al. 1987). It is likely that age may only be an important factor in patients without extrarenal complications (Table 2.5).

Table 2.5. Mortality in ARF according to age and to failure of other organ systems (from Laville et al. 1985)

No. of extrarenal complications	Mortality		Age (years)			
	n	%	0–29	30–49	50–69	>70
			(% mortality)			
0	56	21.4	0	21.4	22.7	28.6
1	33	60.6	66.7	66.7	57.1	60.0
2	34	76.5	75.0	81.8	73.3	75.0
⩾3	24	87.5[a]	66.7	100.0	80.0	100.0
Total	147	54.7	43.8	60.5	52.5	53.1[b]

[a] $p<0.001$.
[b] $p>0.005$ (χ^2 test).

In general, survival is greatly affected by the number and the nature of associated complications. Poor prognostic indicators include respiratory failure requiring artificial ventilation, cardiac failure (Benoit et al. 1982; Brivet et al. 1983), and the number of extrarenal complications (Table 2.5). Interestingly, in the study by Laville et al. (1985), the number of associated complications decreased in older patients, in whom they found no change in mortality compared to younger patients. These authors were able to improve the survival of their patients by a high caloric intake, the figures being significant only in ARF of medical origin but not in surgical or post-traumatic cases.

Drug-Induced ARF in Renal Units

During a one-year period (1983–1984), we recorded prospectively drug-associated ARF in 398 patients, registered in 58 French nephrology units (Kleinknecht et al. 1986a). These cases represented 18.3% of the total number of patients with ARF hospitalized during the same period. In comparison, the corresponding figures were only 5% 20 years ago (Kleinknecht and Ganeval 1973). Drugs involved were primarily antibiotics (mainly aminoglycosides), glafenin (a cyclooxygenase inhibitor), non-steroidal anti-inflammatory drugs (NSAIDs) (mainly clometacin and diclofenac), and contrast media (Table 2.6). Renal biopsy, performed in 81 instances, showed acute tubular necrosis in 42 and acute interstitial nephritis in 20 patients. Hypotension, sodium depletion and/or cardiac failure were predisposing factors in 198 cases. Hypersensitivity reactions were reported in 69 patients, haemolysis in 12 and rhabdomyolysis in 11 patients.

Fifty patients (12.7%) died, 251 recovered fully or regained previous renal function, and in 93 (23.4%) permanent renal damage occurred. Death was more

Table 2.6. Drug-associated acute renal failure: main offending drugs. A prospective collaborative study of the Société de Néphrologie (Kleinknecht et al. 1986a)

Drugs	n	Drugs	n
Antibiotics	136 (34.2%)	*Diuretics*	18 (4.5%)
Aminoglycosides	107	*Chemotherapy*	14 (3.5%)
Penicillins	8	Cisplatinum	4
Cephalosporins	7	Mitomycin	2
Cotrimoxazole	5	Others	8
Rifampicin	4	*Other drugs*	39 (9.8%)
Others	5	Captopril	9
Glafenin and derivatives	79 (19.8%)	Paracetamol	5
NSAIDs	62 (15.6%)	Dextran	3
Contrast media	50 (12.6%)	Colchicine	2
		Others	20

frequent in patients treated by chemotherapy (28.6%) or receiving contrast media (24%), compared with those in whom renal failure was caused by antibiotics (19.1%) or NSAIDs (4.8%). No patient died in the glafenin group. Advanced age, oliguria, a high maximal serum creatinine level and pre-existing cardiac, hepatic or renal insufficiency were of bad prognosis. In general, the survival rate of drug-induced ARF is much better than that of any other type of ARF, excluding acute glomerulonephritis.

The incidence of residual renal damage increases sharply in patients with acute interstitial nephritis (60%) compared to those with acute tubular necrosis (16%) (Kleinknecht et al. 1986b); overall, in total, it was 23.4%, higher than that found in previous studies in France (Chapman 1978) and in the United States (Pru et al. 1982), where the reported figures range between 8% and 16%. Some authors have stressed that the resolution time may extend for up to several months, especially in patients with antibiotic-induced ARF (Appel and Neu 1977). Since the period of follow-up was 3 to 6 months in most of our patients, it is possible that some of them may have recovered later, and that the incidence of renal sequelae was overestimated. Nevertheless, others have found a high proportion of residual renal impairment in drug-induced acute interstitial nephritis, particularly in

Table 2.7. Drug-induced acute renal failure. Personal series, 1984–1987 (n = 44)

Drugs		n
1.	*Analgesics*	23 (52.3%)
	Glafenin	16
	NSAIDs	6
	Paracetamol	1
2.	*Converting enzyme inhibitors*	12 (27.3%)
	Captopril	6
	Enalapril[a]	6
3.	*Antibiotics*	4 (9.1%)
	Gentamicin	2
	Penicillins	2
4.	*Contrast media*	4 (9.1%)
5.	*Diuretics*	1 (2.3%)

[a] Including four patients receiving also NSAIDs and/or diuretics.

patients with renal epithelioid cell granulomas (Kleinknecht et al. 1988). It is unknown whether or not early prednisone therapy may hasten recovery and improve renal prognosis.

We recently reviewed the records of 44 patients hospitalized with drug-induced ARF in our service presenting over the past four years (Table 2.7). We found that analgesics, including NSAIDs, are now the most common drugs involved, followed by angiotensin-converting enzyme inhibitors, whereas the incidence of antibiotic-induced ARF fell compared to the collaborative multicentre trial conducted earlier (Kleinknecht et al. 1986a).

ARF with Multiorgan System Failure in ICU Units

Several recent studies have emphasized the critical role of the associated failure of other organ systems (Cameron 1986; Finn 1988). For example, data from the EDTA-European Renal Association (Wing et al. 1983) indicate that the mortality rate was only 8% if ARF occurred in the absence of other serious problems, but increased abruptly to 65% or more when complicated by uncontrolled sepsis, pulmonary, circulatory and/or liver failure. Moreover, an accurate prognostic index can be obtained by counting the number of organ systems in failure (Cameron 1986).

The main features of ARF in multidisciplinary, surgical and medical ICUs have recently been assessed in a large multicentre study involving 38 intensive care units (Bobrie and Patois 1987). Of 3647 patients 685 (18.8%) had ARF. The following results were found: (a) patients with ARF were older than those without ARF (67% vs 47% of cases, respectively, were more than 55 years old); (b) mortality was higher in patients with ARF (44.9% vs 18.5% in total patients hospitalized in ICUs); (c) factors influencing a poor prognosis included a high simplified acute physiologic score (SAPS), a poor previous health status assessed 3 months prior to hospitalization, associated mechanical ventilation (60% mortality vs 30% in non-ventilated patients), and the presence of oliguria (53% mortality vs 35% in non-oliguric patients); (d) age did not influence mortality, whereas mortality increased with age in patients without ARF. Prognosis according to the number of organs failing could not be given by the authors, who concluded that SAPS was a simple and safe prognostic index for patients with ARF hospitalized in ICUs.

Hospital-Acquired ARF in the ICU

Hospital-acquired ARF is an increasingly recognized condition, ranging between 2% and 5% of all patients admitted to general medical and surgical services (Hou et al. 1983; Shusterman et al. 1987), and increasing up to 23% in surgical ICUs (Wilkins and Faragher 1983). These large variations of incidence may be due to: differences in referral of patients, or in the definition of ARF, according to the various studies; inclusion in some series of patients with prerenal failure or acute-on-chronic renal failure (Hou et al. 1983; Deturck et al 1988); and the inclusion of patients with early ARF or prehospital-acquired ARF (Wilkins and Faragher 1983).

Recently, over a 6-year period, Deturck et al. (1988) collected 38 patients with hospital-acquired ARF out of 7054 patients (0.53%) admitted to a pulmonary ICU in France. Cases with prerenal azotaemia or early ARF, occurring within the first 48 hours of admission, were excluded. The most frequent cause of ARF was acute circulatory failure, especially septic shock. Iatrogenic factors accounted for 42% of all episodes, including sepsis related to intravenous or pleural catheters, and the use of nephrotoxic antibiotics or contrast media. Overall mortality was as high as 79%. Shock, oliguria, and a high peak serum creatinine carried a poor prognosis. The development of secondary ARF was neither correlated with the patient's disease on admission, nor with age, SAPS or pre-existing chronic respiratory disease.

A similar, high mortality (88%) was also found in a British surgical ICU (Wilkins and Faragher 1983), but was not observed in American medical and surgical services in which 25% to 35% of patients with hospital-acquired ARF appear to die (Hou et al. 1983; Shusterman et al. 1987). About half these cases had an iatrogenic origin. The incidence of permanent renal damage in survivors is unknown. Shusterman et al. (1987) pointed out that the development of ARF led to an approximate doubling in the length of stay, thus having a significant impact on hospital costs. Prevention of this type of ARF may rely on reducing the incidence of nosocomial infections, the judicious use of diuretics to prevent excessive volume depletion, the avoidance of nephrotoxic antibiotics, and the prevention of contrast-induced ARF by volume expansion or by using, whenever possible, non-invasive radiological techniques with a low dose of contrast media in patients at high risk.

Overall Incidence of ARF and Survival Costs

The overall incidence of ARF is unknown. Ten years ago, Chapman (1978) estimated that ARF occurred in France in 52 patients per million population per year. Lower figures (22–30 patients) were found later in France and the United Kingdom (Wing et al. 1983) and in the United States (Kjellstrand et al. 1988). This is certainly an underestimate since many patients are treated, either in isolation, in a renal unit or in an intensive care unit; other patients with milder disease may be managed outside these specialized units, in general medical and surgical services (Cameron 1986). A frequency of 60–70 cases of ARF per million population was found in Belgium, Federal Republic of Germany and Spain according to the EDTA–ERA report (Wing et al. 1983) and perhaps better reflects the real situation (Kanfer et al. 1983); an intermediate frequency was found in the Netherlands and in Switzerland.

Between 50% and 75% of these patients will die, and the remainder survive. No accurate figures for survival cost are available. Cameron (1986) estimated that this cost might be particularly high in cases of multiple organ failure, since these patients survive on average 20–30 days before dying. If only 25% of patients survive, the expenditure for each survivor might exceed 2 500 000 French francs or £250 000 (Cameron 1986).

Chronic renal failure follows ARF in approximately 10% of cases, and 40% to 50% of these cases need further chronic dialysis, i.e. 1% of all patients with ARF initiated on dialysis (Chapman 1978; Kjellstrand et al. 1988). Thus each year, in France, about 30 such patients will need chronic dialysis or transplantation, thereby increasing the cost of therapy. This emphasizes the importance of averting the establishment of ARF, particularly of acute tubular necrosis, keeping in mind that this disease is most often iatrogenic and preventable.

References

Appel GB, Neu HC (1977) The nephrotoxicity of antimicrobial agents. N Engl J Med 296: 722–728
Benoit O, Lebleu J, Noël Ch (1982) Aspects actuels de l'insuffisance rénale aiguë. Sem Hop Paris 58: 2499–2503
Bobrie G, Patois E (1987) Facteurs pronostiques de l'insuffisance rénale aiguë en réanimation multidisciplinaire. Réan Soins intens Med Urg (Paris)3: 284 (abstract)
Brivet F, Delfraissy JF, Balavoine JF, Blanchi A, Dormont J (1983) Insuffisance rénale aiguë: l'âge n'intervient pas dans le pronostic. Néphrologie 4: 14–17
Cameron JS (1986) Acute renal failure – the continuing challenge. Q J Med 59: 337–343
Chapman A (1978) Etiologie et pronostic actuel de l'insuffisance rénale aiguë en France: Résultats d'une enquête. In: Cartier F (ed) L'insuffisance rénale aiguë. L'Expansion Scientifique Française, Paris, pp 37–54
Degaichia A, Vonlanthen M, Agrafiotis A, Rottembourg J, Degoulet P, Jacobs C (1981) Insuffisances rénales aiguës de cause médicale. Aspects cliniques et thérapeutiques chez 142 malades traités dans un service de néphrologie. In: Kuss R, Legrain M (eds) Séminaires d'Uro-Néphrologie. Masson, Paris, pp 187–201
Deturck R, Durocher A, Saulnier F, Mathieu D, Wattel F (1988) Insuffisance rénale aiguë organique d'apparition secondaire en réanimation. Réan Soins intens Med Urg 4: 285–288
Finn WF (1988) Recovery from acute renal failure. In: Brenner BM, Lazarus JM (eds) Acute renal failure, 2nd edn. Churchill, New York, pp 875–918
Glaser P, Guesde R, Rouby JJ, Lhuissier D (1981) Insuffisance rénale aiguë en réanimation. Analyse des facteurs étiologiques et pronostiques chez 351 malades hémodialysés. In: Kuss R, Legrain M (eds) Séminaires d'Uro-Néphrologie. Masson, Paris, pp 202–216
Hou SH, Bushinsky DA, Wish JB, Cohen JJ, Harrington JT (1983) Hospital-acquired renal insufficiency: a prospective study. Am J Med 74: 243–248
Kanfer A, Kourilsky O, Sraer JD, Richet G (1983) Acute renal failure. In: Tinker J, Rapin M (eds) Care of the critically ill patient. Springer-Verlag, Berlin, pp 433–455
Kindler J, Rensing M, Sieberth HG (1985) Prognosis and mortality of acute renal failure. In: Sieberth HG, Mann H (eds) Continuous arteriovenous hemofiltration (CAVH). Karger, Basel, pp 129–142
Kjellstrand CM, Berkseth RO, Klinkmann H (1988) Treatment of acute renal failure. In: Brenner BM, Lazarus JM (eds) Acute renal failure, 2nd edn. Churchill, New York, pp 1501–1540
Kleinknecht D, Ganeval D (1973) Preventive hemodialysis in acute renal failure: its effect on mortality and morbidity. In: Friedman EA, Eliahou HE (eds) Proceedings of the conference on acute renal failure. DHEW Pub (NIH), 74–608, Washington DC, pp 165–182
Kleinknecht D, Landais P, Goldfarb B (1986a) Les insuffisances rénales aiguës associées à des médicaments ou à des produits de contraste iodés. Résultats d'une enquête coopérative multicentrique de la Société de Néphrologie. Néphrologie 7: 41–46
Kleinknecht D, Landais P, Goldfarb B (1986b) Analgesic and non-steroidal anti-inflammatory drug-associated acute renal failure: a prospective collaborative study. Clin Nephrol 25: 275–281
Kleinknecht D, Vanhille Ph, Druet Ph (1988) Les néphrites interstitielles aiguës granulomateuses d'origine médicamenteuse. Presse Méd 17: 201–205

Lámeire N, Matthys E, Vanholder R et al. (1987) Causes and prognosis of acute renal failure in elderly patients. Nephrol Dial Transplant 2: 316–322
Laville M, Islam S, Zanettini MC et al. (1985) Survie des malades en insuffisance rénale aiguë: influence de la nutrition et des complications associées. Néphrologie 6: 171–176
Le Gall JR, Mignon FC, Rapin M et al. (1976) Acute gastroduodenal lesions related to severe sepsis. Surg Gynecol Obstet 142: 377–380
Llano F (1984) Fracaso renal agudo: revisión de 202 casos. Aspectos pronósticos. Nefrologia 4: 181–190
McInnes EG, Levy DW, Chaudhuri MD, Bhan GL (1987) Renal failure in the elderly. Q J Med 64: 583–588
Pertuiset N, Ganeval D, Grünfeld JP (1984) Acute renal failure in pregnancy: an update. Semin Nephrol 4: 232–239
Pru C, Ebben J, Kjellstrand C (1982) Chronic renal failure after acute tubular necrosis. Kidney Int 21: 176
Shusterman N, Strom BL, Murray TG, Morrison G, West SL, Maislin G (1987) Risk factors and outcome of hospital-acquired acute renal failure. Clinical epidemiologic study. Am J Med 83: 65–71
Wilkins RG, Faragher EB (1983) Acute renal failure in an intensive care unit: incidence, prediction and outcome. Anaesthesia 38: 628–634
Wing AJ, Broyer M, Brunner FP et al. (1983) In: Combined report on regular dialysis and transplantation in Europe. XIII. 1982. Acute (reversible) renal failure. Proc Eur Dial Transplant Assoc 20: 64–71

Discussion

Some of the participants were not familiar with the French analgesic compound glafenin. Professor Kleinknecht explained that it was a 4,7-aminochloroquinoline derivative and acted through the inhibition of prostaglandin formation.

Professor Better was very impressed with these data. He agreed that acute tubular necrosis associated with trauma, pigment (bilirubin, myoglobin) and pregnancy was much less frequent, but yet when they did occur in Kleinknecht's series they were associated with a high mortality. Professor Better also emphasized the nephrotoxic effects of low-molecular-weight dextran. Moreover, he was disturbed by the high mortality rate in patients with obstructive uropathy. So often this condition can be missed when an inexperienced ultrasonographer examines the patient with acute renal failure and this observer-dependency of the technique remains a considerable drawback to its use in the intensive care unit.

Attention then turned to the prevention of gastrointestinal bleeding in patients with acute renal failure in the intensive care unit. Dr Bihari emphasized that on at least three occasions, speakers had made reference to the fact that this particular complication no longer seemed to be a problem in the management of patients with renal failure. Whether the disappearance of severe gastrointestinal haemorrhage as a cause of death in this condition was related to alkalinization of the gastric aspirate with antacids or H_2 antagonists, or whether it was related to improvements in resuscitation and support of the circulation remained to be determined. Nevertheless, the costs of therapy with H_2 antagonists were quite substantial and a number of participants referred to the emerging studies which suggested that treatment with antacids and H_2 antagonists seemed to predispose to an increased incidence of nosocomial pneumonias. Professor Kleinknecht referred to the studies of Jean-Roger Le Gall which demonstrated that the incidence of stress ulceration in patients with acute renal failure was more likely to reflect the presence of untreated sepsis rather than reflect the severity of the renal failure alone. Professor Better suggested that early enteral feeding was a more appropriate means of reducing the incidence of stress ulcers and Dr Noone re-affirmed that achlorhydria was indeed associated with an increased risk of pulmonary infection.

Professor Cameron turned the discussion to the distinction between acute interstitial nephritis and acute tubular necrosis. He wondered whether the histopathologist could be so confident in making the distinction. Professor Kleinknecht admitted that there were some patients who were difficult to classify into one or other of the disease groups and Dr Solez confirmed these histopathological difficulties. Dr Solez emphasized that it is possible to see an inflammatory infiltrate in the renal tubules in acute tubular necrosis but usually the severity of this inflammatory infiltrate was less extensive than that seen with acute interstitial nephritis. He stressed that this issue of tubulitis was obviously of importance in the transplanted kidney and may be important in the native kidney in terms of mechanisms underlying the pathogenesis of acute renal failure.

Chapter 3

Acute Renal Failure and Sepsis: A Microbiologist's View

P. Noone

Introduction

Recently a review of acute renal failure in the intensive care unit made several important observations (Cameron 1986). First, and perhaps most important, that in spite of 30 years of advance in the treatment of renal failure, mortality rates for acute renal failure in critically ill patients seem to be fixed at around 50%–70%. However, it is clear that many of the patients who fail to survive have more than renal failure. In those cases with renal failure alone, following surgery a trauma mortality is only 10% or less. But as other organ systems begin to fail, mortality rates climb sharply. Two organ systems failing increases mortality to 50%; whereas three organ systems or more failing is associated with a mortality rate greater than 75%.

A second important observation is that whilst patients may survive longer than previously (in terms of days or weeks), because of dialysis and other intensive care measures, this increases costs markedly but does not affect longer-term outcome. Finally, Cameron emphasizes that sepsis is a very important factor in the development of organ failure. In particular intra-abdominal sepsis can be crucial, often because it may be difficult to detect. Ultrasonography, CAT scanning and radioactive gallium screening may be helpful in locating intra-abdominal abscesses but *re-exploration of the suspect abdomen is essential* – even repeatedly. Cameron quotes the experiences of Milligan et al. (1978) who showed that of 86 re-explorations in 40 patients, 66 revealed remediable problems.

Coratelli et al. (1987) also state that sepsis is the major cause of death in up to 70% of patients with acute renal failure and is the usual cause of multiple organ failure. They estimate that Gram-positive infections account for 30% of such cases, but Gram-negative rods for 70% of cases. Fry et al. (1980) and Manship et al. (1984) also noted sepsis as the major cause of organ failure in their ITU practice. Peng-Fei Shen and Shi-Chun Zhang (1987) confirm the same trend in

China. In their experience multiple organ failure complicating acute renal failure is triggered, principally, by uncontrolled sepsis.

Hence, sepsis is perhaps the key factor in the development of renal failure and multiple organ failure in critically ill patients. Both Gram-negative and Gram-positive organisms and yeasts can cause systemic infection with renal failure. The clinical pictures overlap considerably but there is little doubt that in the past 40 years, aerobic Gram-negative rod infection has proved to be the major microbial problem in hospitalized patients, especially the immunocompromised, both in terms of morbidity and mortality.

Epidemiology

Finland and his collaborators (McGowan et al. 1975) have most clearly charted the change in nosocomial infections from Gram-positive to Gram-negative organisms and by the 1970s there was worldwide recognition of this epidemiological shift. In 1978 Reinarz estimated that there were some 240 000 episodes of Gram-negative rod septicaemia in the USA annually with a mortality of 50 000 patients. The 1984 Nosocomial Infection Surveillance carried out by the CDC showed 33.5 cases of infection per 1000 discharges in the 51 US hospitals studied with aerobic Gram-negative rods causing over 51% of the infections (Horan et al. 1984). A similar British Survey carried out in 1981 of 43 British hospitals revealed that 19% of all patients were infected although only 9% had hospital-acquired infection. Aerobic Gram-negative rods were second only to *Staphylococcus aureus* in causing wound infections and pneumonia in these patients (Meers et al. 1981).

The aerobic Gram-negative rods involved in such GNR infections include *Escherichia coli*, *Klebsiella*, *Enterobacter*, *Serratia*, *Pseudomonas aeruginosa*, other pseudomonads, *Proteus*, *Citrobacter* and *Acinetobacter*. Although *E. coli* is usually a colonic commensal it does indeed cause sepsis if it escapes from the bowel lumen to sterile areas and is a major pathogen associated with bowel trauma, perforation, operation, inflammation and ischaemia, causing peritonitis, cholecystitis, hepatic abscess, and of course cystitis and pyelonephritis. It is less common as a cause of pneumonia. *Klebsiella*, *Enterobacter*, *Serratia*, *P. aeruginosa* and *Acinetobacter* on the other hand, are free living and occur much less commonly than *E. coli* as gut commensals in healthy people. However, they are ubiquitous in moist circumstances, many of them being able to survive and multiply at ambient temperatures, often with minimal nutritional supplies. They also show a great ability to become resistant to antimicrobial agents – both antibiotics and disinfectants. In hospital the debilitated patient is surrounded by Gram-negative rods – in the food, the water supply, on the hands of attending staff – and can easily become colonized, a process aided by antimicrobial therapy which removes protection afforded by commensal flora. In hospitalized patients the gut from mouth to rectum is probably the major reservoir of these organisms in any clinical setting and can easily lead to autogenous invasive infection with surgery, invasive investigation, invasive therapy, immunocompromising treatments (cytotoxins, radiotherapy, steroids), intubation, intravenous catheters and intravesical catheters. Of course, cross infection is facilitated by the hands of attendants allowing the colonizing Gram-negative rods in one patient to become an invasive pathogen in his/her more compromised neighbour. Cross infection in this manner has been shown with *Klebsiella* (Adler et al. 1970), *Serratia* (Mutton et al. 1981), *Acinetobacter* (French et al. 1980) and *P. aeruginosa* (Noone et al. 1983). Hand washing in ITU can be perfunctory or even overlooked altogether (Albert and Condie 1981).

In the CDC surveillance study (Horan et al. 1984), aerobic Gram-negative rods not only accounted for two-thirds of the 12 218 isolates from nosocomial urinary infection but more disturbingly for 55.7% of the 4567 isolates causing lower respiratory tract infection with three species – *P. aeruginosa*, *Klebsiella* and *Enterobacter* – accounting for 37.9%. The modern ITU practice of using H_2 blockers and antacids prophylactically to eliminate gastrointestinal haemorrhage of course helps upper gut colonization with aerobic organisms. This has considerable implications for cross infection and for secondary pneumonia in intubated patients.

Gram-Negative Septicaemia

Classically a patient with Gram-negative rod bacteraemia presents clinically with fever and rigors, but this is by no means inevitable and hypothermia can occur especially in the elderly. Indeed the early clinical clues for detecting aerobic Gram-negative rod bacteraemia can stem from its complications including hypotension, falling urine output, acidosis, thrombocytopenia, bleeding, jaundice, changes in mental state, hyperventilation, and occasionally the skin lesions of ecthyma gangrenosum. Gram-negative rod bacteraemia and indeed endotoxaemia associated with focal sepsis can precipitate organ failure in the kidney, lung, liver, heart and adrenals.

Endotoxin

Although all Gram-negative rods contain endotoxin as an integral part of their cell wall, virulence factors and the ability to survive, invade and multiply in tissues varies considerably even within the same species. Virulence factors include the characteristics of adherence to mucosal surfaces, resistance to non-specific serum lysing and opsonizing antibodies, antiphagocytic properties and the elaboration of extracellular factors such as toxins and enzymes (*P. aeruginosa* can be especially notable in this respect).

Figure 3.1 shows the structure of the Gram-negative rod cell wall. Outside the cytoplasmic membrane there is a solid membrane of mucopeptide or peptidoglycan (a much thinner layer than found in Gram-positive organisms) and then outside that the outer membrane of lipoprotein and polysaccharide. The latter is specific and is the basis for "O" (somatic) antigen typing schemes. Outside the outer membrane many bacteria have a capsule or envelope of polysaccharide

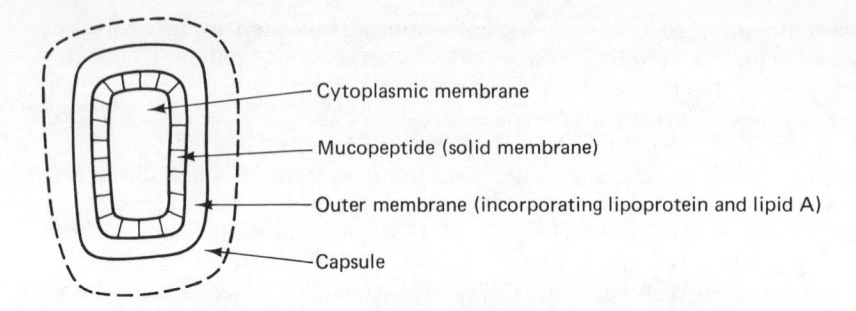

Fig. 3.1. Structure of the Gram-negative rod cell wall.

nature, the basis of the K antigen in *E. coli*, the serotyping antigen of *Klebsiella* and the Vi antigen of *Staphylococcus typhi*. It confers antiphagocytic properties.

As far as GNR septicaemia and septic shock are concerned the crucial part of the cell wall is the so-called core region of the outer membrane. Although the O-antigen part varies between species, the inner core glycolipid (or lipid A) is common to all and is the key component in triggering all the pathophysiological events associated with endotoxaemia. In this it is not unique and it is worth noting that cell wall antigens of Gram-positive bacteria including the M protein of group A Steptococci, can trigger similar effects.

Pathophysiology of Gram-Negative Septicaemia

Endotoxin can trigger all the pathophysiological effects induced by whole Gram-negative rod cells – living or dead. The effects are complex and still not fully understood (Fig. 3.2). There is also a problem of translating the effects produced in one mammalian species to another. It does seem that man is one of the more susceptible species, especially to pyrogenic effects.

Endotoxin switches on at least four different physiological systems. Hageman Factor (Factor XII) is activated and this in turn activates the complement cascade, coagulation, fibrinolysis and the kallikrein–kinin system.

Complement activation results in the release of factors causing the migration of phagocytic cells into the tissues. Anaphylotoxins are also released which lead to increased vascular permeability and an enhanced inflammatory action. Coagulation is mediated through activation of pre-PTA (plasma thromboplastin antecedent) to PTA. A chain of events leads to fibrinogen being converted into fibrin with resultant clotting. Uncontrolled coagulation accompanying a major bacterial challenge leads to consumption of platelets (thrombocytopenia) and clotting factors II, V and VIII and thrombosis. The term DIC (disseminated intravascular coagulation) is used to describe this state. This uncontrolled clotting can be accompanied by paradoxical bleeding because of the removal of clotting factors. Thrombosis, bleeding, tissue ischaemia, necrosis and haemolysis can all take place leading to organ failure (kidney, lung or liver).

Endotoxin can also lead to greatly increased fibrinolysis via activation of plasminogen pro-activator. Plasmin, produced through this mechanism, can in turn trigger the complement cascade. Excessive fibrinolysis enhances the pathological effects of coagulopathy and is part of the DIC phenomenon. It is worth

```
                    ┌──────────┐  ╫→ Prostaglandin    ○ (Vasodilatation)
                    │ Endotoxin│       (blocked by NSAID)
                    └────┬─────┘
                         ▼
Complement  ◄────── Activated ──────────────────► Kallikrein
 cascade            Hageman factor                    │
    │              ╱          ╲                       │
    ▼            PTA         Plasminogen           Bradykinin
┌──────────┐      │              │                    │
│Inflammation│    ▼              ▼                    ▼
└──────────┘ ┌─────────┐    ┌──────────┐        Increased vascular
             │Coagulation│  │Fibrinolysis│          permeability
             └────┬─────┘   └─────┬────┘                │
                  └────────┬──────┘                     ▼
                           ▼                      ┌────────────┐
                        ┌─────┐                   │Hypotension │
                        │ DIC │                   └────────────┘
                        └─────┘
```

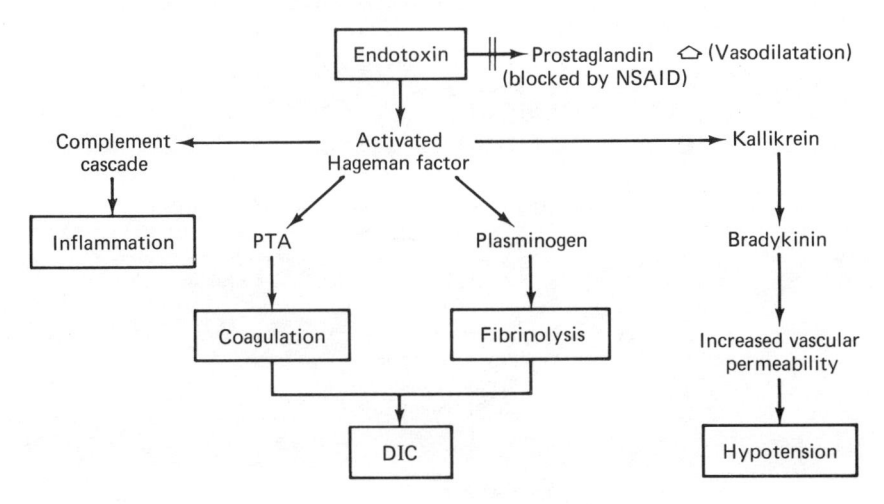

Fig. 3.2. The pathophysiology of Gram-negative septicaemia.

noting that in patients with severe liver disease, the clotting and bleeding abnormalities of DIC associated with Gram-negative rod bacteraemia and/or endotoxaemia are usually exacerbated. Other factors which worsen bleeding and clotting in Gram-negative rod sepsis include direct endotoxin damage of the intima of blood vessels and the interaction of bacterial antigen–host antibody complexes with leucocytes resulting in the release of substances which can inactivate clotting.

Pathophysiology of Renal Failure

For a considerable time there was some controversy about how endotoxin was associated with hypotension but it would appear to be secondary to the activation of the bradykinin system by activated Hageman factor. Bradykinin is vasoactive causing vasodilation and increased vascular permeability. Decreased vascular resistance ensues with consequent hypovolaemia, hypotension and hypoperfusion of the organs including kidney, lungs, liver and heart.

In the case of the kidney, hypoperfusion of the kidney perhaps together with a direct stimulating effect of endotoxin itself leads to activation of the renin system with depressed levels of angiotensin-converting enzyme (ACE) and raised levels of angiotensin and renin (Hilgenfeldt et al. 1987). This exacerbates renal ischaemia with falling glomerular filtration (GF) and tubular necrosis (itself exacerbated by vascular obstruction and interstitial tissue oedema brought on by coagulopathy and bradykinin release) (Fig. 3.3).

Patients with liver disease and jaundice are more vulnerable to renal failure during endotoxaemia and have a higher mortality. Coratelli et al. (1987) showed a clear relationship; mortality rates of 85% were seen in patients with serum bilirubin levels above 20 mg% as opposed to 33% in those with bilirubin levels less than 10 mg%.

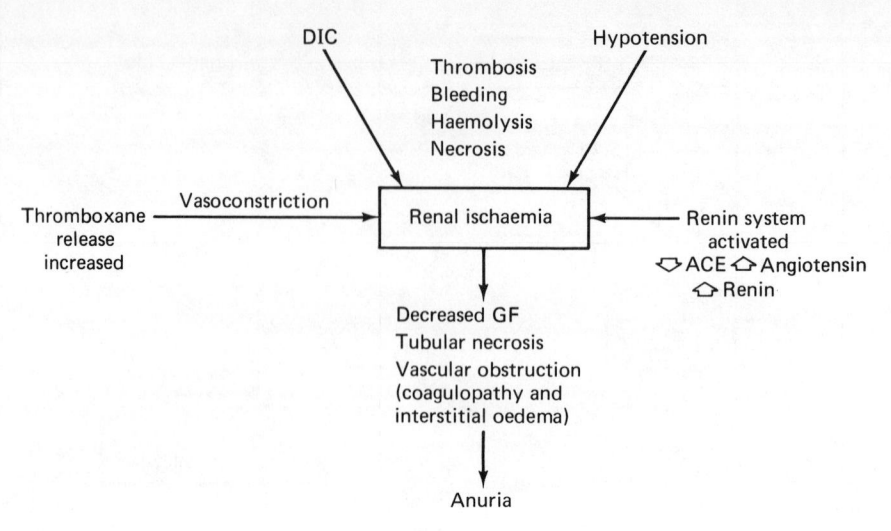

Fig. 3.3. Factors involved in renal failure in Gram-negative septicaemia.

Renal hypoperfusion stimulates prostaglandin production designed to enhance perfusion and glomerular filtration rate. This protective mechanism is switched off by the NSAID group of drugs – nowadays available off-prescription – which are commonly taken by elderly patients and all patients suffering chronic painful musculoskeletal conditions. Renal failure is therefore more likely with Gram-negative rod sepsis in such patients.

Raised plasma thromboxane levels have been associated with an increase in pulmonary vascular resistance in the early phase of septic shock (Oettinger et al. 1987). This may be important in the development of adult respiratory distress syndrome.

All the problems associated with Gram-negative rod endotoxaemia and systicaemia (DIC, renal failure, shock, ARDS) have been reported also with Gram-positive and fungal infections (Turner and Naumburg 1987; Ramsay et al. 1985). Clinically this is important as it necessitates empirical antimicrobial therapy directed against a wide range of micro-organisms in the critically ill patient with life-threatening sepsis where there is no microbiological information available.

Management

The management of sepsis in the critically ill is crucial. Prompt recognition and early effective therapy can reduce its duration, severity and complications. It is important to identify infecting pathogens accurately, not only to obtain precise antimicrobial susceptibilities but also for useful epidemiological information which may indicate how sepsis occurred, from what source, if there has been cross infection or a breakdown in hygiene standards and to allow one to take effective action.

Surveillance cultures are normally of limited value for routine clinical purposes, but when there is clinical suspicion of sepsis multiple blood cultures, deep aspirated respiratory secretions, urine, wound swabs etc. are essential.

Where deep sepsis is a possibility (e.g. following intra-abdominal surgery, or multiple trauma) the diagnosis should be pursued actively with whatever imaging techniques are available and if necessary with surgery.

Antibiotics

Antimicrobial choice must be aimed primarily against aerobic Gram-negative rods, although metronidazole is a mandatory concomitant where there is deep sepsis, or sepsis following gut surgery or damage, and anaerobes may be present.

Aminoglycosides (gentamicin, netilmicin, amikacin) have been the mainstay of treatment of life-threatening Gram-negative infection. They are reliably active against Enterobacteriaceae and *P. aeruginosa*, although gentamicin resistance is an increasing problem in Southern Europe, the Far East, Latin America and parts of the USA. There are nonetheless a number of other problems with their use.

First, it is imperative to give an adequate dose to achieve therapeutic concentrations. This is of particular importance in pneumonia. Amikacin has a better pharmacokinetic profile than gentamicin as well as a more reliable antibacterial spectrum (Holloway 1985) and may be less nephrotoxic (Kahlmeter and Dahlager 1984). The newer concept of giving aminoglycosides in a once-a-day larger dosage may improve efficacy and reduce toxicity.

Second, all aminoglycosides have ototoxic and nephrotoxic potential. The latter is obviously relevant in the critical care situation. There is substantial evidence from animal studies that endotoxin-affected or ischaemic kidneys are more susceptible to the nephrotoxic effect of aminoglycosides (Zager and Prior 1986). Bergeron et al. (1987) have also shown that hydrocortisone has a nephrotoxic potentiating effect in rats. This illustrates the fact that a patient with endotoxaemia may be receiving combinations of agents which individually may not have great nephrotoxicity but in combination could be more deleterious.

Whilst recognizing the nephrotoxic potential of aminoglycosides it is worth emphasizing again that uncontrolled sepsis is itself highly nephrotoxic. The septic process should be halted as rapidly as possible. Aminoglycosides are potent agents and act rapidly. In a recent comparative study of amikacin and netilmicin administered to 202 patients with hospital-acquired major Gram-negative rod infection we noted an overall nephrotoxicity (serum creatinine increasing by 50% above baseline values during or immediately following therapy) of 8%. On the other hand, however, the number of patients who showed significant improvement of renal function (serum creatinine falling by 50% or more from abnormal pre-treatment values) was 20 of 58 (34%). In a recent prospective study of ITU infections, we treated 34 patients, out of 98 who stayed in ITU more than 3 days, with aminoglycosides. There was 69% successful elimination of pathogens (aerobic Gram-negative rods) and 3 out of 26 showed evidence of nephrotoxicity (50% or more rise in serum creatinine).

Nevertheless there has been a move towards using newer broad-spectrum beta-lactam antibiotics (especially cephalosporins) as first-line therapy for severe infection in the critically ill. Of course these antibiotics may avoid intrinsic nephrotoxicity but they may have other side effects ranging from a tendency to enhance bleeding problems (e.g. carbenicillin, moxalactam), hepatic dysfunction, suppression of protective commensal flora and gastrointestinal upset including pseudomembraneous colitis.

There is also the problem of resistance emerging during treatment or overgrowth with hospital-acquired resistant organisms (Sanders and Sanders 1983). *P. aeruginosa* (Bragman et al. 1986), *Serratia, Enterobacter cloacae* and *Acinetobacter* are particularly adept at creating such problems. Although not especially pathogenic to the healthy these are major pathogens in the immunocompromised and critically ill.

In addition to this there are questions about the efficacy of new antibiotics as sole therapy. One of our own studies showed cefotaxime to be significantly inferior to netilmicin in treating aerobic Gram-negative rod sepsis (excluding *P. aeruginosa*) in the lungs and intra-abdominally (Sage et al. 1987). The latest reported EORTC study (1987) of bacteraemia in neutropenic hosts, showed that ceftazidime and "short course" amikacin (3 days) was very significantly inferior to a full course of both agents.

There are the new quinolones especially ciprofloxacin and ofloxacin which look highly promising for treating aerobic Gram-negative rod sepsis. Our own experience is good in leukaemic patients. However, further full-scale comparative trials are needed to evaluate these agents.

In spite of the increasing array of available antibiotics and improving diagnostic techniques, patients in ITU continue to die from hospital-acquired infection and its complications. There must be an increased emphasis on prevention.

Prophylaxis

Much has been done to improve the microbial safety of ventilators by the use of filters (Holdcroft et al. 1973) and the protection of humidifiers with chlorhexidine and heat, but intubation itself in the presence of upper gut aerobic Gram-negative rod colonization (facilitated by H_2 blockers, antacids and by antibiotic administration) is associated with an increased incidence of pneumonia.

There are a number of widely agreed measures for preventing cross infection in ITU. Chief of these are (a) adequate staffing (at least one nurse per patient per shift) and (b) adequate hand washing between patient contacts. As indicated, Gram-negative rods (as well as *S. aureus*) and yeasts are carried transiently (and occasionally more permanently) on the hands. This can prove dangerous during procedures such as aspiration of the lungs, handling intravascular lines, wound drains, and intravesical catheters.

Nevertheless the greatest reservoir of aerobic Gram-negative rods (and yeasts) is the patient's own gastrointestinal tract from mouth to rectum. The normal commensal flora of the patient's gut tends with time to be replaced by hospital-acquired Gram-negative rods, a process enhanced by administration of antibiotics.

A recent controversial scheme for preventing ITU infection by eliminating patient carriage of aerobic Gram-negative rods has been put forward by Stoutenbeek et al. (1987). The patient is given non-absorbable antibiotics (including an oral paste) for the duration of stay in ITU. This is similar to the practice adopted with neutropenic and liver transplant patients. Cefotaxime was also given for an initial 4 days systemically to prevent (domiciliary) acquired infection, giving time for the oral agents to work. Respiratory sepsis seems to be prevented by this strategy in multiple trauma patients, with reduced mortality, but plans to treat all ITU patients this way (Ledingham et al. 1988) are more worrying, chiefly because of the risks of selection of resistant organisms such as *Acinetobacter*, *Serratia* and *Pseudomonas* (Noone 1988).

Other methods for reducing Gram-negative rod pneumonia include sucralfate administration instead of H_2 blockers and oral antacids, which by preserving a low gastric pH inhibits colonization of the stomach and pharynx (Driks et al. 1987).

All these techniques will have to be studied in further detail but the aim of preventing aerobic Gram-negative rod sepsis in the patients must be one of our principal strategies for reducing renal and multiple organ failure.

References

Adler JL, Shulman JA, Terry PM, Feldman DB, Skaling P (1970) Nosocomial colonisation with kanamycin resistant *Klebsiella pneumoniae* types 2 & 11 in a premature nursery. J Pediatr 77: 376–385

Albert RK, Condie F (1981) Hand washing patterns in medical intensive-care units. N Engl J Med 24: 1465–1466

Bergeron MG, Bergeron Y, Beauchamp D (1987) Influence of hydrocortisone sulfate on intrarenal accumulations of gentamicin in endotoxaemic rats. Antimicrob Agents Chemother 31: 1816–1821

Bragman S, Sage R, Booth L, Noone P (1986) Ceftazidime in the treatment of serious *Pseudomonas aeruginosa* sepsis. Scand J Infect Dis 18: 425–429

Cameron JS (1986) Acute renal failure in the intensive care unit today. Intensive Care Med 12: 64–70

Coratelli P, Passaranti G, Giannattasio M, Amerio A (1987) Acute renal failure after septic shock. Adv Exp Med Biol 212: 233–243

Driks MR, Craven DE, Celli BR, Manning M, Burke RA, Gavin GM, Kunches LM, Farber HW, Wedel SA, McCabe WR (1987) Nosocomial pneumonia in intubated patients given sucralfate as compared with antacids or histamine type 2 blockers. N Engl J Med 317: 1376–1382

EORTC International Antimicrobial Therapy Co-operative Group (1987) Ceftazidime combined with a short or long course of amikacin for empirical therapy of Gram negative bacteraemia in cancer patients with granulocytopenia. N Engl J Med 317: 1692–1698

French GL, Casewell MW, Roncossmi AJ, Knight S, Phillips I (1980) A hospital outbreak of antibiotic resistant acinetobacter anitrations: epidemiology and control. J Hosp Infect 1: 125–131

Fry DE, Pearlstein L, Fulton RL, Pohl HC Jr (1980) Multiple system organ failure. The role of uncontrolled infection. Arch Surg 115: 136–140

Hilgenfeldt U, Kienapfel G, Kellerman W, Schott R, Schmidt M (1987) Renin–angiotensin system in sepsis. Clin Exp Hypertens [A]9: 1493–1504

Holdcroft A, Lumley J, Gaya H (1973) Why disinfect ventilators? Lancet I: 240–241

Holloway WJ (1985) Management of sepsis in the elderly. Am J Med (Suppl. 6B) 80: 143–148

Horan TC, White JW, Jarvis WR, Emori TG, Culver DH, Munn VP, Thornsberry C, Olson DR, Hughes JM (1984) Nosocomial infection surveillance. Communicable Dis Rep 35: 1755–2855

Kahlmeter G, Dahlager JI (1984) Aminoglycoside toxicity and review of clinical studies published between 1978–82. J Antimicrob Agents Chemother (Suppl A) 13: 9–22

Ledingham I McA, Alcock SR, Eastway AT et al. (1988) Triple regimen of selective decontamination of the digestive tract, systemic cefotaxime and microbiological surveillance for prevention of acquired infection in intensive care. Lancet I: 785–790

Manship L, McMillin RD, Brown JJ (1984) The influence of sepsis and multisystem organ failure on mortality in the surgical intensive care unit. Am Surg 50: 94–101

McGowan JE, Barnes MW, Finland M (1975) Bacteraemia at Boston City Hospital: occurrence and mortality during 12 selected years (1935–1972) with special reference to hospital acquired cases. J Infect Dis 132: 316–335

Meers PD, Ayliffe GAJ, Emmerson AM et al. (1981) Report on the National Survey of Infection in Hospitals (1980). J Hosp Infect Suppl. 2: 1–51

Milligan SL, Luft FC, McMurray SD, Kleit SA (1978) Intra-abdominal infection in acute renal failure. Arch Surg 113: 467–472

Mutton KJ, Brady LM, Harkness JL (1981) *Serratia* cross infection in an intensive therapy unit. J Hosp Infect 2: 85–97

Noone P (1988) Selective decontamination in intensive therapy units. Lancet I: 1388 (letter)

Noone MR, Pitt TL, Bedder M, Howlett AM, Rogers KB (1983) *Pseudomonas aeruginosa* colonisation in an intensive therapy unit and role of cross infection and host factors. Br Med J 286: 341–344

Oettinger W, Berger D, Berger HG (1987) The clinical significance of prostaglandins and thromboxane as mediators of septic shock. Klin Wochensholis 65: 61–68

Peng-Fei Shen, Shi-Chun Zhang (1987) Acute renal failure and multiple organ system failure. Arch Surg 122: 1131–1133

Ramsay AG, Olesmicky L, Pirani CL (1985) Acute tubulo-interstitial nephritis from *Candida albicans* with oliguric renal failure. Clin Nephrol 24: 310–314

Reinarz JA (1978) Nosocomial infections. Clin Symp 30: 1–32

Sage R, Nazareth B, Noone P (1987) A prospective randomised comparison of cefotaxime vs. netilmicin vs. cefotaxime plus netilmicin in the treatment of hospitalised patients with serious sepsis. Scand J Infect Dis 19: 331–337

Sanders CC, Sanders WE Jr (1983) Emergence of resistance during therapy with the newer beta-lactam antibiotics: role of inducible beta-lactamases and implications for the future. Rev Infect Dis 5: 639–648

Stoutenbeek CP, Van Saene HKF, Zandstra DF (1987) The effect of oral non-absorbable antibiotics on the emergence of resistant bacteria in patients in an intensive care unit. J Antimicrob Chemother 19: 513–520

Turner MC, Naumburg EG (1987) Acute renal failure in the neonate. Clin Pediatr 26: 189–190

Zager RA, Prior RB (1986) Gentamicin and Gram negative bacteraemia. J Clin Invest 78: 196–204

Discussion

All participants agreed that the prevention of infection in patients with acute renal failure of any cause was a major priority in the intensive care unit. Dr Bihari emphasized that the modern hypothesis of the pathogenesis of multiple organ failure depended on a concept of a "gut leak – liver prime" phenomenon. This concept developed by Frank Cerra and others was related to the development of a leaky gut, the consequence of ischaemia, malnutrition, and bacterial overgrowth followed by bacterial and endotoxin translocation into the portal circulation. The delivery of bacteria and endotoxin to Kupffer cells within the liver results directly in the activation of the reticulo-endothelial cell system within the liver and spill over into the systemic circulation of endotoxin, bacteria and various vasoactive mediators. Selective decontamination of the gastrointestinal tract was an obvious approach to the problem and Dr Bion informed the meeting that this technique was about to be instituted in his unit in patients undergoing liver transplantation. The Utrecht group had also used the regimen for 5 years in about 200–300 patients who required ventilation for longer than 48 hours. This technique in their hands had been associated with a reduction in respiratory infection with Gram-negative rods from more than 20% to less than 10%. Dr Noone emphasized that simple measures of hygiene such as hand washing were to be encouraged before the introduction of such complicated and potentially hazardous therapy such as selective decontamination. All participants agreed that further studies of SDD were required and that this technique might well be a fundamental advance in the care of the complicated case of acute renal failure.

Attention turned to the use of the aminoglycosides in the critically ill and Dr Bihari referred to the recent literature concerning the increased volume of distribution of gentamicin in patients with serious illnesses. He emphasized the importance of a large (3–5 mg kg^{-1}) loading dose of gentamicin in order to achieve adequate peak levels. Dr Noone confirmed the importance of this large loading dose and went on to comment that many physicians now use aminoglycosides on a once-a-day basis, even in patients with relatively normal renal function. This is done so that a large, once-a-day dose can be given to achieve a peak level of at least 6 mg l^{-1} so as to obtain adequate penetration of pulmonary and other tissues. Several participants suggested that other antibiotics such as the third generation cephalosporins and imipenem should be used in the intensive care unit so as to avoid the nephrotoxicity of aminoglycosides and the necessity of measuring blood levels. Dr Linton reported the results of a study performed within his own unit, in which 100 patients were prescribed aminoglycosides. Of these 100 patients, in whom two blood samples were collected for the measurement of blood levels, only 9% of the samples were ordered and collected at the appropriate time, and when the results were obtained, only a quarter of the observations were acted on in an appropriate manner. Dr Linton emphasized that although there was disagreement about the importance of peak and trough measurements, this controversy was irrelevant since it appeared in clinical practice that doctors do not know, or ignore the results of measurements when they are obtained from the laboratory. Most participants agreed that since the monitoring of aminoglycoside levels in the intensive care unit was so difficult, these drugs were best avoided and other broad-spectrum antibiotics used.

Chapter 4

Acute Renal Failure at a Crossroads

K. Solez and L. C. Racusen

Acute renal failure in the intensive care (intensive therapy) unit, whilst the subject of this symposium, is but a microcosm of the field of acute renal failure in general. In many respects the field is at a crossroads, or a turning point. It is nearly 50 years since the first complete descriptions of acute renal failure appeared in English (Beall et al. 1941; Bywaters and Beall 1941; DeNavasquez 1940; Dunn et al. 1941; Mayon-White and Solandt 1941) and nearly 40 years since the publication of Oliver's classic microdissection studies (Oliver et al. 1951; Oliver 1953). In the course of our professional careers since the early 1970s, there have been at least 16 meetings or symposia devoted to acute renal failure or nephrotoxicity, not counting the present gathering (Table 4.1). The emphasis has gradually shifted from characterization and dialytic treatment to prevention, early diagnosis, and specific pharmacological therapies. The first prospective human trials of intervention with atrial natriuretic peptide, calcium channel blockers, thyroxine, and oxygen free radical scavengers are just now getting underway, after many years of studies confined to the laboratory. It is likely that in the next few years an agent will be found which is as effective in reversing early acute renal failure as tissue plasminogen activator is in reversing early myocardial infarction (Thrombolysis in Myocardial Infarction Study Group 1985). A new International Acute Renal Failure Working Group has been formed, with links to the International Society of Nephrology, to strengthen international communication between physicians and scientists with an interest in acute renal failure, including many in the Third World countries where septic abortion, snake bite, and haemorrhagic fever are still common antecedents.

In industrialized countries the background causes of acute renal failure have changed substantially over the past 20 years. Nephrotoxic therapeutic agents and sepsis now represent the most common antecedent conditions in hospitalized patients (Porter and Bennett 1980; Hou et al. 1983). The classic use of urinary sodium and other urinary indices to separate "acute tubular necrosis" (ATN) from prerenal states has been challenged (Pru and Kjellstrand 1984; Zarich et al.

Table 4.1. Acute renal failure/nephrotoxicity symposia

1973	London, UK (Flynn)
1973	Brooklyn, NY (Friedman, Eliahou)
1975	Rottach-Egern, FRG (Thurau)
1977	Rouen, France (Fillastre)
1979	Sydney, Australia (Duggin)
1981	Rouen, France (Fillastre)
1981	Pinehurst, NC (Porter)
1981	Tel Aviv, Israel (Eliahou)
1981	Guildford, UK (Bach)
1982	Baltimore, Md (Solez, Whelton)
1984	San Antonio, Texas (Stein)
1984	Guildford, UK (Bach)
1985	Antwerp, Belgium (DeBroe, Porter)
1986	Sapporo, Japan (Tanabe, Hook, Endou)
1987	Guildford, UK (Bach)
1988	Edmonton, Canada (Solez, Racusen)

1985). It has been suggested that acute renal failure as is now encountered in the modern intensive care unit is such a heterogeneous condition that the old diagnostic criteria no longer apply. In fact, this is probably not the case. If one examines the seven types of acute renal failure characterized by a low urine sodium and "prerenal" indices (Table 4.2) it is likely that in each entity the renal dysfunction is due to decreased renal perfusion, just as is assumed in the concept of prerenal azotaemia. What separates the other conditions listed from classic prerenal azotaemia is that the renal dysfunction cannot be reversed by administration of fluid or restoration of normal blood pressure and cardiac output, probably because there is a not-readily-reversible element of intrarenal vasospasm and/or redistribution of extracellular fluid present. But the original concept underlying the use of urinary indices – that in the absence of diuretic use "prerenal" indices indicate an intact tubular system while "ATN" indices indicate tubular damage – has never been demonstrated as being incorrect. Most patients encountered in the intensive care unit with sepsis, burns, or liver failure are too seriously ill to undergo a renal biopsy, so the intactness of their tubules cannot be assessed histologically. In the hepatorenal syndrome, biopsies obtained immediately after death show sparse tubular lesions consistent with "ATN" (Solez 1984). However, by the time of death these patients have often demonstrated a rise from their previously very low levels of urine sodium and FE_{Na} indicating some terminal element of superimposed "ATN". This demonstrates that it is necessary to follow serial indices to obtain an accurate picture of events.

Table 4.2. Types of acute renal failure other than classic prerenal azotaemia characterized by a low urine sodium

1.	Hepatorenal syndrome
2.	Burns
3.	Radiographic contrast material nephrotoxicity
4.	Sepsis
5.	Rhabdomyolysis
6.	Cyclosporin nephrotoxicity
7.	Transplant rejection

In most of the conditions in Table 4.2, there is almost immediate return of function once the underlying cause of renal failure is removed. This is in contrast to true "ATN" in which a period of often several weeks is required before tubular integrity is restored and normal renal function returns. Rapid return of function in non-"ATN" states is perhaps best illustrated in renal allografts. Successful treatment of early acute rejection or cessation of cyclosporin dosing in cyclosporin nephrotoxicity leads to nearly instantaneous return of function.

It has long been assumed that "ATN" in the transplanted kidney and "ATN" in the native kidney are essentially the same disease. However, recent studies by Olsen et al. (1989) have demonstrated striking morphological differences between the two conditions. Transplant "ATN" has significantly fewer tubular casts and significantly more deposition of calcium oxalate crystals than in native kidney "ATN". The thinning or absence of proximal tubular brush border which is a prominent feature of native kidney "ATN" (Solez et al. 1979; Jones 1982) is virtually absent in transplant "ATN". Also largely missing is the picture of "tubular cell unrest" with great cell-to-cell variation in size and shape which characterizes native kidney "ATN". On the other hand, transplant "ATN" demonstrates occasional foci of true tubular necrosis, whereas native kidney "ATN" generally shows no necrotic cells but is characterized by gaps along the tubular basement membrane where tubular cells have been shed and not replaced.

Recent studies have shown that cell shedding by the kidney is a considerably more interesting phenomenon than previously imagined. For comparable degrees of renal failure the rate of tubular cell shedding is many-fold greater in transplant "ATN" than in native kidney "ATN" (Racusen et al. unpublished). In most types of "ATN" in human patients and in animals a substantial proportion of the cells shed in the urine are fully viable cells which can be readily grown in tissue culture (Racusen et al. 1988). The factors which cause these living cells to detach from the tubular basement membrane and pass into the tubular fluid are unknown, but the observation that many of the cells which detach are alive is potentially of fundamental importance in the design of intervention strategies to abort the onset of acute renal failure or to lessen its severity once it is established. An analogy can be drawn with an equally important observation recently made in the brain showing that many brain cells remain viable after what had been considered a lethal period of brain ischaemia (Petito et al. 1987). Drugs that prevent calcium influx in part by blocking glutamate receptors in the brain offer the possibility of aborting what would otherwise be catastrophic injury to brain cells (Choi 1987). Agents which prevent cell detachment in the kidney may be shown to be of similar benefit in protection of kidney function and cellular integrity.

The relationships between tubular cell shedding in the urine, cell detachment within the kidney, and renal dysfunction are likely to be complicated. While the *presence* of substantial numbers of tubular cells in the urine indicates tubular injury, the *rate* at which the tubular cells appear in the urine is probably more a reflection of urine and tubular fluid flow rate than of the rate at which cells are detaching. In the oliguric kidney detached cells in obstructed nephrons may take a long time to reach the final urine, if they do so at all. In this situation cells may be fully viable at the time they detach, but necrotic or perhaps not even identifiable as cells when they reach the bladder. When viewed in this way the greater number of tubular cells reaching the urine in transplant "ATN" versus native kidney "ATN" may reflect the fewer tubular casts and lesser degree of tubular obstruction present in transplant "ATN". However, it must be admitted that the now well-established correlations between morphological tubular cell injury and renal functional impairment in "ATN" (Solez and Whelton 1984) are best demonstrated within individual models or clinical types. It is quite possible that there is indeed more tubular injury with cell detachment in transplant "ATN" compared with native kidney "ATN" for comparable degrees of renal functional impairment. This does not negate the value of studying renal morphology or tubular cell excretion in the urine. It simply means that one cannot assume that the same relationships will hold between severity of tubular injury or cell excretion and renal functional impairment in all models or clinical types of "ATN" since the character of the tubular injury varies.

We have previously observed (Solez et al. 1979) that tubular injury continues throughout the course of "ATN" in man. This is likely to be related to the defect in autoregulation observed in "ATN" making the kidney vulnerable to new hypotensive insults (Adams et al. 1980). Although little studied in previous investigations of clinical "ATN" the additional insults leading to fresh tubular injury may be important in prolonging the course of "ATN". Analysis of tubular cell shedding patterns may help to determine whether the additional insult is most commonly hypotension and/or dehydration brought about by haemodialysis. The intriguing notion that haemodialysis may actually in this sense cause superadded tubular injury and lengthen the course of "ATN" in some cases is clearly worthy of further study.

References

Adams PL, Adams FF, Bell PD, Navar LG (1980) Impaired renal blood flow autoregulation in ischemic acute renal failure. Kidney Int 18: 68–76
Beall D, Bywaters EGL, Belsey RHR, Miles JAR (1941) A case of crush injury with renal failure. Br Med J i: 432
Bywaters EGL, Beall D (1941) Crush injuries with impairment of renal function. Br Med J i: 427
Choi DW (1987) Ionic dependence of glutamate neurotoxicity. J Neurosci 7(2): 369–379
DeNavasquez S (1940) The excretion of haemoglobin with special reference to the transfusion kidney. J Pathol Bacteriol 51: 413
Dunn JS, Gillespie M, Niven JSF (1941) Renal lesions in two cases of crush syndrome. Lancet II: 549
Hou SH, Bushinsky DA, Wish JB, Cohen JJ, Harrington JT (1983) Hospital acquired renal insufficiency: A prospective study. Am J Med 74: 243–248
Jones DB (1982) Ultrastructure of human acute renal failure. Lab Invest 46: 254–264
Mayon-White R, Solandt OM (1941) A case of limb compression ending fatally in uraemia. Br Med J i: 434
Oliver J (1953) Correlations of structure and function and mechanisms of recovery in acute tubular necrosis. Am J Med 15: 535
Oliver J, MacDowell M, Tracy A (1951) The pathogenesis of acute renal failure associated with traumatic and toxic injury: Renal ischemia, nephrotoxic damage, and the ischemuric episode. J Clin Invest 30: 1307
Olsen S, Burdick JF, Keown PA, et al. (1989) Primary acute renal failure ("acute tubular necrosis") in the transplanted kidney: morphology and pathogenesis. Medicine 68: 173–187
Petito CK, Feldmann E, Pulsinelli WA, Plum F (1987) Delayed hippocampal damage in humans following cardiorespiratory arrest. Neurology 37: 1281–1286
Porter GA, Bennett WM (1980) Nephrotoxin-induced acute renal failure. In: Brenner BM, Stein JH (eds) Acute renal failure. Churchill Livingstone, New York

Pru C, Kjellstrand CM (1984) The FE$_{Na}$ test is of no prognostic value in acute renal failure. Nephron 36: 20
Racusen LC, Fivush B, Zapata BS, Solez K (1988) Culture of viable tubular cells (TC) from urine of patients with "acute tubular necrosis" (ATN). Lab Invest 33: 364 (abstr)
Solez K (1984) The pathology and pathogenesis of human "acute tubular necrosis". In: Solez K, Whelton A (eds) Acute renal failure: correlations between morphology and function. Marcel Dekker, New York, pp 17–42
Solez K, Whelton A (eds) (1984) Acute renal failure: correlations between morphology and function. Marcel Dekker, New York
Solez K, Morel-Maroger L, Sraer J-D (1979) The morphology of "acute tubular necrosis" in man: analysis of 57 renal biopsies and a comparison with the glycerol model. Medicine (Baltimore) 58: 362–370
The TIMI Study Group (1985) The thrombolysis in myocardial infarction (TIMI) Trial. N Engl J Med 312: 932–936
Zarich S, Fang LST, Diamond JR (1985) Fractional excretion of sodium: Exceptions to its diagnostic value. Arch Intern Med 145: 108–112

Discussion

The discussion was initiated by Dr Neild who drew an analogy between the nephrotoxicity associated with cyclosporin and the pathogenesis of the endothelial injury seen in acute renal failure. Dr Neild emphasized that the transplanted kidney can make a rapid recovery from acute tubular necrosis. Biopsy evidence in this condition suggests a substantial amount of necrosis yet two weeks later the cellular architecture is largely restored. He emphasized that in general, there are many casts to be found in the urine in the first 48 hours after acute renal failure in the transplanted kidney, and yet by day 5 these casts have disappeared. Calcium oxalate deposition in the substance of the transplanted kidney may be one cause for the crystal formations seen in transplant-related acute tubular necrosis. Whether this deposition of calcium oxalate is made worse by cyclosporin is unknown, but is probably unlikely. Dr Neild and Dr Solez both emphasized that the nephrotoxicity associated with cyclosporin was more likely to be of a vascular origin. Dr Parsons was concerned about the presence of polymorphs in the biopsy material that was presented. He wondered whether the presence of polymorphs reflected acute bacterial invasion of the kidney and Dr Solez replied that the accumulation of leucocytes in the vasa recta and the renal medulla is a feature of all types of acute tubular necrosis even in pure animal models. Intratubular polymorphs were more suggestive of renal infarction, e.g. transplant rejection, or some sort of vasculitic process together with intravascular coagulation. Dr Solez reiterated that it was always impossible to know whether one was missing bacterial infection. There seem to be technical problems associated with the culture of renal biopsy tissue and it is rare to get a positive bacterial culture.

Chapter 5

Acute Renal Failure in Old Age

J. F. Macias

In this review, acute renal failure (ARF) is defined as a syndrome characterized by the abrupt interruption of renal function to the extent that the kidney is unable to maintain control of the internal milieu. The term "old age" refers to people aged 65 and over. Having established this definition of ARF in old age it is important to recognize the increased incidence of the syndrome in elderly patients. There are a number of explanations for this higher incidence, but, in my opinion, three are outstanding: (a) the high incidence of systemic illnesses, (b) polypharmacy in the elderly, (c) the renal aging process itself (Kafetz 1983).

Among the systemic illnesses, hypertension, cardiac insufficiency, arteriosclerosis, diabetes, myeloma, prostatic enlargement and urinary tract infection all predispose to the development of ARF in certain situations (Frocht and Fijlit 1984). The likelihood of developing ARF is even greater if additional risks, such as fluid deprivation or exploration with contrast media, are required in patients with these pathologies. The role of polypharmacy should not be underestimated since drugs, such as diuretics, laxatives, analgesics and NSAIDs, are often prescribed to, and taken by, the aged.

Various evolutionary changes borne by the kidney as it ages predispose elderly individuals to the development of ARF; these include a fall in both GFR (glomerular filtration rate) and RBF (renal blood flow). If these changes are forgotten it is quite easy to induce nephrotoxic ARF in old people. Another factor is the inability to retain Na when the elderly person is salt deprived (Epstein and Hollenberg 1976). Low aldosterone levels and a certain degree of incompetence of the ascending limb of Henle's loop in the reabsorption of Na, can account for this feature of the aging kidney (Macias et al. 1978). Furthermore, an elderly person's high osmolar threshold for thirst also facilitates volume depletion. It is mandatory for persons caring for aged patients always to bear these two features of the aging kidney in mind. Similar aetiological factors play a role in the development of ARF in both young and elderly patients. ARF is classically divided into prerenal (acute reversible renal hypoperfusion), established ARF (acute tubular necrosis in the vast majority of cases) and post-renal (or obstructive ARF). We found that dehydration and electrolyte imbalance could account for 23% of established ARF in our series (Macias-Nunez and Sanchez-Tomero 1987), in comparison with 50% in Kumar et al.'s (1978) experience.

Established ARF may be provoked by agents acting primarily upon tubular cells acutely injuring the interstitium, by intratubular obstruction or by some effect on the glomerular tuft. Obviously, all these situations which lead to prerenal oliguria can proceed to acute established ARF if the underlying cause of the problem is not corrected. Myoglobinuria following arterial embolectomies, non-steroidal anti-inflammatory drugs, rapidly progressive idiopathic glomerulonephritis, mesangiocapillary glomerulonephritis, vasculitis and the proliferative variety of systemic lupus erythematosus are perhaps the more specific causes of this variety of ARF in the aged. Another important aetiology is septic shock. As many as 25% of cases of ARF in the elderly managed in our renal unit at the University Hospital of Salamanca have some form of sepsis underlying their postsurgical ARF. Cardiogenic shock may also play a role since many more elderly patients with septic shock are unable to maintain a hyperdynamic circulation for a prolonged period of time.

Post-renal or obstructive ARF accounts for 17%–38% of cases of ARF in the elderly. Superimposition of urinary tract infection on obstructive ARF introduces the problems of sepsis and worsens the patient's prognosis.

More often than not, the cause of ARF in a particular individual is "multifactorial", i.e. there is usually a deficiency in fluid replacement before surgery followed by dehydration, hypotension, infection, incorrect antibiotic administration (aminoglycosides especially) and finally, ARF.

The renal indices for diagnosing ARF are slightly different in the elderly compared with younger patients. For instance, a urinary Na concentration lower than 70 mmol l^{-1} in an elderly patient with clinical and biochemical findings of acute renal failure may suggest the presence of a prerenal element (acute reversible renal hypoperfusion). On the other hand, when urinary Na concentration is greater than 70 mmol l^{-1} one should think in terms of acute tubular necrosis (ATN). These values are in contrast to those generally accepted in younger patients.

Prognosis is ominous in the elderly. The influence of age is regarded by some authors as a negative factor in the outcome of ARF. Others believe that it is not age as such, but rather the aetiology which governs prognosis. In our experience pre-existing illnesses, particularly respiratory insufficiency with arterial hypoxaemia has a very bad prognosis.

Regardless of age, the prognosis of "multiple organ failure" has been mentioned, although a specific study focusing on the mortality of elderly patients is lacking. As previously stated, in any patient with two malfunctioning organs (the kidney and any other), mortality dramatically increases. In surgical series the effect of multiple organ failure in worsening prognosis after emergency operations of all types ranges from 23% (one organ, kidney) to 100% (3–5 organs). When lung dysfunction with the need for ventilation appears in the course of ATN, survival is almost negligible (Rasmussen and Ibells 1982; Macias-Nunez and Sanchez-Tomero 1987).

In view of the poor prognosis of ARF in the elderly, we believe that prophylactic manoeuvres are of paramount importance. The maintenance of an adequate extracellular volume and drug dosage schemes suitable for the patient's GFR are vital. We advise at least two litres of fluid per day in sick elderly patients. Before surgical operations it is even more important to provide them with fluid. If oral intake must be avoided (before surgery of the gastrointestinal tract, for example) administration of two litres of isotonic saline is useful in preventing the occurrence of ARF.

Treatment does not differ from that of younger patients. Regardless of age we have found total parenteral nutrition (TPN) helpful particularly in cases of ARF due to septic shock. Anecdotally, we have found an improvement in survival in patients treated with TPN (30% survival) compared with those who were not (9.6% survival), but, as always, this difference in survival may reflect only a difference in the severity of illness.

References

Epstein M, Hollenberg NK (1976) Age as a determinant of sodium conservation in man. J Lab Clin Med 87: 411–417
Frocht A, Fillit H (1984) Renal disease in the geriatric patient. J Am Geriatr Soc 32: 28–43
Kafetz K (1983) Renal impairment in the elderly: a review. J R Soc Med 76: 398–401
Kumar R, Hill CM, McGeown MG (1978) Acute renal failure in the elderly. Lancet I: 90–91
Macías JF, Garcia-Iglesias C, Bondía A, Rodriguez JL, Corbacho L, Tabernero JM, de Castro S (1978) Renal handling of sodium in old people: a functional study. Age Ageing 7: 178–181
Macías-Núñez JF, Sánchez-Tomero JA (1987) Acute renal failure in old people. In: Macías-Núñez JF, Cameron JS (eds) Renal function and disease in the elderly. Butterworths, London, pp 461–484
Rasmussen HH, Ibells LLS (1982) Acute renal failure: multivariate analysis of causes of risk factors. Am J Med 73: 211–219

Discussion

Dr Macias was closely questioned concerning the differences between the two groups of patients – those treated with and those who did not receive parenteral nutrition. The Spanish regimen for parenteral nutrition included amino acids together with lipid and glucose. Nitrogen was administered at 0.2–0.3 g per kg of body weight, and about 150 non-protein kilocalories were given with each gram of nitrogen. Dr Macias admitted that in his studies of acute renal failure in the elderly, the patients who did not receive parenteral nutrition were not studied concurrently. These patients formed a group that were treated in the 1970s whereas patients who were fed parenterally formed a second group treated from 1979 onwards. Dr Solez remarked that since the original report by Abel et al. concerning the importance of amino acid therapy in improving survival from acute renal failure, few investigators had managed to demonstrate much of an effect using nutrition alone. Dr Linton drew attention to a meta-analysis of controlled clinical trials of essential amino acids and hyperosmotic glucose in the treatment of acute renal failure which had appeared recently in the journal *Renal Failure*. He claimed that this meta-analysis had looked closely at four appropriately controlled, randomized clinical trials of amino acids and had had great difficulty in demonstrating any worthwhile effect of such therapy on hospital survival rates. He finished by emphasizing that there was very little hard evidence to suggest that feeding with amino acids was in fact beneficial, despite the fact that when the survival rate from multi-system failure associated with renal failure is so low, one might expect even a minor benefit to become obvious. Dr Macias replied that his regime using carbohydrates, fats and amino acids was not comparable, because the American regime did not include fat and the use of hyperosmotic glucose, more than 30%, was not beneficial in Dr Macias' experience.

Professor Cameron moved the discussion to some consideration of the time taken for elderly patients to die or to recover their renal function. He thought that many nephrologists were seeing young patients survive 2, 3 or 4 weeks before dying from multi-system failure and that this prolonged intensive care survival results in the utilization of very expensive resources. He wondered whether the elderly were more economic and graceful and died earlier. Dr Macias replied that the situation was the same with the elderly patient in so far as the median length of survival in intensive care of patients who subsequently died was somewhere between 4 and 6 weeks. That is the elderly were just as expensive to treat! Dr Macias also emphasized that a normal serum creatinine in an elderly patient does not necessarily mean that that patient has normal renal function. All participants agreed that the serum creatinine alone was a poor guide to the glomerular filtration rate and this had to be borne in mind when using such nephrotoxic drugs as aminoglycosides and non-steroidal anti-inflammatory compounds. Conservation of sodium also appears to be impaired in elderly patients and Dr Ledingham suggested that the renin–angiotensin system might become increasingly sluggish with old age.

Professor Better asked whether the elderly were more likely to develop ototoxicity associated with gentamicin and diuretic poisoning. Dr Macias replied that ototoxicity related to the use of diuretics was more common in the elderly and Professor Cameron referred to a review published in the *Journal of Microbial Chemotherapy* which summarized all the trials of aminoglycosides relating the different compounds to the incidence of side effects. Apparently ototoxicity was much less frequent with netilmicin, whereas it was much more common with amikacin. The elderly do seem to be more at risk from ototoxicity, but again, this may reflect the small body mass and the normal serum creatinine of an elderly person which may conceal a large reduction in glomerular filtration rate.

Section II
Some Aspects of Renal Physiology

Chapter 6

Cortical and Juxtamedullary Glomerular Blood Flow After Temporary Ischaemia

M. Steinhausen, M. Fretschner, E. Gulbins and N. Parekh

Temporary ischaemia is one of the most common models used to investigate the pathophysiology of acute renal failure (Arendshorst et al. 1975; Eisenbach and Steinhausen 1973). Sixty minutes of unilateral occlusion of the renal artery induces complete anuria for one to three days with restitution of kidney function 10–40 days later (comparable to observations in man after surgical shock) (Steinhausen 1984). The cause of prolonged anuria after temporary ischaemia is often discussed. Some investigators have proposed a continuous reduction in renal blood flow as an important factor contributing to the prolonged anuria (Finn and Chevalier 1979), but it has been demonstrated that blood flow to the cortex and the papilla is not decreased for long periods following ischaemia (Böttcher and Steinhausen 1976; Parekh and Veith 1981). Tubular leakage and blockage of tubules by protein cylinders are considered by others to be the most important causes of prolonged anuria (Parekh et al. 1984; Steinhausen and Parekh 1984; Tanner and Steinhausen 1976; Yagil et al. 1988). In some studies it has also been proposed that an isolated reduction of the medullary blood flow may be an important factor in the pathogenesis of acute renal failure. Karlberg et al. (1983) reported a reduction of about 88% of the blood flow to the inner stripe and the inner zone of the medulla. The blood flow to the cortex and the outer stripe of medulla was reduced by only about 40% and 44% (Karlberg et al. 1983). Brezis et al. (1984) demonstrated that the thick ascending limb of Henle's loop is highly vulnerable to hypoxia (Brezis et al. 1984). Mason et al. (1984) proposed medullary blood congestion as an important factor in acute renal failure (Mason et al. 1984; Mason 1986). However, there are enormous technical problems in the measurement of medullary blood flow. In the mammalian kidney the tip of the papilla is the only part accessible to direct intravital microscopy (Zimmerhackl et al. 1985b; Böttcher and Steinhausen 1976). In this area only small parts of the vasa recta are visible. The other parts of the medulla cannot be visualized by intravital microscopy. To improve visualization of the renal microcirculation in vivo, we developed the model of the split hydronephrotic kidney (Steinhausen et al. 1983, 1986b, 1987a). We have recently improved this technique to enable measurement of both cortical and juxtamedullary glomerular blood flow in the same kidney (Steinhausen et al. unpublished). This technique has now been used to clarify whether medullary blood flow is reduced after temporary ischaemia or not.

Methods

Experiments were performed on female (Munich) Wistar rats (240–280 g). The technique of producing a split hydronephrotic kidney has been described in detail by Steinhausen et al. (1983, 1986b). Hydronephrosis was induced by permanent ligation of the left ureter via a flank incision under pentobarbital anaesthesia (Nembutal^R, Ceva, Bad Segeberg, FRG, 60 mg kg^{-1}, i.p.). The present experiments were performed 2–3 months later on the hydronephrotic kidney under thiobutabarbital anaesthesia (Inactine^R, BYK, Konstanz, FRG, 100 mg kg^{-1}, i.p.). Under controlled body temperature (37–37.5 °C) and with continuous monitoring of systemic blood pressure by a catheter in the left carotid artery, isotonic saline solution was infused into the jugular vein (0.2 ml min^{-1} kg^{-1}). Before further interventions the rats were tracheostomized. The hydronephrotic kidney was exposed by a flank incision and split along the greater curvature. The dorsal half of the kidney was sutured to a semicircular wire attached to the bottom of a Plexiglas bath. The bath was filled with an isotonic and isocolloidal solution (Haemaccel^R, Behringwerke, Marburg/Lahn, FRG) regulated at 37 °C. For intravital microscopy a Leitz Ultropac water-immersion objective (UO–55) combined with a television and a video recorder was used. The luminal diameters of the vessels were measured directly from the television screen. To assess the overall blood flow in the kidney, 0.05 ml lissamine-green dye was injected intravenously and the arrival time of lissamine-green in the chosen glomeruli was measured. Arrival times of 2.7 s or less were considered to represent a normal blood flow (Steinhausen and Tanner 1976).

To find a juxtamedullary glomerulus, the preparation had to be scanned first at low magnification using a 11× or a 22× objective. We identified a juxtamedullary glomerulus by the length of the efferent arteriole (see Table 6.1). Further characteristics of the juxtamedullary glomeruli were their size and the large luminal diameters of the afferent and efferent arterioles. After surgical procedures kidneys were allowed to equilibrate to the tissue bath conditions for at least 1 hour. The intraluminal diameters of the (a) arcuate artery, (b) afferent arteriole of a cortical and a juxtamedullary glomerulus, and (c) efferent arteriole of a cortical and a juxtamedullary glomerulus were measured over a period of 180 min.

Diameter measurements were done on a digitalized video frame from the coordinates of the vessel wall with the aid of a computer.

Blood flow velocity was measured in efferent arterioles of both glomeruli with an RBC velocity-tracking correlator using the method of Wayland and Johnson (1967) (Model 102 B, IPM San Diego, CA). The glomerular blood flow was calculated from blood flow velocity and luminal diameter.

Table 6.1. Mean and SEM values of length of vas efferens, luminal diameters, and glomerular blood flow of cortical and juxtamedullary vessels of the split hydronephrotic kidney under control conditions for both groups

	Group 1 ($n=5$)	Group 2 ($n=5$)
Length of vas efferens (μm)		
cortical	283 ± 77	254 ± 22
juxtamedullary	4957 ± 1573[a]	3472 ± 392[a]
Luminal diameter (μm)		
Arcuate arteries	61.1 ± 3.3	55.4 ± 3.2
Afferent arterioles		
cortical	12.4 ± 1.1[a]	10.5 ± 0.5
juxtamedullary	19.5 ± 2.0[a]	17.5 ± 1.2[a]
Efferent arterioles		
cortical	12.9 ± 1.1	13.1 ± 0.84
juxtamedullary	33.9 ± 3.0[a]	27.9 ± 5.0[a]
Glomerular blood flow (nl min^{-1})		
cortical	40.6 ± 10.5	38.5 ± 11.5
juxtamedullary	356.1 ± 140.8[a]	250.6 ± 64.1[a]

[a] Cortical against juxtamedullary <0.05.

Temporary ischaemia of the left kidney was induced by an aortic ligation distal to the right and proximal to the left renal artery for one hour. Before clamping the abdominal aorta two control measurements (C1, C2) were performed at an interval of 10 min. The vessel diameters and the glomerular blood flow rate were measured 4, 10, 30, 60, 90, 120, 150 and 180 min after opening the clamp.

The rats were divided into two groups: group 1 ($n=5$) received an infusion of saline solution (0.2 ml kg^{-1} min^{-1}) throughout the experiment; group 2 ($n=5$) was given a continuous infusion of Haemaccel (0.2 ml kg^{-1} min^{-1}) after opening the aortic clamp. At the end of each experiment prazosin (10^{-6} mol l^{-1}) and nitrendipine (2.8×10^{-6} mol l^{-1}) were added to the bath.

Statistics. The data are presented as mean ± SEM. Comparison of mean values against control were made using analysis of variances. Probability values of less than 5% were considered significant.

Results

Control values of vascular diameters, the length of cortical and juxtamedullary arterioles and the glomerular blood flow are listed in Table 6.1. All values of juxtamedullary glomeruli are significantly higher than for cortical glomeruli. The glomerular blood flow was significantly decreased only during the initial post-ischaemic period (Fig. 6.1). Four minutes after the end of the ischaemia the flow was decreased by about 60% as compared with the preischaemic control (C1, C2). In the following 30 min the glomerular blood flow increased slowly; 180 min after reperfusion the cortical and juxtamedullary blood flow were not signifi-

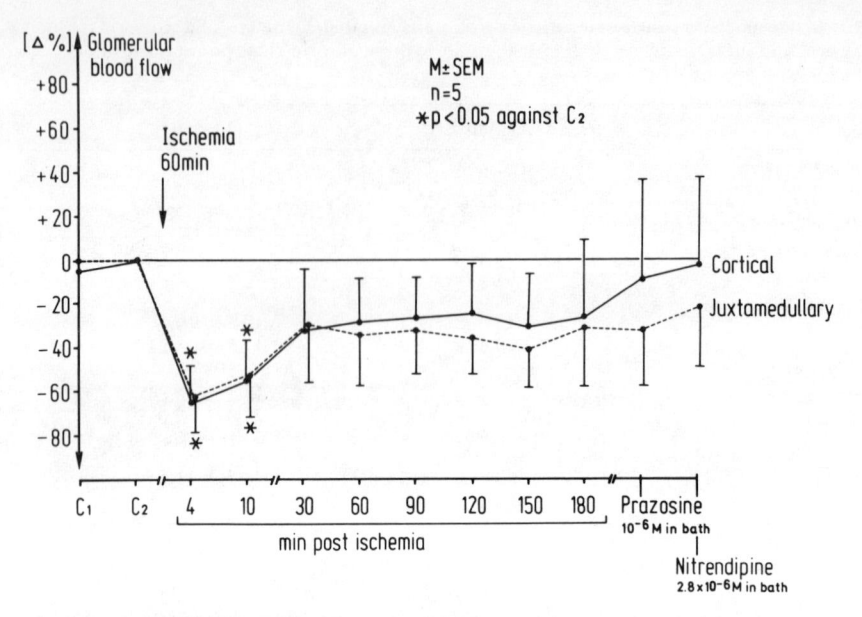

Fig. 6.1. Relative changes in glomerular blood flow measured in efferent arterioles of cortical and juxtamedullary glomeruli in split hydronephrotic kidney of rats under control conditions and after temporary ischaemia (group 1).

cantly decreased. During the whole postischaemic period there was no significant difference between the juxtamedullary and the cortical blood flow.

A small, but not significant improvement to cortical and juxtamedullary blood flow was seen with the alpha blocker prazosin as well as the calcium antagonist nitrendipine. Intravenous infusion of an isotonic and isocolloidal solution (Haemaccel^R) prevented the reduction of glomerular blood flow (Fig. 6.2).

The luminal diameters of the first group without Haemaccel infusion differed significantly from preischaemic controls only in the initial postischaemic period (Fig. 6.3). The most significant reduction of the luminal vessel diameter was observed in the arcuate artery 10 min (-25%) and 30 min (-20%) after opening the aortic clamp. Ten minutes after the end of ischaemia the luminal diameter of the cortical afferent arteriole was decreased by about 12%. After this initial decrease the arteriole diameter was not significantly less than the preischaemic values. The diameter of the juxtamedullary afferent arteriole was not significantly reduced.

The intravenous infusion of the isotonic and isocolloidal solution induced a vasodilation of the preglomerular vessels (Fig. 6.4). The luminal diameters of cortical and juxtamedullary efferent arterioles were not significantly decreased during the postischaemic period (Fig. 6.5). The small reduction in vessel diameters was prevented by the infusion of Haemaccel (Fig. 6.6). A difference in diameter changes between cortical and juxtamedullary efferent arterioles was not observed.

In neither group was the arterial blood pressure significantly reduced after the end of ischaemia. No significant difference between the arterial blood pressure of rats with and without infusion was observed (Fig. 6.7).

Cortical and Juxtamedullary Glomerular Blood Flow After Temporary Ischaemia

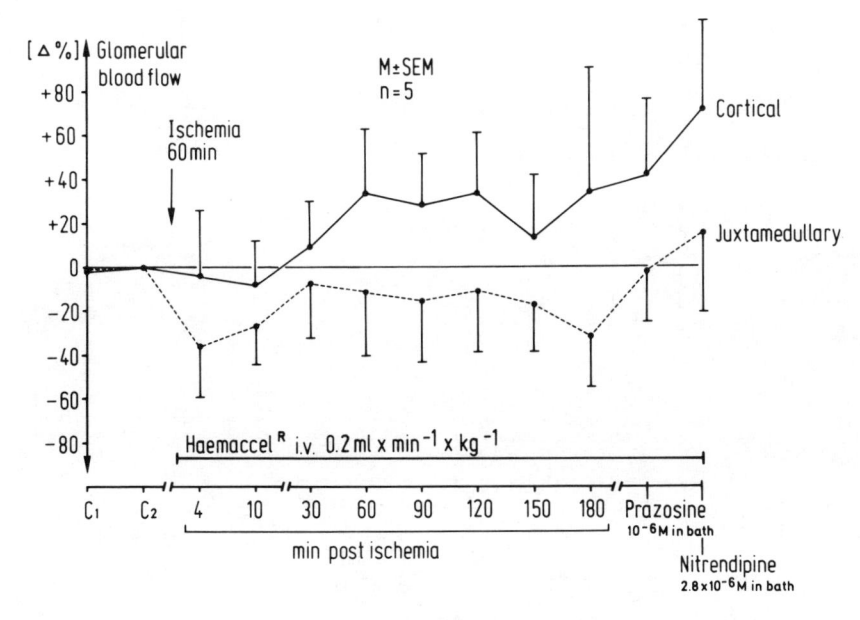

Fig. 6.2. Relative changes in glomerular blood flow as shown in Fig. 6.1. These animals received an infusion of Haemaccel after the end of ischaemia (group 2).

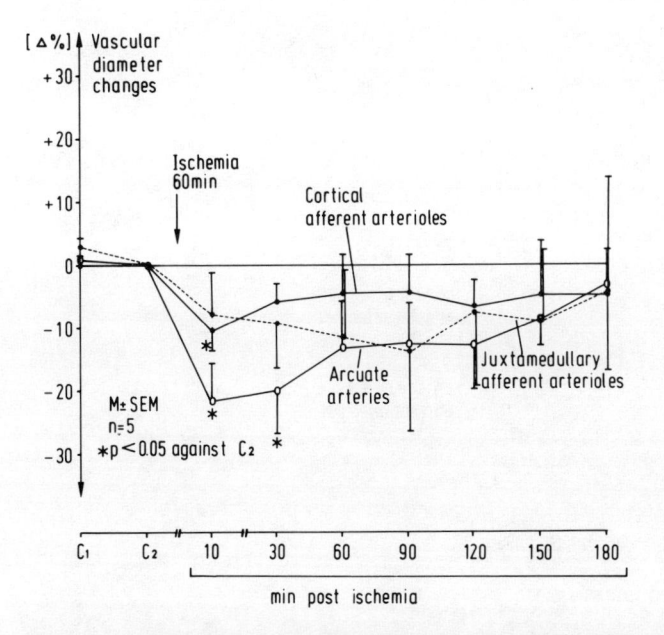

Fig. 6.3. Relative changes in luminal diameters of preglomerular vessels after temporary ischaemia without postischaemic infusion of an isotonic and isocolloidal solution (group 1).

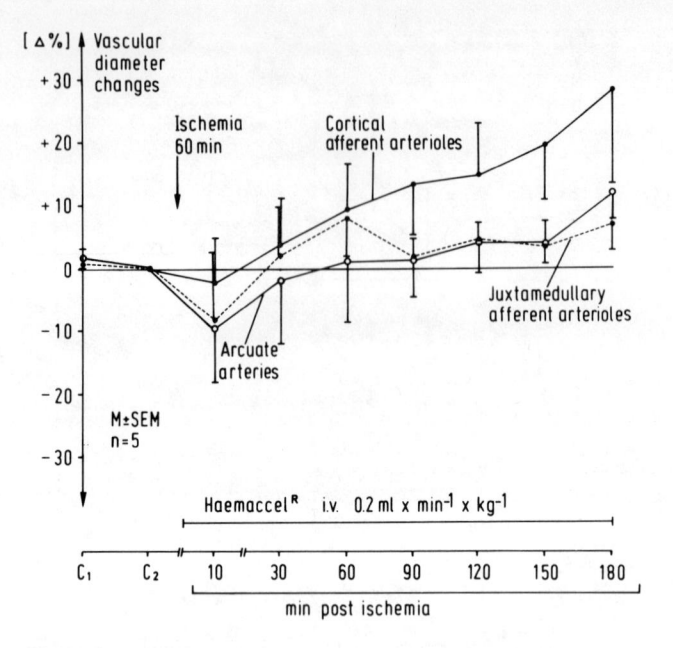

Fig. 6.4. Relative changes in luminal diameters of preglomerular vessels as in Fig. 6.3. These animals received an infusion of Haemaccel (group 2).

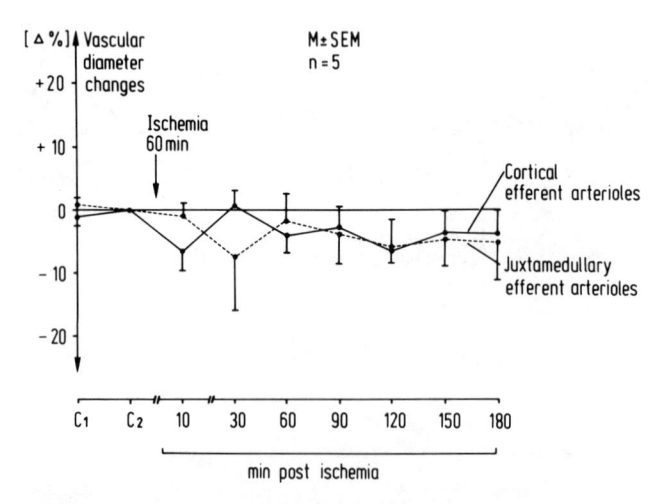

Fig. 6.5. Relative changes in luminal diameters of efferent arterioles without postischaemic infusion of an isotonic and isocolloidal solution (group 1).

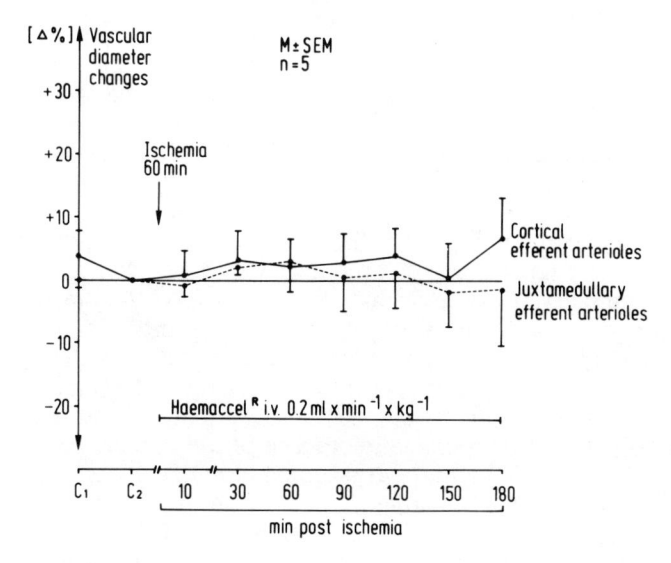

Fig. 6.6. Relative changes in luminal diameters of efferent arterioles with postischaemic Haemaccel infusion (group 2).

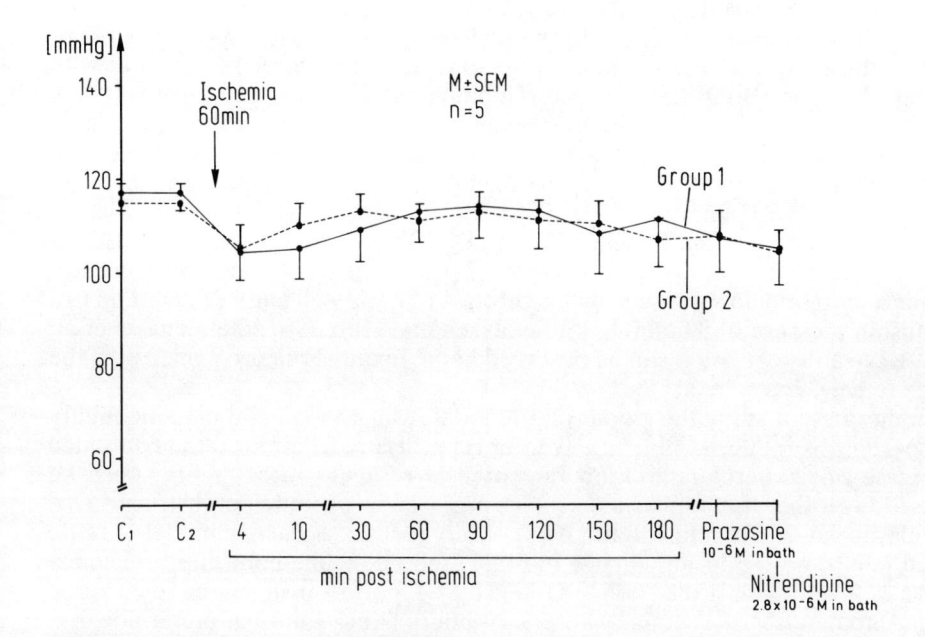

Fig. 6.7. Changes in mean arterial blood pressure after temporary ischaemia without (group 1) and with postischaemic infusion of an isotonic and isocolloidal solution (group 2).

Discussion

In the present study no differences between cortical and juxtamedullary blood flow under postischaemic conditions were obtained. In contrast to these results, Karlberg et al. (1983) demonstrated with a ^{86}Rb extraction method a significant difference between the cortical and medullary blood flow 10 minutes after clamping the renal artery. Unfortunately, the authors did not perform further measurements after the first decrease of the renal blood flow. The early difference between cortical and juxtamedullary blood flow, seen only with the Rb technique may be explained by differences in tubular damage and different tubular Rb uptake. Norlén et al. (1978), using microspheres to measure renal blood flow, reported a reduced renal blood flow after cold ischaemia for 12 and 16 hours. The reduction was more pronounced in the deep cortex and the juxtamedullary glomeruli than in the superficial glomeruli of the cortex. After cold ischaemia for 2 hours the regional and the total renal blood flow were not significantly altered (Norlén et al. 1978). Also using microspheres Mason et al. (1984) observed a 65% reduction in the perfusion of juxtamedullary nephrons and a 35% reduction in superficial nephrons after acute ischaemia (cf. Thiel et al. 1982). They have proposed that hypoxia induces erythrocyte aggregation, vascular congestion and blood stasis (Mason 1986). Many of these differences are probably a consequence of the different methods employed in measurement. The problem with the microsphere technique lies in the underestimation of the medullary blood flow by an unequal distribution of microspheres within the kidney (Bankir et al. 1979).

Although the hydronephrotic kidney is a non-filtering kidney, we have assumed it is possible to transfer the results of these experiments to the normal kidney. The walls of the vessels in the hydronephrotic kidney appear histologically, ultrastructurally and electrophysiologically unaltered compared with normal kidneys (Bührle et al. 1986; Nobiling et al. 1986). The relatively low cortical blood flow in the split hydronephrotic kidney is probably a result of stretching the vascular walls during hydronephrosis. The response of the split hydronephrotic kidney to many pharmacological interventions, especially to angiotensin II (Steinhausen et al. 1986a, 1987a), dopamine (Steinhausen et al. 1986b), calcium antagonists (Fleming et al. 1987a,b; Steinhausen et al. 1987b) etc. seems to be comparable to that of the filtering kidney. The cortical glomerular blood flow of the hydronephrotic kidney is well autoregulated up to a perfusion pressure of 80 mmHg (Steinhausen and Holz 1987; Steinhausen et al. 1989). No autoregulation can be observed in the juxtamedullary glomeruli of the same female Wistar rats.

In the present study the glomerular blood flow in cortical and juxtamedullary glomeruli was reduced only initially after reperfusion. Therefore, the continued decrease of glomerular filtration rate, typical of acute renal failure, must be caused by other pathophysiological changes such as tubular obstruction or tubular leakage. Churchill et al. (1977) observed in an ischaemic model of acute renal failure no significant change in renal blood flow one hour after ischaemia and a 20% reduction after 4 hours. Others have reported an increased renal blood flow 4 hours after ischaemia, whereas 20 hours later, a normal blood flow has been observed (Frega et al. 1976). Parekh and Veith (1981) obtained in the same model of acute renal failure comparable results with a reduction of renal blood flow by about 25% over ten days. By contrast, however, Finn and Chevalier (1979) reported a reduction of the blood flow by about 60% over 4 weeks after temporary ischaemia.

It has been proposed that postischaemic vasoconstriction may be caused by the tubuloglomerular feedback mechanism (Köhler 1987). A feedback system over the macula densa system does not exist in the hydronephrotic kidney but an increased angiotensin II activity after ischaemia in the kidney is well known. It can be assumed that the initial postischaemic vasoconstriction is caused by angiotensin II, especially since angiotensin II induces intense vasoconstriction of the vessels in the hydronephrotic kidney (Steinhausen et al. 1987a), (the renin content in the hydronephrotic kidney corresponding to that in control kidneys) (Nobiling et al. 1986).

In recent studies with cyclosporin A (Zimmerhackl et al. 1988) and leukotriene D4 (Gulbins et al. 1988) we have observed constriction of the larger preglomerular arterioles. The arcuate arterioles constricted much more than afferent or efferent arterioles. This is consistent with the results of the present study with stronger vasoconstriction of the arcuate artery than the afferent arteriole. Therefore, leukotriene D4 may be an important factor in some kinds of ischaemic renal failure, especially those with anaphylactic or inflammatory pathogenesis. Results from Hagmann and Keppler (1982) support this assumption. They reported an increased synthesis and a decreased metabolism of leukotrienes in septic shock. They antagonized the lethal effects of endotoxin with leukotriene-antagonists (Hagmann and Keppler 1982, Hagmann et al. 1984, 1985; Scheuber et al. 1987). Under conditions such as septic shock this type of renal vasoconstriction may be responsible for the first phase of an ischaemic acute renal failure.

Summary

The present results demonstrate during the initial phase after 60 minutes of renal ischaemia a similar decrease in the vessel diameters of cortical and juxtamedullary arterioles. The changes of glomerular blood flow rates after temporary ischaemia were not significantly different between cortical and juxtamedullary arterioles. In both types of glomerulus the renal blood flow was reduced only initially after ischaemia; a postischaemic infusion of an isocolloidal solution could prevent this blood flow reduction. Reduced blood flow seems to be an important factor only in the initial phase of acute renal failure.

Acknowledgements. The authors would like to acknowledge the technical assistance of Rudolf Dussel in the experiments reported here.

References

Arendshorst WJ, Finn WF, Gottschalk CW (1975) Pathogenesis of acute renal failure following temporary renal ischemia in the rat. Circ Res 37: 558–568

Bankir L, Trinh Trang Tan MM, Grünfeld JP (1979) Measurements of glomerular blood flow in rabbits and rats: erroneous findings with 15 μm microspheres. Kidney Int 15: 126–133

Böttcher W, Steinhausen M (1976) Microcirculation of the renal papilla of rats under control conditions and after temporary ischemia. Kidney Int 10: 74–80
Brezis M, Rosen S, Silva P, Epstein FH (1984) Selective vulnerability of the medullary thick ascending limb to anoxia in the isolated perfused rat kidney. J Clin Invest 73: 182–190
Bührle CP, Hackenthal E, Helmchen U, Lackner K, Nobiling R, Steinhausen M, Taugner R (1986) Methods in laboratory investigation. The hydronephrotic kidney of the mouse as a tool for intravital microscopy and in vitro electrophysiological studies of renin-containing cell. Lab Invest 54: 462–472
Churchill S, Zarlengo MD, Carvalho JS, Gottlieb MN, Oken DE (1977) Normal renocortical blood flow in experimental acute renal failure. Kidney Int 11: 246–255
Eisenbach GM, Steinhausen M (1973) Micropuncture studies after temporary ischemia of rat kidneys. Pflugers Arch 343: 11–25
Finn WF, Chevalier RL (1979) Recovery from postischemic acute renal failure in the rat. Kidney Int 16: 113–123
Fleming JT, Parekh N, Steinhausen M (1987a) Calcium antagonists preferentially dilate preglomerular vessels of hydronephrotic kidney. Am J Physiol 253: F1157–F1163
Fleming JT, Garthoff B, Mayer D, Rosen B, Steinhausen M (1987b) Comparison of the effects of antihypertensive drugs on pre- and postglomerular vessels of the hydronephrotic kidney. J Cardiovasc Pharmacol 10 [Suppl 10]: 149–153
Frega NS, Dibona DR, Guertler B, Leaf A (1976) Ischemic renal failure. Kidney Int 10: 17–25
Gulbins E, Fretschner M, Parekh N, Rauterberg EW, Steinhausen M (1988) Leukotrienwirkungen (LTD_4) auf die renale Mikrozirkulation. 12. Jahrestagung der Deutschen Gesellschaft für Mikrozirkulation, Bern
Hagmann W, Keppler D (1982) Leukotriene antagonists prevent endotoxin lethality. Naturwissenschaften 69: 594–595
Hagmann W, Denzlinger C, Keppler D (1984) Role of peptide leukotrienes and their hepatobiliary elimination in endotoxin action. Circ Shock 14: 223–235
Hagmann W, Denzlinger C, Keppler D (1985) Production of peptide leukotrienes in endotoxin shock. FEBS Lett 180: 309–313
Karlberg L, Norlén BJ, Öjteg G, Wolgast M (1983) Impaired medullary circulation in postischemic acute renal failure. Acta Physiol Scand 118: 11–17
Köhler H (1987) Nierenfunktion und Schock. In: Kilian J, Messmer K, Ahnefeld FW (eds) Schock. Springer-Verlag, Berlin, Heidelberg, New York, pp 163–172
Mason J (1986) The pathophysiology of ischemic acute renal failure: a new hypothesis about the initiation phase. Renal Physiol 9: 129–147
Mason J, Torhorst J, Welsch J (1984) Role of the medullary perfusion defect in the pathogenesis of ischemic renal failure. Kidney Int 26: 283–293
Nobiling R, Bührle CP, Hackenthal E, Helmchen U, Steinhausen M, Whalley A, Taugner R (1986) Ultrastructure, renin status, contractile and electrophysiological properties of the afferent glomerular arteriole in the rat hydronephrotic kidney. Virchows Arch [A] 410: 31–42
Norlén BJ, Engberg A, Källskog Ö, Wolgast M (1978) Intrarenal hemodynamics in the transplanted rat kidney. Kidney Int 14: 1–9
Parekh N, Veith U (1981) Renal hemodynamics and oxygen consumption during postischemic acute renal failure in the rat. Kidney Int 19: 306–316
Parekh N, Esslinger HU, Steinhausen M (1984) Glomerular filtration and tubular reabsorption during anuria in postischemic acute renal failure. Kidney Int 25: 33–41
Scheuber PH, Denzlinger C, Wilker D, Beck G, Keppler D, Hammer DK (1987) Cysteinyl leukotrienes as mediators of staphylococcal enterotoxin B in the monkey. Eur J Clin Invest 17: 455–459
Steinhausen M (1984) Intravital microscopic observations of acute renal failure as a tool for simultaneously analyzing structure and function. In: Solez K, Whelton A (eds) Acute renal failure: correlations between morphology and function. Marcel Dekker, New York, pp 169–175
Steinhausen M, Holz FG (1987) Autoregulation of glomerular blood flow during converting-enzyme inhibition by captopril. Biomed Biochim Acta 46: 1005–1009
Steinhausen M, Parekh N (1984) Renal microcirculation and acute renal failure. Klin Exp Urol 8: 24–35
Steinhausen M, Tanner GA (1976) Microcirculation and tubular urine flow in the mammalian kidney cortex. Sitzungsberichte der Heidelberger Akademie der Wissenschaften. Mathematische naturwissenschaftlich Klasse, 3 Abhandlung. Springer, Berlin Heidelberg New York
Steinhausen M, Snoei H, Parekh N, Baker R, Johnson PC (1983) Hydronephrosis: a new method to visualize vas afferens, efferens, and glomerular network. Kidney Int 23: 794–806

Steinhausen M, Kücherer H, Parekh N, Weis S, Wiegman DL, Wilhelm KR (1986a) Angiotensin II control of the renal microcirculation: effect of blockade by saralasin. Kidney Int 30: 56–61

Steinhausen M, Weis S, Fleming J, Dussel R, Parekh N (1986b) Responses of in vivo renal microvessels to dopamine. Kidney Int 30: 361–370

Steinhausen M, Sterzel RB, Fleming JT, Kühn R, Weis S (1987a) Acute and chronic effects of angiotensin II on the vessels of the split hydronephrotic kidney. Kidney Int 31: 64–73

Steinhausen M, Fleming JT, Holz F, Parekh N (1987b) Nitrendipine and the pressure-dependent vasodilation of vessels in the hydronephrotic kidney. J Cardiovasc Pharmacol 9: 39–43

Steinhausen M, Blum M, Fleming JT, Holtz FG, Parekh N, Wiegman DL with technical assistance of Dussel R (1989) Visualization of renal autoregulation in the split hydronephrotic kidney of rats. Kidney Int 35: 1151–1160.

Tanner GA, Steinhausen M (1976) Tubular obstruction in ischemia-induced acute renal failure. Kidney Int 10: 67–73

Thiel G, de Rougemont D, Kriz W, Mason J, Torhorst J, Wolgast M (1982) The role of reduced medullary perfusion in the genesis of acute ischemic renal failure. Nephron 31: 321–323

Wayland H, Johnson PC (1967) Erythrocyte velocity measurement in microvessels by a two slit-photometric method. J Appl Physiol 22: 333

Yagil Y, Myers BD, Jamison RL (1988) Course and pathogenesis of postischemic acute renal failure in the rat. Am J Physiol 255: 257–264

Zimmerhackl B, Parekh N, Kücherer H, Steinhausen M (1985a) Influence of systemically applied angiotensin II on the microcirculation of glomerular capillaries in the rat. Kidney Int 27: 17–24

Zimmerhackl B, Dussel R, Steinhausen M (1985b) Erythrocyte flow and dynamic hematocrit in the renal papilla of the rat. Am J Physiol 249: F898–F902

Zimmerhackl LB, Fretschner M, Steinhausen M (1988) Cyclosporin (CyA) vermindert den renalen Blutfluss (RBF) durch Vasokonstriktion der A. arcuata bei der hydronephrotischen Ratte (HR). 19. Kongress der Gesellschaft für Nephrologie, Göttingen

Discussion

Immediately following his presentation, Dr Steinhausen was asked whether there was afferent and efferent vasodilatation with acetylcholine. He confirmed that this was the case, but he had no data on the effects of bradykinin. Dr Schrier mentioned that the cremaphore used in the Sandoz IV preparation of cyclosporin, which is a modified castor oil, had been shown to produce the same changes in renal blood flow as cyclosporin itself. Whilst this was true for acute studies, this did not appear to be the case with chronic dosing. After multiple doses cyclosporin appears to have a very different effect from the cremaphore on its own. Dr Steinhausen confirmed that the solvent for CyA is critical. Cremophore solvent itself may alter renal blood perfusion. He used two different solvents to dissolve CyA: cremophore and ethanol–Tween in combination with rat plasma. Using either solvent CyA caused similar responses. In contrast, solvents alone did cause a slight increase in blood flow and did not demonstrate significant vasoconstriction. Blood flow did not decrease in the control groups. Therefore results indicate that CyA itself and not the solvent caused the vasoconstriction of arcuate arteries in the split hydronephrotic kidney.

Dr Bihari turned the discussion towards the concept of vasomotion in the normal microcirculation. He referred to Professor Konrad Messmer's work on this subject and asked Dr Steinhausen whether vasomotion occurred in the glomerular capillary microcirculation. Dr Steinhausen replied that in his model of the hydronephrotic rat kidney, isolated and perfused, there was no evidence of vasomotion. Dr Epstein pursued this question of whether there were periodic variations in microflow in the isolated, perfused, hydronephrotic rat kidney. He referred to previous studies of the rat kidney in vivo which were thought to demonstrate periodic variations in microcirculatory blood flow in the rat kidney cortex. Dr Steinhausen stood firm and reiterated his opinion that vasomotion was unlikely to be an important feature of microcirculatory blood flow in the kidney in stable conditions. However, vasomotion could be induced in the hydronephrotic kidney by infusing a calcium agonist (Bay K 8644). This calcium agonist has also been shown to cause an extremely high vessel tone in the hydronephrotic kidney.

Chapter 7

Are Atrial Pressures Involved in the Regulation of Sodium and Water Balance? Studies in Conscious Animals

G. Kaczmarczyk, E. Schmidt, K. Falke and H. W. Reinhardt

Introduction

The maintenance of sodium and water balance is an essential requirement for proper cell function. Some (but probably not all) variables related to the adjustment of sodium balance after the expansion of the extracellular fluid volume are depicted in Fig. 7.1. The relations of hormonal, physical and neural factors are complex and for any investigation into this subject, some basic experimental considerations are required: separation of acute from chronic conditions; separation of mechanisms involved in sodium excretion from mechanisms involved in sodium retention; consideration of the quantitative involvement of single parameters with respect to others; relations between conscious and anaesthetized conditions; consideration of pre-existing conditions of sodium and water balance and, last but not least, awareness of the redundancy of regulation systems involved in such an essential challenge as providing sodium and water homeostasis.

In the present paper the involvement of the pressures in the atria of the heart as one of the afferent mechanisms for maintaining sodium and water homeostasis is discussed. This is of some considerable importance in patients requiring intensive care since disturbances in cardiac filling pressures are frequent, and often difficult to identify in the presence of mechanical ventilation.

Since Gauer's observation (Gauer et al. 1951) that in anaesthetized animals an increase in left atrial pressure (balloon inflation) leads to a brisk diuresis, it has been generally accepted that atrial receptors are involved in the control of body fluid volume – although no data on sodium excretion are available. Left and right atrial pressures are frequently measured in order to obtain information concerning the plasma volume (and at the same time, total body fluid volume). Nevertheless, very often there is a great difference between the measured pressures and the actual status of salt and water balance.

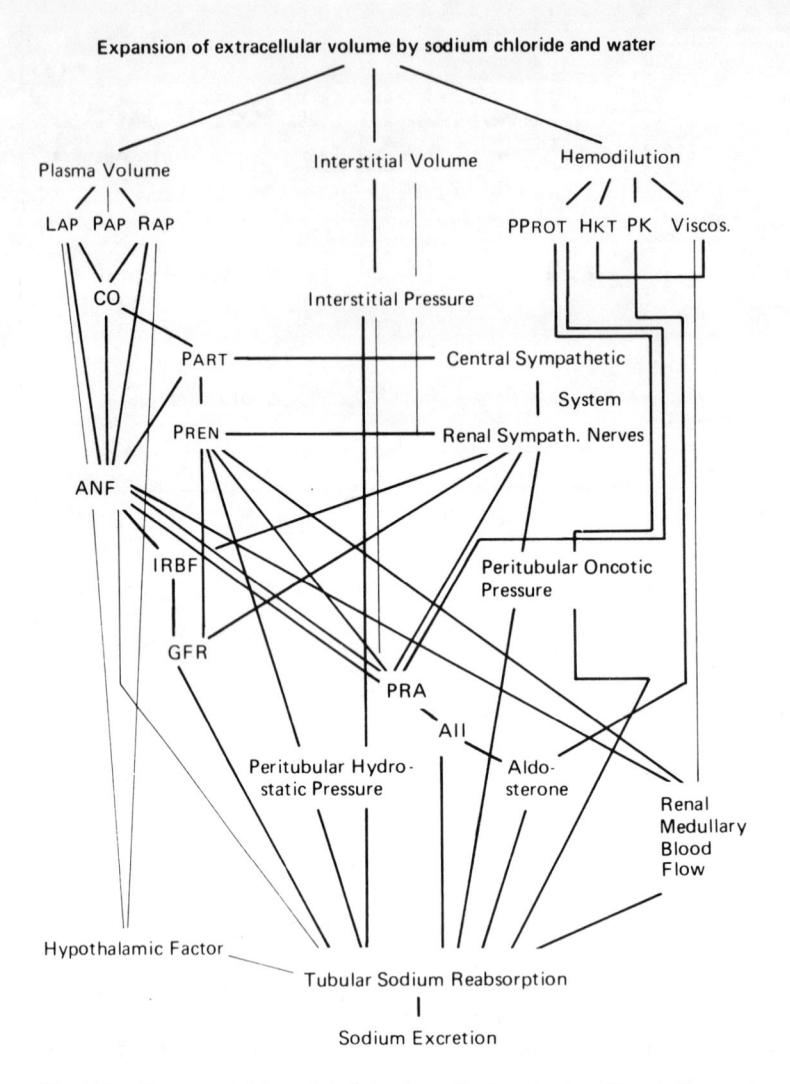

Fig. 7.1. Some variables related to the adjustment of sodium balance after expansion of the extracellular fluid volume.

Activation of atrial receptors is due to changes in atrial transmural pressure (transmural pressure is atrial pressure minus intrathoracic pressure). During spontaneous ventilation intrathoracic pressure is negative, reaching its lowest value during inspiration, and left and right atrial transmural pressures are positive. It has been shown that in conscious, spontaneously breathing dogs an increase in left atrial pressure and therefore left atrial transmural pressure inhibits the release of antidiuretic hormone (ADH) (Kaczmarczyk et al. 1983) and decreases plasma renin activity (Reinhardt et al. 1980). In contrast, during mechanical ventilation intrathoracic pressure increases (via an increased airway pressure) during inspiration and, as positive end-expiratory pressure is applied frequently, also during expiration: in this situation, average atrial transmural pressures decrease. Reducing airway pressure by changing the ventilation protocol has been shown to improve renal function immediately (Steinhoff et al. 1982). Thus in general the sodium and water-retaining effects of mechanical ventilation are thought to be due to the concomitant decrease of atrial transmural pressures, although other mechanisms (such as a decrease in cardiac output and arterial blood pressure, and an increase in renal venous pressure) may also be involved. Several investigators have demonstrated that mechanical ventilation is accompanied by activation of mechanisms inducing sodium and water retention: plasma ADH increases (Hemmer et al. 1980; Annat et al. 1983) (although this has recently been questioned) (Payen et al. 1987), the renin–angiotensin system is activated (Annat et al. 1983). In the critically ill patient, these events are the undesirable side effects of otherwise necessary mechanical ventilation, and these side effects frequently cannot be overcome even by the use of diuretics.

How are Atrial Pressures Related to Renal Sodium and Water Excretion?

Results presented below stem from an intact animal model, in which controlled conditions were provided as follows:

Conscious, female beagle dogs (body wt (bw) 12–14 kg) were studied.

These animals were chronically instrumented (left and/or right atrial catheters, arterial catheter or carotid loops, other implants as necessary for the special experimental protocol, i.e. renal electromagnetic flowmeter or nylon purse string around the mitral annulus (Fig. 7.2)).

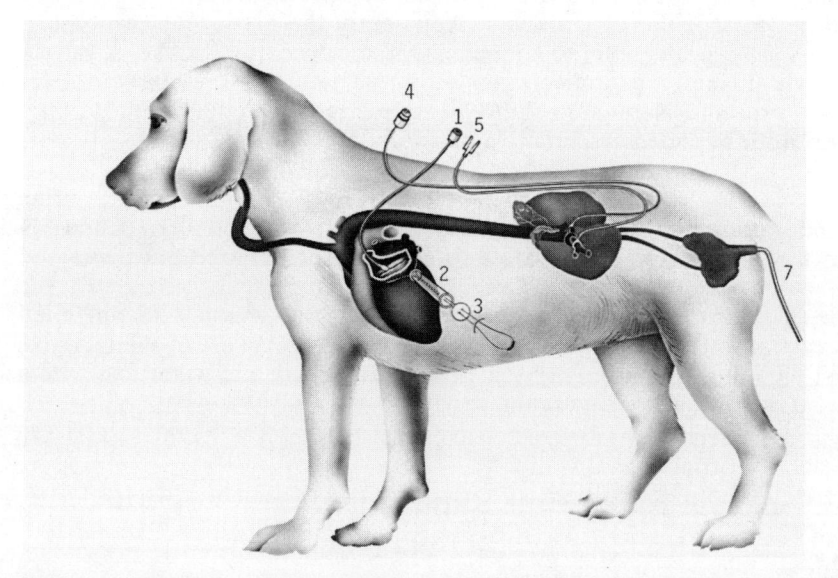

Fig. 7.2. Chronically instrumented dog. Left atrial catheter (*1*), nylon purse string (*2*) led out through the thoracic wall (*3*), renal flowmeter and cuff (*4,5*), bladder catheter (*7*).

Standardized dietary conditions were maintained (self-prepared diet with a constant daily sodium and water intake on a body weight basis, complete intake guaranteed by tube feeding at a constant time of the day (9 a.m.)).
Standardized environmental conditions (room temperature, light and dark) were provided.
Studies were performed in intact animals and in those with chronic cardiac denervation (after Randall et al. 1980).

"Atrial Natriuresis"

In this animal model, an increase in renal sodium excretion during left atrial distension was first described in 1977 (Fig. 7.3). The left atrial pressure was increased by pulling a nylon purse string which had been previously (4 weeks recovery from thoracotomy) positioned around the mitral annulus and led out through the thoracic wall. Pressure was increased by 10 cmH$_2$O, such an increase occurring under physiological conditions (e.g. postprandial after the intake of a high sodium diet) (Kaczmarczyk et al. 1979). In these studies renal blood flow and GFR did not change, whilst an increase in urine volume was regularly observed (Kaczmarczyk et al. 1978).

In the first instance, these results seemed to support the "volume receptor hypothesis". In addition the data seemed to extend this mechanism to sodium regulation – the other essential part of total body fluid regulation. The question of why this "atrial natriuresis" had not been found earlier, could be answered by comparing, for example, results in conscious animals with or without a previously performed non-hypotensive haemorrhage (10 ml (kg bw)$^{-1}$ h^{-1}) (Fig. 7.4). "Atrial natriuresis" was attenuated completely whereas urine volume still increased in some of the experiments. Apparently the natriuretic response is much more sensitive and easier to attenuate than the diuretic response. A variety of experimental conditions under which atrial natriuresis is present or not (as anaesthesia, preceding sodium loss, etc.) was described (Reinhardt et al. 1982). Atrial natriuretic peptide is apparently not involved in "atrial natriuresis" (Goetz et al. 1986).

However, it was also evident, that the effect of left atrial distension on urine volume and sodium excretion was only very transient; if the left atrial distension was performed for longer periods, urine volume and sodium excretion decreased again and reached control values, whereas plasma renin activity increased at the same time (Fig. 7.5). The prolonged increase in left atrial pressure no longer led to an increase of water and sodium excretion, most likely because of a decrease in the interstitial fluid compartment by the previous sodium and water loss with a concomitant increase in plasma renin activity.

Plasma Volume Expansion Experiments

In another protocol, plasma volume and left atrial pressure were increased by infusing 0.25 ml min^{-1} (kg bw)$^{-1}$ 0.9% saline or a "plasma expander" (Fig. 7.6).

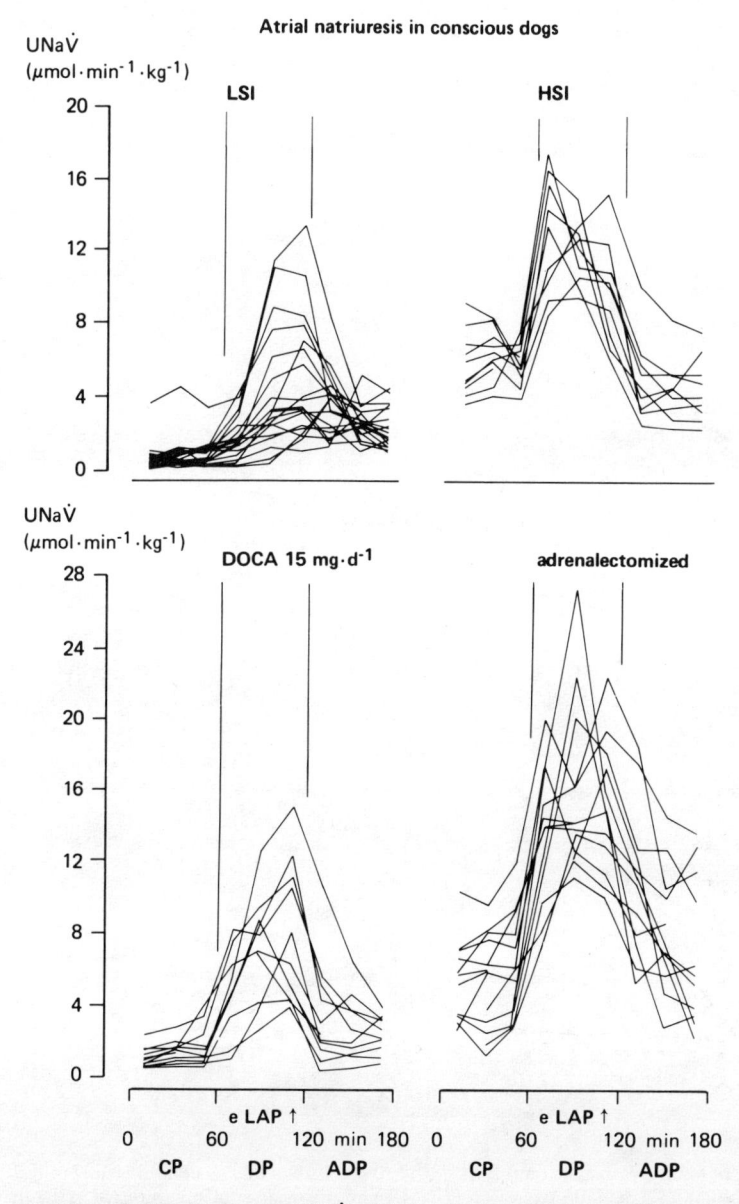

Fig. 7.3. Sodium excretion ($UNa\dot{V}$) during a 60 min control period (CP), during a 60 min left atrial distension ($eLAP\uparrow$, DP) and during a 60 min period after left atrial distension (ADP). *LSI*, low dietary sodium intake (0.5 mmol Na (kg bw)$^{-1}$ day^{-1}); *HSI*, high dietary sodium intake (14.5 mmol Na (kg bw)$^{-1}$ day^{-1}); *DOCA*, chronic application of desoxycorticosterone acetate (15 mg day^{-1}, and low sodium intake); *adrenalectomized*, chronically maintained on high sodium intake after surgical adrenalectomy 4 weeks before. Each line represents a single experiment in one dog. (Data from Kaczmarczyk et al. 1978; Reinhardt et al. 1977, 1980.)

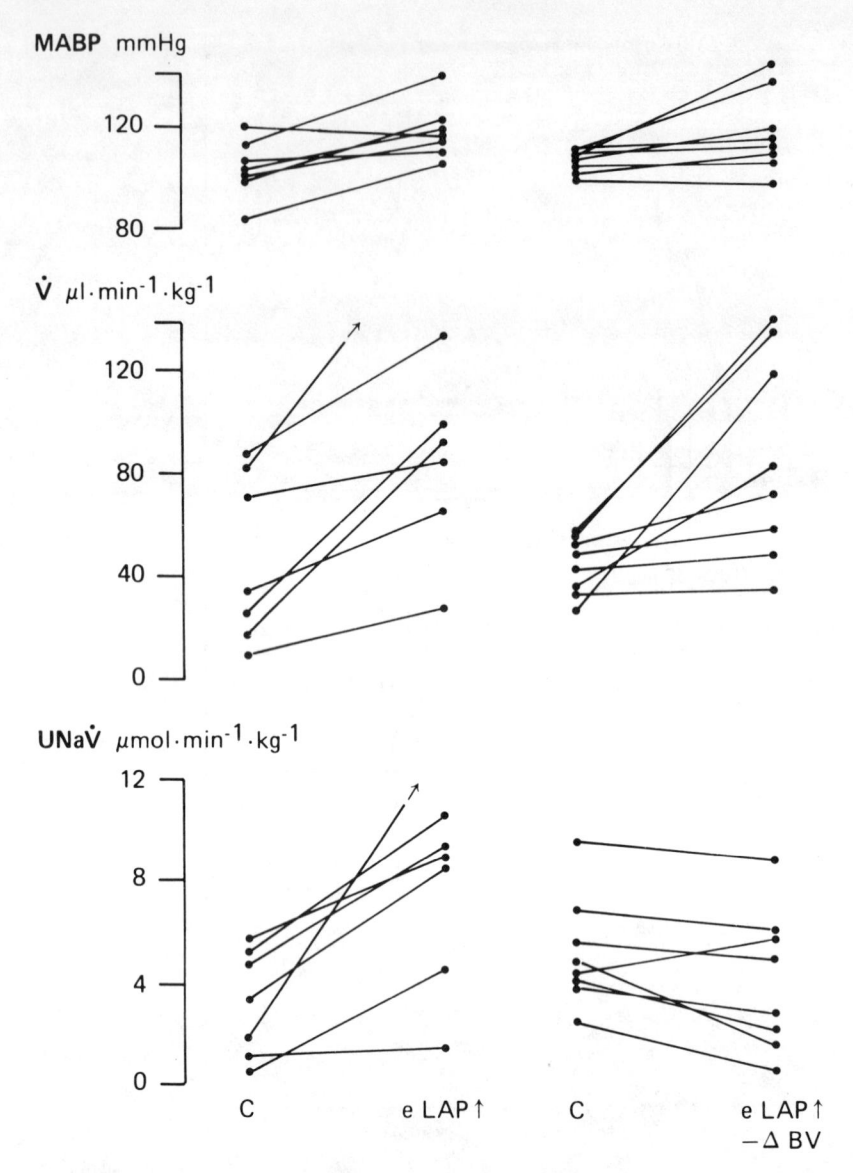

Fig. 7.4. The effect of left atrial distension (*eLAP* ↑ , by 10 cmH$_2$O by means of a reversible mitral stenosis) on urine volume ($\dot{V}$), sodium excretion ($UNa\dot{V}$) and mean arterial pressure (*MABP*) in conscious dogs, kept chronically on a high sodium intake (HSI, 14.5 mmol Na (kg bw)$^{-1}$ day^{-1}) before (*left side*) and after a non-hypotensive haemorrhage (*right side*) ($-\Delta$BV, 10 ml (kg bw)$^{-1}$ 60 min^{-1}). Each line represents a single experiment in one dog.

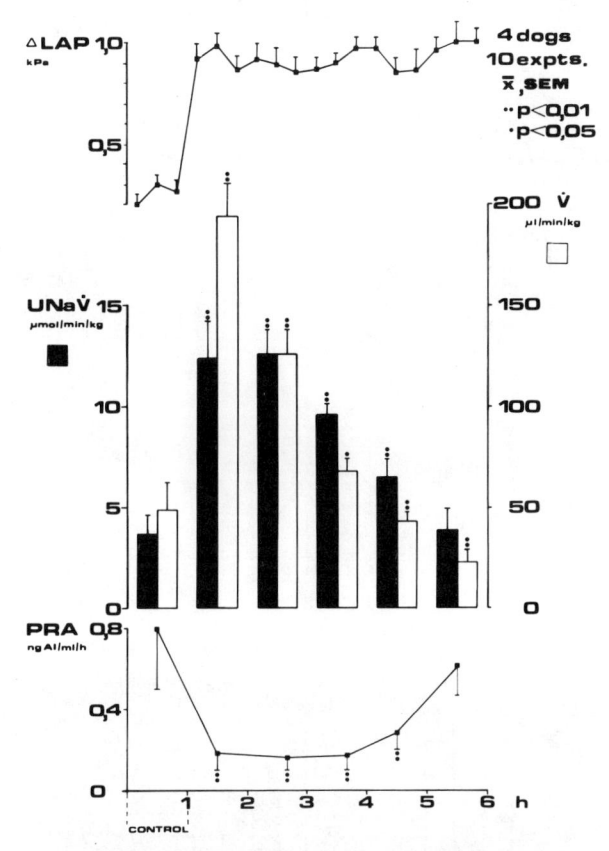

Fig. 7.5. Effect of a 5 hour period of left atrial distension (ΔLAP) on urine volume ($\dot{V}$), sodium excretion ($UNa\dot{V}$) and plasma renin activity (PRA) in conscious dogs kept chronically on a dietary sodium intake of 14.5 mmol Na (kg bw)$^{-1}$ day^{-1}.

The dogs had been kept previously on a high dietary sodium intake (14.5 mmol Na (kg bw)$^{-1}$ day^{-1}).

From these experiments, it was evident that an increase in left atrial pressure *per se* did not result in an increase in sodium excretion. However, sodium excretion promptly increased when isotonic saline was given (previous high sodium intake provided), although the left atrial pressure did not increase. This discrepancy between an increase in left atrial pressure and sodium excretion was observed in dogs on a high as well as in dogs on a low sodium intake (Fig. 7.7). If we assume that dietary sodium intake decreases renal nerve sympathetic activity (Di Bona and Sawin 1985) which also has been shown to be decreased by left atrial distension in anaesthetized animals (Karim et al. 1972), this decrease of renal sympathetic activity – if present at all in conscious animals – apparently does not induce renal sodium excretion, probably as the (renal?) interstitial volume is not expanded.

From these results, the unique role of the atrial receptors in the involvement of regulation of body fluid homeostasis is difficult to sustain.

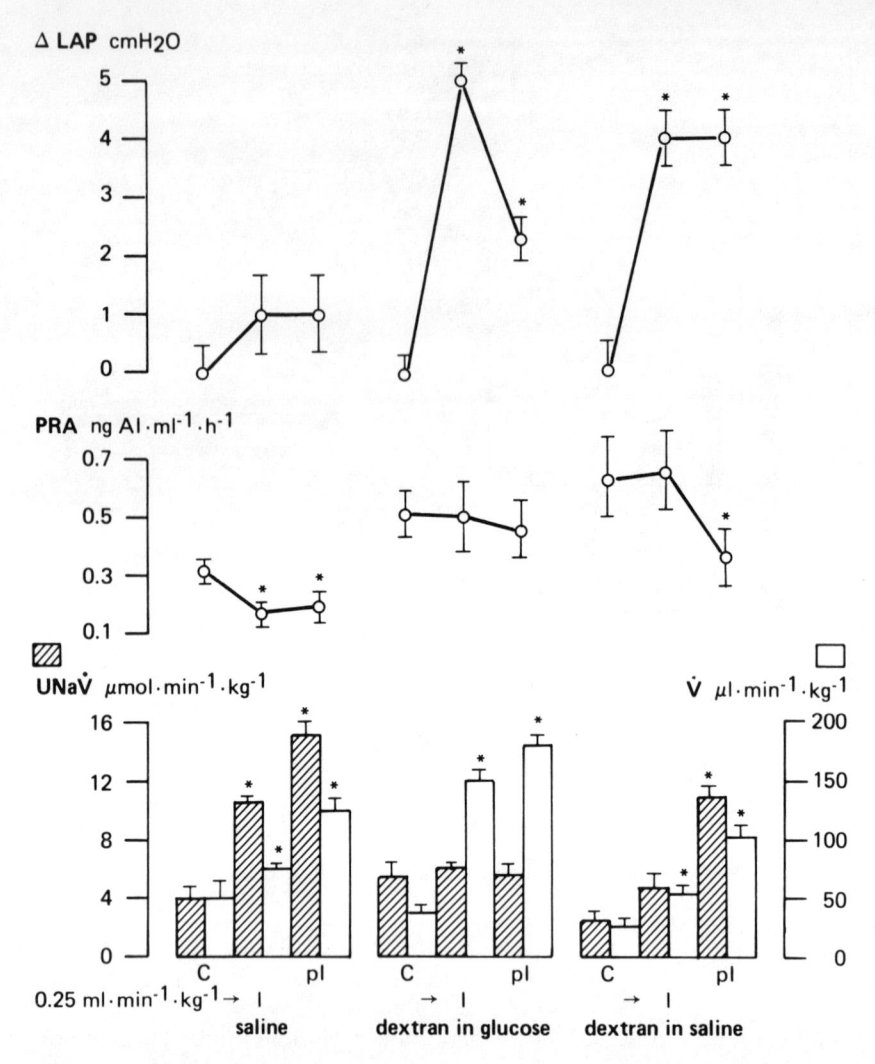

Fig. 7.6. Changes in left atrial pressure (ΔLAP), plasma renin activity (PRA), sodium excretion ($UNa\dot{V}$) and urine volume ($\dot{V}$), during a 60 min control period (C), during a 60 min infusion period (I) and during 60 min after infusion (pI). $\bar{x} \pm$ SEM, saline: 4 dogs, 16 experiments; dextran (mol. wt. 40 000) in glucose: 3 dogs, 9 experiments; dextran in saline: 4 dogs, 16 experiments; $*p<0.05$ refers to control period (C).

Chronic Cardiac Denervation Experiments

Another experimental approach is to examine cardiac denervated animals in order to see whether the afferent signals from the atria are essentially integrated in body fluid control mechanisms. From these experiments two pieces of information were obtained:

1. "Atrial natriuresis" is abolished in cardiac denervated dogs (Fig. 7.8), although atrial natriuretic peptide is released (Goetz et al. 1986).

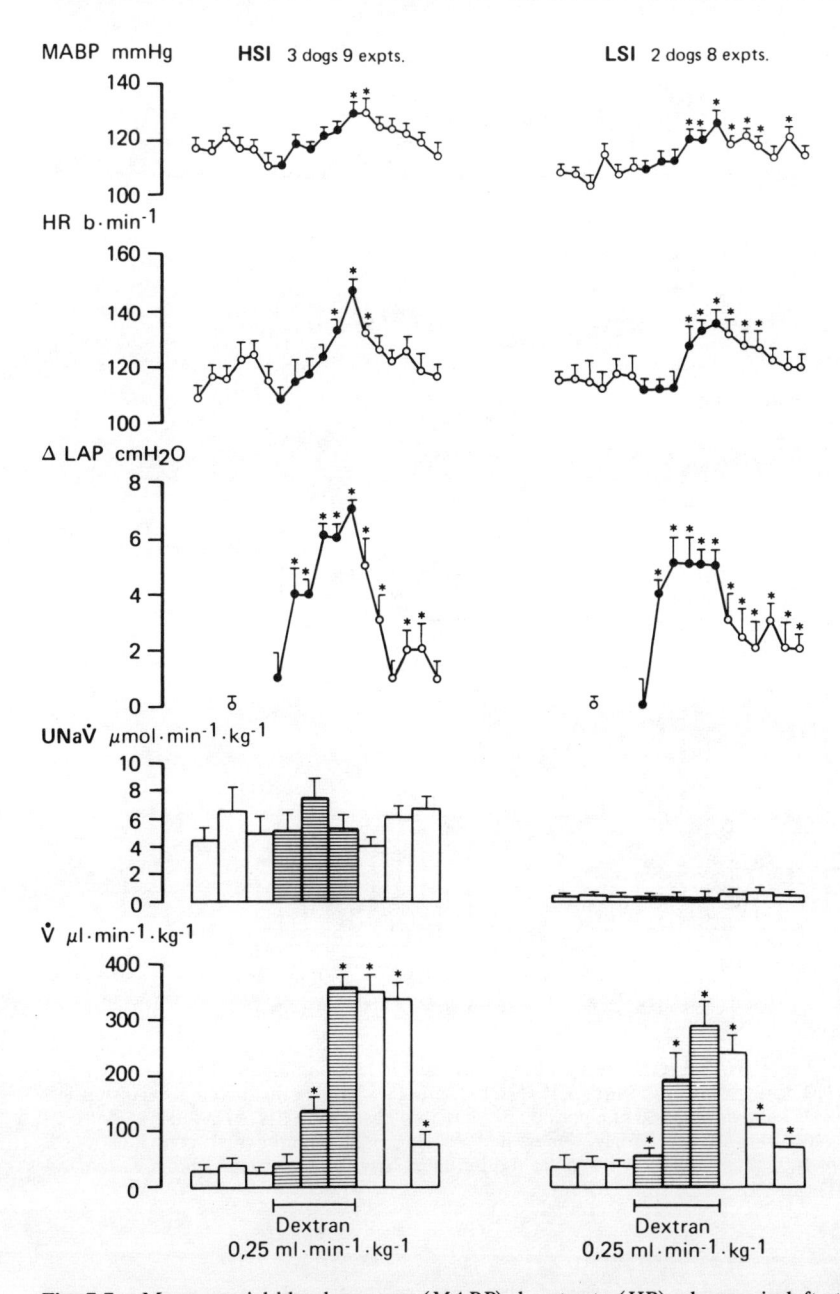

Fig. 7.7. Mean arterial blood pressure (*MABP*), heart rate (*HR*), changes in left atrial pressure (ΔLAP), sodium excretion ($UNa\dot{V}$) and urine volume ($\dot{V}$) in dogs chronically kept on a high sodium intake (*HSI*, 14.5 mmol Na (kg bw)$^{-1}$ day^{-1}) and in dogs kept chronically on a low sodium intake (*LSI*, 0.5 mmol Na (kg bw)$^{-1}$ day^{-1}). 60 min control period (CP), 60 min infusion period (IP, 0.25 ml min^{-1} kg^{-1} dextran in glucose) and 60 min after infusion period (AIP, 20 min urine collection periods). *$p<0.05$ refers to control period before infusion.

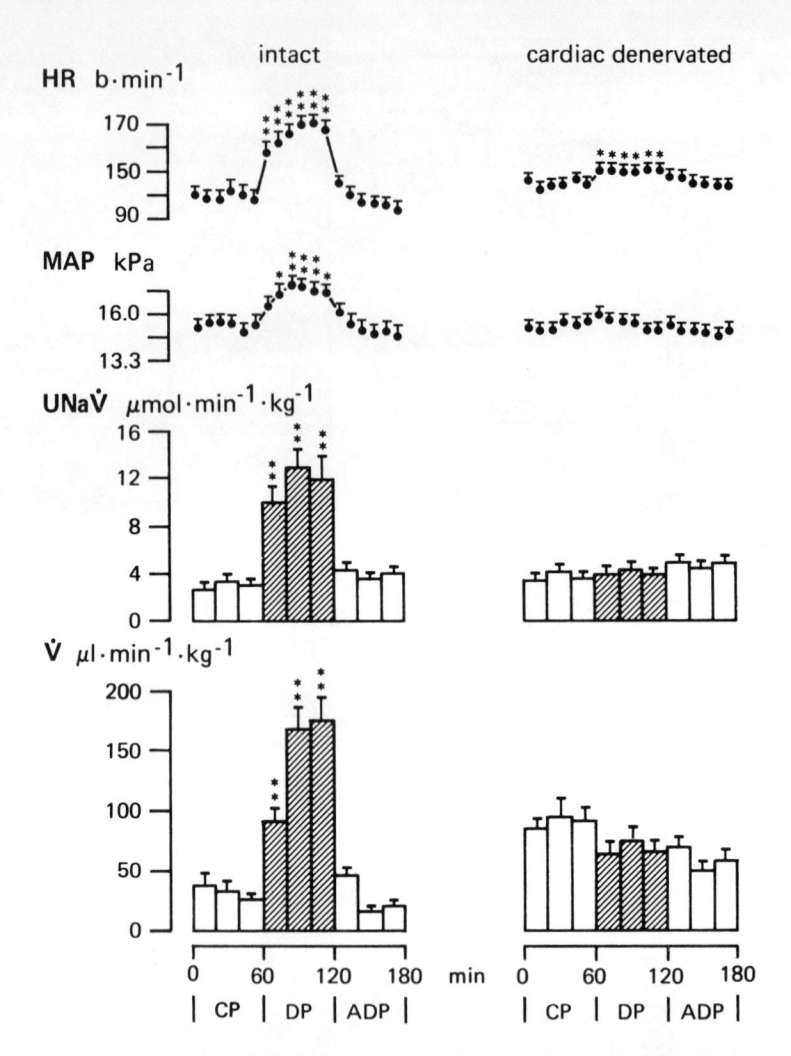

Fig. 7.8. Heart rate (*HR*), mean arterial blood pressure (*MAP*), sodium excretion (*UNaV̇*) and urine volume (*V̇*) during a 60 min control period (*CP*), during a 60 min period of left atrial distension by 10 cmH$_2$O (*DP*) and during a 60 min period after left atrial distension (*ADP*) in intact (6 dogs, 19 experiments) and chronically cardiac denervated (4 dogs, 20 experiments) conscious dogs. **$p<0.005$, *$p<0.05$ refers to *CP*. No significant differences between the groups. (From Kaczmarczyk et al. 1981).

2. When isotonic saline is infused to increase left atrial pressure, cardiac denervated dogs excrete the saline load as fast as intact dogs (Fig. 7.9). Indeed, there is a positive correlation between renal sodium excretion and an increase in left atrial pressure in the cardiac denervated dog (Fig. 7.10).

Thus, under these conditions, left atrial pressure only represents the expansion of the extracellular volume, and the signal from the heart is not required to get rid of the extra sodium load.

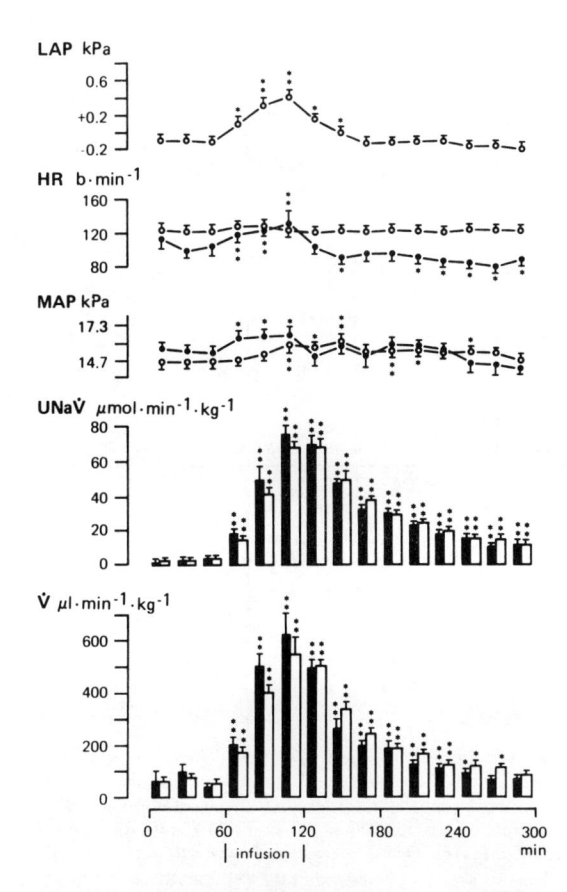

Fig. 7.9. Left atrial pressure (*LAP*), heart rate (*HR*), mean arterial blood pressure (*MAP*), sodium excretion (*UNaV̇*) and urine volume (*V̇*) in intact (4 dogs, 8 experiments) and chronically cardiac denervated (same 4 dogs, 15 experiments) conscious dogs before, during and after a 60 min infusion period with 1 ml min^{-1} (kg bw)$^{-1}$ isotonic saline i.v. **$p<0.005$, *$p<0.05$ refers to control period. *Black columns*, *solid symbols*, intact dogs; *open columns*, *open symbols*, chronically cardiac denervated dogs. No significant differences between the groups. (From Kaczmarczyk et al. 1981).

Fig. 7.10 summarizes the relations between an increase in left atrial pressure and renal sodium excretion during the three different infusion protocols.

In summary, we have come to the conclusion that proper adjustment of sodium and water balance after expansion of the extracellular fluid volume may be achieved without the presence of the cardiac nerves. Atrial pressures may represent the status of the extracellular volume, but the renal response is brought about by signals arising from outside the atria. If the atrial pressure is increased without concomitant expansion of the extracellular volume, the increase in sodium excretion is transient, easy to attenuate or even to abolish totally.

All these studies refer to the renal excretion ability of an extra load of sodium and water, but the question remains as to how important are the cardiac nerves in a situation in which there is a decrease in transmural pressure produced either by chronic sodium and water deficit or an acute sodium and water loss. There are only a few reports on this subject in the literature; all these were done in acutely

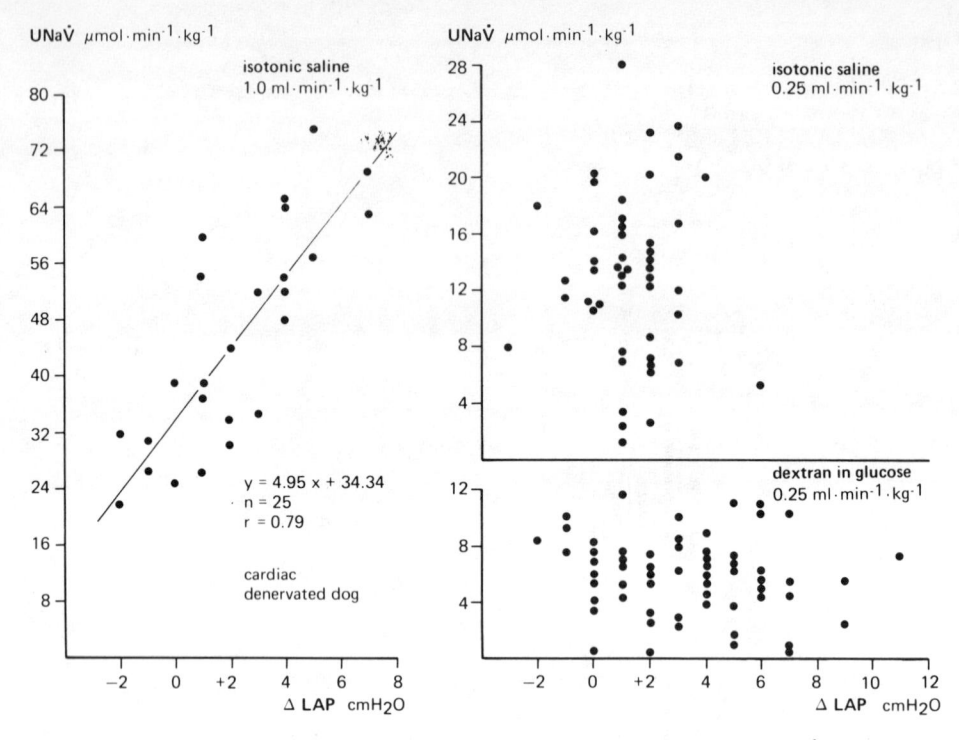

Fig. 7.10. Increase in left atrial pressure (ΔLAP) and renal sodium excretion ($UNa\dot{V}$) in conscious dogs. *Left*, 5 experiments in one dog (HSI): three urine collection periods during i.v. infusion of 1.0 ml saline min^{-1} (kg bw)$^{-1}$, two collection periods thereafter. *Right, upper part*, 16 experiments in 4 dogs (HSI) (4 experiments each): three urine collection periods during i.v. infusion of 0.25 ml saline min^{-1} (kg bw)$^{-1}$. *Right, lower part*, 20 experiments in 5 dogs (HSI) and 11 experiments in 3 dogs (LSI). HSI, high dietary sodium intake, 14.5 mmol Na (kg bw)$^{-1}$ day^{-1}; LSI, low dietary sodium intake, 0.5 mmol Na (kg bw)$^{-1}$ day^{-1}.

stressed, anaesthetized animals, with few exceptions (Goetz et al. 1976). In a chronic balance study, we investigated 24 hour sodium excretion over a period of 9 days after having produced an acute sodium loss by means of peritoneal dialysis. Using local anaesthesia, a peritoneal catheter was implanted, 1000 ml of 5% glucose instilled into the peritoneal cavity, left in place for 60 min and taken off thereafter (for details see Kaczmarczyk et al. 1986b). The sodium content of the fluid was measured and the sodium deficit (between 5 and 6 mmol (kg bw)$^{-1}$) calculated. After this procedure, the central venous pressure was measured daily over a period of 60 min having the dog in a type of Pavlov sling. Central venous pressure was decreased in intact as well as in cardiac denervated dogs over a period of four days (Fig. 7.11) after peritoneal dialysis, indicating possible stimulation of atrial receptors.

Renal sodium excretion decreased immediately after the peritoneal dialysis and remained at low values over the following days (Fig. 7.12). Both groups of dogs, intact and cardiac denervated, showed the same ability to reduce sodium excretion in response to the sodium loss and to retain sodium, when it was offered again with the diet (Fig. 7.12). At the same time, a strong activation of the renin–angiotensin system was observed, which was almost identical in both groups

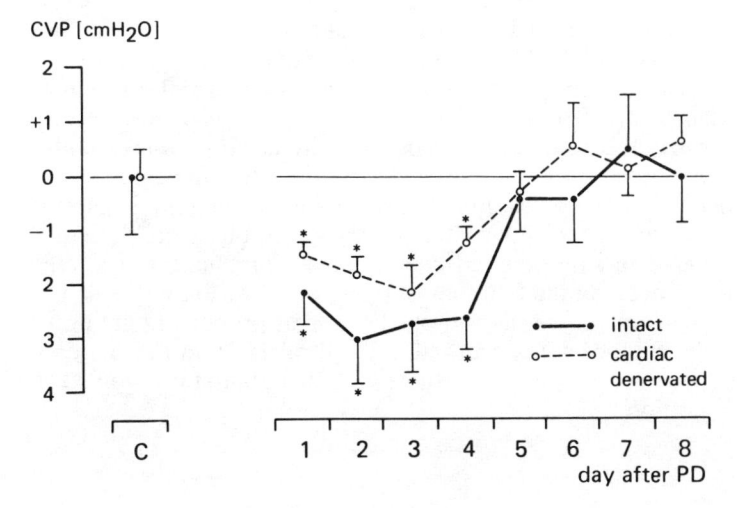

Are Atrial Pressures Involved in the Regulation of Sodium and Water Balance?

Fig. 7.11. Changes of central venous pressure (*CVP*) before and after peritoneal dialysis (*PD*) in intact (*n*=6) and chronically cardiac denervated (*n*=6) dogs. *$p<0.05$ refers to control (*C*) value before *PD*.

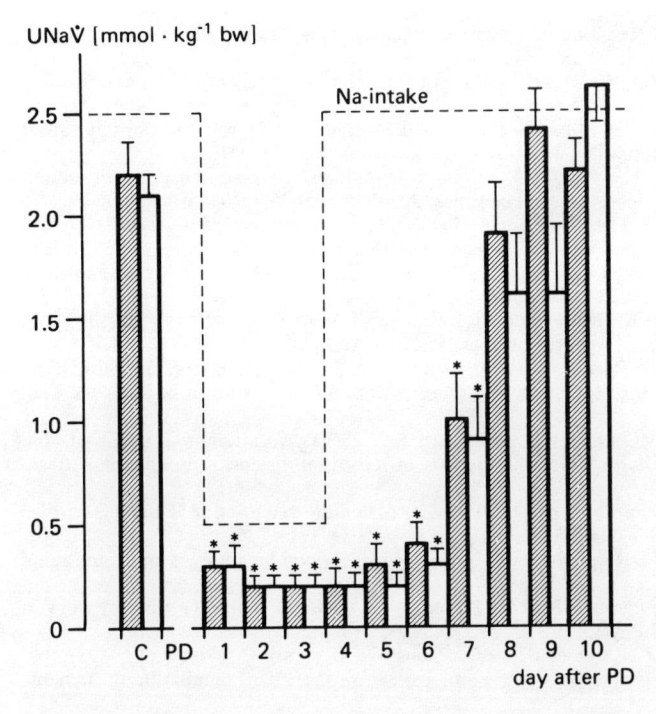

Fig. 7.12. Daily renal sodium excretion after a peritoneal dialysis ($-\Delta$Na 5–6 mmol (kg bw)$^{-1}$) in intact (*n*=6, *hatched bars*) and cardiac denervated (*n*=6, *open bars*) dogs. The *broken line* indicates the daily dietary sodium intake. *$p<0.05$ refers to control (*C*) values. No significant differences between the groups.

(Kaczmarczyk et al. 1986a). From these experiments it was concluded that chronic cardiac denervation did not impair the ability of appropriate adjustment of sodium balance after a sodium loss resulting in a decrease in atrial transmural pressure (Kaczmarczyk et al. 1986a).

In summary, we conclude from these studies, that the atrial pressures under acute conditions may represent the intravascular volume. But the status of the *extracellular volume compartment determines renal sodium excretion*. Sodium is excreted in response to the extracellular volume expansion, but atrial pressures are only one signal, which may become redundant, and sodium homeostasis may be regulated from other areas in the body, most likely from the kidney itself. As far as the effects of mechanical ventilation on the loss of proper regulation of body sodium and water balance are concerned, it is speculated that the decrease in atrial transmural pressure *per se* is not the essential parameter involved in sodium and water retention.

References

Annat G, Viale JP, Bui Xuan B, Aissa OH, Benzoni D, Vincent M, Gharib C, Motin J (1983) Effect of PEEP ventilation on renal function, plasma renin, aldosterone, neurophysins and urinary ADH, and prostaglandins. Anesthesiology 58: 136–141
Di Bona GF, Sawin LL (1985) Renal nerve activity in conscious rats during volume expansion and depletion. Am J Physiol 248: F15–F23
Gauer OH, Henry JP, Sieker HO, Wendt WE (1951) Heart and lungs as a receptor region controlling blood volume. Am J Physiol 167: 786 (abstr)
Goetz KL, Bloxham DD, Bond GC, Sharma JN (1976) Persistance of the renal response to atrial tamponade after cardiac denervation. Proc Soc Exp Biol Med 152: 423–427
Goetz KL, Wang BC, Geer PG, Leadley Jr RJ, Reinhardt HW (1986) Atrial stretch increases sodium excretion independently of release of atrial peptides. Am J Physiol 250: R946–R950
Hemmer M, Viquerat CE, Suter PM, Vallotton MB (1980) Urinary antidiuretic hormone excretion during mechanical ventilation and weaning in man. Anesthesiology 52: 395–400
Kaczmarczyk G, Eigenheer F, Gatzka M, Kuhl U, Reinhardt HW (1978) No relation between atrial natriuresis and renal blood flow in conscious dogs. Pflügers Arch 373: 49–58
Kaczmarczyk G, Schimmrich B, Mohnhaupt R, Reinhardt HW (1979) Atrial pressure and postprandial volume regulation in conscious dogs. Pflügers Arch 381: 143–150
Kaczmarczyk G, Drake A, Eisele R, Mohnhaupt R, Noble MIM, Stubbs J, Reinhardt HW (1981) The role of the cardiac nerves in the regulation of sodium excretion in conscious dogs. Pflügers Arch 390: 125–130
Kaczmarczyk G, Christe W, Mohnhaupt R, Reinhardt HW (1983) An attempt to quantitate the contribution of antidiuretic hormone to the diuresis of left atrial distension in conscious dogs. Pflügers Arch 396: 101–105
Kaczmarczyk G, Gaul E, Reinhardt HW (1986a) Ability of sodium retention in conscious cardiac denervated dogs under chronic conditions. Union of Physiol Sci 161
Kaczmarczyk G, Mohnhaupt R, Reinhardt HW (1986b) Renal sodium handling in intact and renal denervated dogs. Pflügers Arch 407: 382–387
Karim F, Kidd C, Malpus CM, Penna PE (1972) The effects of stimulation of left atrial receptors on sympathetic nerve activity. J Physiol (Lond) 227: 243–260
Payen DM, Farge D, Beloucif S, Leviel F, De La Coussaye JE, Carli P, Wirquin V (1987) No involvement of antidiuretic hormone in acute antidiuresis during PEEP ventilation in humans. Anesthesiology 66: 17–23
Randall WC, Kaye MP, Thomas JX, Barber MJ (1980) Intrapericardial denervation of the heart. J Surg Res 29: 101–109
Reinhardt HW, Kaczmarczyk G, Eisele R, Arnold B, Eigenheer F, Kuhl U (1977) Left atrial pressure and sodium balance in conscious dogs on a low sodium intake. Pflügers Arch 370: 59–66

Reinhardt HW, Eisele R, Kaczmarczyk G, Mohnhaupt R, Oelkers W, Schimmrich B (1980) The control of sodium excretion by reflexes from the low pressure system independent of adrenal activity. Pflügers Arch 384: 171–176

Reinhardt HW, Kaczmarczyk G, Mohnhaupt R, Simgen B (1982) The control of sodium metabolism to maintain osmo- and volume homeostasis. Klin Wochenschr 60: 1240–1244

Steinhoff H, Falke K, Schwarzhoff W (1982) Enhanced renal function associated with intermittent mandatory ventilation in acute respiratory failure. Intensive Care Med 8: 69–74

Discussion

The discussion commenced with a consideration of the role of renal neural tone in the natriuresis observed in these experiments. Dr Kaczmarczyk emphasized that the same response was seen following elevations of left atrial pressure in dogs in whom the kidneys had been denervated. Whatever the mechanism of natriuresis in these animals atrial natriuretic peptide did not seem to be an important mediator of the response. Dr Myers referred to some work in human cardiac transplant recipients in whom head-up water immersion produces a brisk diuresis. This diuresis coincides exactly with a sharp increase in atrial natriuretic peptide, and there is a simultaneous increase in production of cyclic GMP by the kidney. Thus, in the human it seems that there is a remarkable correlation between left atrial pressure, atrial natriuretic peptide and natriuresis in the denervated cardiac transplant recipient and this difference suggests a fundamental species difference. Similarly, in patients who require mechanical ventilation, there appeared to be quite a good correlation between right atrial transmural pressure and right atrial concentrations of atrial natriuretic peptide.

Dr Myers was also concerned about the concentration of dextran used in the reported experiments. He emphasized that a hyperoncotic colloid infusion may indeed have an antinatriuretic effect. The mechanism of this was not well understood, but probably had something to do with peritubular forces. This difference in treatment might underlie some of the salt retention seen in some of the dogs studied.

Section III
Pathogenesis of Acute Renal Failure in the Intensive Therapy Unit

Chapter 8

Endothelial and Mesangial Cell Dysfunction in Acute Renal Failure

G. H. Neild

Introduction

During a period of acute renal failure (ARF) oliguria can persist for days although there may be only minor morphological evidence of tubular injury.

In both clinical and experimental examples of ARF, a reduction in renal blood flow (RBF) leading to renal ischaemia is a major factor during the initiation of injury. The reason why oliguria persists when renal blood flow is restored is unclear. In the maintenance phase of ARF, both vascular and tubular elements play a role. RBF may be totally restored, but blood flow and pressure in the glomerulus may remain insufficient for effective glomerular filtration to occur. In addition oliguria is maintained by a combination of intraluminal tubular obstruction and back-leak of tubular fluid through the injured tubules into the renal interstitium (Brezis et al. 1986; Levinsky 1977; Myers and Moran 1986).

Generally in man there are many factors that summate in the induction of ARF. To date, most experimental models of acute tubular necrosis (ATN) have involved a massive single insult, which bears little relationship to the onset of ATN in man. Recently, multifactorial models have been introduced, in which different systems regulating blood flow are altered, and which perhaps more faithfully simulate the human situation (Vari et al. 1988; Heyman et al. 1988).

In this review I will discuss vascular factors in the induction and maintenance of ARF, as represented in the left hand side of Fig. 8.1. There are two major considerations – vascular tone and vascular pathology. Although these will be discussed separately they are closely related.

Although many of the mediators are still unknown there are tantalizing clues to their identity. Why should volume or salt loading generally protect and even more so why should volume contraction, or states in which the kidney behaves as if it is ischaemic such as hepatorenal syndrome and cyclosporin nephrotoxicity, render the kidney exquisitely susceptible to further nephrotoxic insults?

```
            ACUTE RENAL INJURY
           ↙              ↘
   Vascular Effects    Tubular Effects
    ↙      ↘             ↙      ↘
  Kf↓    RBF↓      Obstruction   Backleak
         ↘    ↙
        Net Filtration
        Pressure ↓
              ↓
            GFR
```

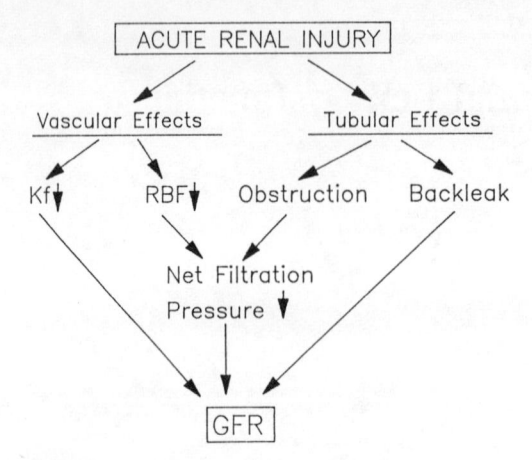

Fig. 8.1. Factors involved in the induction and maintenance of ARF.

Physiology of the Normal Kidney

Glomerular Filtration

The glomerular circulation is not truly capillary as no metabolism occurs. The glomerular capillary can be considered as a hemi-arteriole since on one side it is covered by mesangial cells, which are derived from smooth muscle. The glomerular basement membrane (GBM) is freely permeable to crystalloids and filtration across the membrane is proportional to the hydrostatic pressure inside the capillary.

The hydrostatic pressure inside the glomerular capillary is regulated by two resistance vessels, the afferent and efferent arteriole. For filtration to occur the hydrostatic pressure has to exceed the sum of the capillary oncotic pressure and the tubular fluid pressure in Bowman's space. When renal blood flow is decreased as a consequence of a rise in preglomerular vascular resistance, hydrostatic pressure may be maintained by an increase in efferent arteriolar tone relative to afferent tone. If the hydrostatic pressure falls below a critical level filtration will cease even though blood still flows through the glomerular capillary circulation.

The rate of filtration, i.e. glomerular filtration rate (GFR), also depends on the total capillary surface area available for filtration, as well as the rate of plasma flow. The permeability of the GBM to crystalloids, i.e. the effective hydraulic permeability (k), could in theory change in response to injury, although this can not be measured directly. However, the ultrafiltration coefficient (Kf), which is the product of the total capillary surface area available for filtration and k, can be measured. Thus the ultrafiltration rate for a single glomerulus (SNGFR) may be expressed as the product of Kf and the net ultrafiltration pressure (Brenner et al. 1986b).

It is important to emphasize the role of Kf, since, as will be discussed, reduction in this quantity may play a vital role in the maintenance of the reduced GFR in acute renal failure. Vasoconstrictors such as angiotensin, not only increase efferent arteriolar tone but cause mesangial cell contraction which will reduce the effective capillary surface area, i.e. Kf (Brenner et al. 1986b).

Thus, glomerular ultrafiltration is controlled by arteriolar and mesangial tone. These, in turn, are partly regulated by the juxtaglomerular apparatus (JGA) as part of the tubuloglomerular feedback system (Blantz and Pelayo 1984).

Control of Renal Blood Flow

Cortical Blood Flow

The tone in the arterioles is influenced by several vasoactive systems – including sympathetic nervous system, renin–angiotensin, prostaglandins and thromboxanes (Heller 1987). The potential role of vascular paracrine mediators such as neuropeptides and endothelium-derived factors (Vanhoutte 1988) is still being explored.

Evidence of arteriolar reactivity has come from micropuncture studies of glomerular haemodynamics, from direct observation of vessels, and from isolated vascular segments (Brezis et al. 1986; Edwards 1985). The various renal resistance vessels show quite different reactivity. Thus of constrictor agents, noradrenaline has a similar effect on interlobular arteries and both afferent and efferent arterioles, whereas angiotensin probably acts exclusively on the efferent arteriole (Edwards 1985; Knox and Granger 1985). Of dilator agents, acetylocholine acts on all three vessels, dopamine just on the arterioles, and bradykinin exclusively on the efferent arterioles (Brezis et al. 1986; Edwards 1985). (The bradykinin data come from the rabbit, and since in this species bradykinin is not active as an inducer of endothelium-derived vascular relaxation, the data may be unrepresentative for man.)

In response to changes in perfusion pressure, the kidney like many other organs can autoregulate. With respect to the kidney, both renal blood flow and GFR are kept stable. This autoregulation may also be demonstrated in both denervated and isolated perfused kidneys. As will be discussed later, loss of autoregulation is a regular feature of acute tubular necrosis. The ability of the vascular smooth muscle to respond to changes in perfusion pressure has been termed "myogenic reflex". The description of endothelium-derived relaxant factor (Furchgott and Zawadski 1980; Vanhoutte 1988) and its ability to co-ordinate flow through the resistance vessels (Griffith et al. 1987), and the endothelium-derived constricting factor, endothelin (Yanagisawa et al. 1988), may explain some of the features of this reflex.

The kidneys have one of the highest blood flow rates per unit tissue mass in the body: although they represent less than 0.5% of the body mass, they receive about 20% of the cardiac output. In general, renal blood flow per gram of tissue declines progressively from outer to inner cortex. Glomerular density shows a similar gradient. This ensures that the outer cortical glomeruli have a large flow of plasma to filter.

Medullary Blood Flow

The medullary blood supply is derived entirely from efferent arterioles of the inner cortical glomeruli (Kriz 1982). These arterioles descend into the medulla and divide into the descending vasa rectae, which themselves descend in vascular bundles and at intervals leave to supply the adjacent peritubular capillary plexus. In the region of the thick ascending limb of loop of Henle the plexus is very dense.

The capillary plexus drains upwards via the ascending vasa rectae which empty into the arcuate veins at the cortico-medullary junction. Both descending and ascending vasa rectae are resistance vessels, which regulate medullary blood flow. Ascending vessels have very thin walls and are potentially very susceptible to compression by swollen tubules (Kriz 1982).

There are many methodological problems measuring medullary flow, but by using non-diffusible indicators, such as radiolabelled albumin or red cells, or rubidium ions, the medullary flow has been shown to account on average for 10%–15% of total renal blood flow (Brenner et al. 1986a). Flow in the outer cortex is approximately sixfold greater than outer medulla and twenty-fold greater than inner medulla. Autoregulation occurs in the medulla.

In the kidney there are gradients of oxygen availability. Medullary tissue pO_2 is much lower than arterial pO_2, and in animals medullary pO_2 is in the range of 10 mmHg. The cortico-medullary gradient of pO_2 is maintained by counter-current diffusion of O_2 between arterial and venous branches of the vasa rectae (Brezis et al. 1984a,b). With this arrangement the renal medulla is in a constant state of cellular hypoxia. Direct measurements of the redox state of cytochrome aa_3 (the terminal electron carrier of the mitochondrial chain which transports electrons directly to O_2) show that in well-oxygenated tissue (e.g. resting muscle) the cytochrome is 98% oxidized, whereas in the kidney it is only 80% oxidized, and in the isolated perfused kidney 60% (Brezis et al. 1984a,b). Indirect evidence suggests that the thick ascending limb of the loop of Henle in particular operates on the verge of hypoxia (Brezis et al. 1984b).

New Developments in Regulation of Glomerular Haemodynamics

Endothelium-Derived Relaxant Factor (EDRF)

For several years it has been recognized that a number of vasodilators (such as acetylcholine, bradykinin) are endothelium-dependent (Furchgott and Zawadski 1980; Griffith et al. 1984). In response to such agonists the endothelium releases an EDRF, whose biological action is virtually indistinguishable from nitric oxide (NO) (Palmer et al. 1987). The precursor substrate for this activity is thought to be L-arginine (Schmidt et al. 1988). EDRF is both a potent vasodilator and an inhibitor of platelet aggregation and adhesion (Radomski et al. 1987a,b). In these ways it is very similar to the endothelium-derived prostacyclin, and the two are synergistic (Radomski et al. 1987b). EDRF/NO acts on the target cell by stimulating soluble guanylate cyclase which leads to an increase in intracellular cyclic-GMP (Rapoport et al. 1983). EDRF is thought to have a local paracrine action, acting directly on adjacent smooth muscle cells. It is probable that there are several EDRFs, which may include ammonia and adenosine (Vanhoutte 1988).

EDRF is also released in response to shear stress and transmural pressure and Griffith et al. (1987) have shown that EDRF coordinates blood flow in resistance vessels.

Endothelium-Derived Constricting Factor (EDCF)

Endothelin has recently been characterized as a very potent vasoconstrictor peptide released from the endothelium in response to noradrenaline, thrombin, hypoxia, increased transmural pressure, mechanical stretch. It is a cyclic 21 amino acid peptide with sequence homology to several invertebrate toxins (such as apamin, a bee venom, and neurotoxin, a scorpion venom). It has a prolonged action and when infused into a rat causes a sustained rise in blood pressure for 40–60 minutes.

Its vasopressor action is reversed by isoproterenol and glyceryl trinitrate, but resistant to the following antagonists: alpha-adrenergic, H_1-histaminergic, serotonergic, cyclo-oxygenase, lipoxygenase. Its action is antagonized by calcium-channel blockers such as nicardipine. It appears that it may act as an endogenous agonist of the dihydropyridine-sensitive Ca^{2+} ion channel.

It is conceivable that the sustained reduction in Kf, presumably as a consequence of mesangial cell contraction, may be mediated via endothelin release in response to local ischaemia.

Mesangial Cell Contraction

Mesangial cells are modified smooth muscle cells. They have surface receptors for angiotensin II, contain actomyosin, and contract in response to many vasoconstrictors (see Table 8.1) (Kreisberg et al. 1985; Ausiello et al. 1980; Mene and Dunn 1986; Neuwirth et al. 1987). Evidence for contraction came first from amphibian glomeruli, then vascular casts of dog glomeruli, and time-lapse films of cultured human glomeruli (Kreisberg et al. 1985). More and more, recent work has used mesangial cells in culture but there are several methodological problems, and until recently poor cell markers with which to identify these cells. A major problem has been phenotypic changes with prolonged culture – and in particular loss of contractility (Kreisberg et al. 1985). In addition to this being due to loss of surface receptors or loss of contractile protein it is now thought that the mesangial cells bind so tightly to the culture vessel surface that they cannot contract. Mesangial cells themselves produce a number of vasoactive factors including vasodilatory prostaglandins, thromboxane A_2 and PAF. For example, mesangial cell contraction in response to angiotensin II may be difficult or impossible to demonstrate, until the cells are treated with a cyclo-oxygenase inhibitor, since the angiotensin II stimulates the release of vasodilatory prostaglandins which offsets the contraction (Ausiello et al. 1980).

Table 8.1. Mediators of mesangial contraction

Angiotensin II
Norepinephrine
Thromboxane A_2
Leukotrienes D_4, C_4
Platelet-activating factor
Platelet-derived growth factor
Vasopressin
Histamine

The list of compounds that cause a fall in Kf is longer than for mesangial contraction since some like parathyroid hormone and prostacyclin act by stimulating the renin–angiotensin system, i.e. induce angiotensin-mediated contraction of mesangial cells (Table 8.2). The list of compounds causing mesangial contraction increases. Recently cyclosporin (Lamas et al. 1988a) and adenosine (Lamas et al. 1988b) have been added to the leukotrienes (Simonson and Dunn 1986).

Table 8.2. Mediators of reduction in Kf

Vasoconstrictors
As for mesangial contraction (see Table 8.1)
Parathyroid hormone (PTH)[a]
Prostaglandin E_2[a]
Vasodilators
Prostaglandin E_1, I_2
Acetylcholine, bradykinin
Histamine
Papaverine

[a] Reversed by ACE inhibitors.

On the other hand a number of drugs will inhibit mesangial contractility, such as isoproterenol, dopamine, atriopeptins and nitroprusside and these appear to act by raising intracellular levels of cAMP and cGMP (Mene et al. 1988).

Renal Ischaemia – Changes in Renal Blood Flow in Response to Injury

Reduction in GFR During Induction of Renal Failure

Response to Compromised Renal Perfusion (Prerenal Failure)

The immediate increase in renal vascular resistance in response to hypovolaemia and heart failure is mediated by massive sympathetic activity with secondary activation of the renin–angiotensin system. Although renal blood flow is decreased, glomerular filtration (GFR) may be preserved initially by a disproportionate rise in efferent arteriolar tone, which is mediated in particular by angiotensin. In addition the increased tone in the preglomerular vessels is offset by local, renal production of vasodilatory prostaglandins (Ballerman et al. 1986). For these reasons the use of either angiotensin-converting enzyme inhibitors or inhibitors of cyclo-oxygenase, in patients with renal hypoperfusion, may cause a precipitous decline in GFR and sometimes oliguria.

Following controlled haemorrhage, in experimental models, there is a preferential reduction in outer cortical flow, although neither the quantity nor mechanism is known (Brenner et al. 1986a). This redistribution is present in denervated kidneys. When ischaemia is induced by infusion of norepinephrine or angiotensin, or by renal nerve stimulation there is no redistribution although total blood flow is reduced by 50%.

Changes in sodium balance also affect regional blood flow; in summary, sodium depletion leads to a decrease in absolute and fractional outer cortical perfusion and vice versa with sodium expansion (Brenner et al. 1986a).

The techniques used for measuring regional perfusion all have methodological problems: those normally used are inert gas washout or the more recent freeze-dissection washout, or infusions of radiolabelled microspheres (Brezis et al. 1986).

Regional Variations in Renal Perfusion Leading to Established Renal Failure

Initially, hypoperfusion leads to a relative reduction in flow to the outer cortex (physiological hypoperfusion). However, when more severe, medullary blood flow is reduced and ischaemic damage to the adjacent tubules occurs (Frega et al. 1976; Mason et al. 1984, 1987). Even so there is a disproportionate decrease in GFR compared with blood flow.

In established ATN, there is a reduction in medullary blood flow of greater than 50% (shown by microsphere techniques, hydrogen clearance, Rb extraction) even when blood flow to the outer cortex is restored. The precise role played by endothelial and epithelial cell swelling, rheological, humoral and neural factors is unclear (Brezis et al. 1986), but these factors are reviewed below.

Relationship of GFR to Reduced Blood Flow and Tubular Injury

It is likely that this disproportionate and subsequently, sustained decrease in GFR is partly due to reduction in the effective capillary surface area (Kf). Direct measurements of Kf by micro-puncture and other techniques have confirmed this in several models of ATN, both ischaemic and toxic (e.g. gentamicin-, uranium-induced) (Brezis et al. 1986; Gross and Anderson 1985; Wolfert et al. 1987; Williams et al. 1981). The mechanism is not known although angiotensin, leukotrienes and other locally produced factors (Brenner et al. 1986b; Ballerman et al. 1986; Wolfert et al. 1987) can cause mesangial cell contraction, and possibly direct toxic injury to the mesangial cells may occur. In a recent study of severe ATN, induced in the rat by high doses of mercury salts, the complete cessation of filtration was associated with normal total renal blood flow, but intense afferent arteriolar constriction and a reciprocal decrease in efferent tone (Wolfert et al. 1987), leading to an inadequate capillary pressure for filtration to occur.

In experimental models of ATN induced by ischaemia, there is a reduction in renal blood flow of more than 50% with a rise in renal vascular resistance. Correction of blood flow, by volume expansion or vasodilatation, during the initial phase of injury will lead to recovery of GFR, but if correction occurs after 24–48 hours GFR does not recover. Once ATN is established, renal blood flow may return to normal and the sustained reduction in GFR is out of proportion to the blood flow. Tubular damage and obstruction play a major role in the maintenance phase (Kreisberg and Venkatachalam 1988; Hostetter and Brenner 1988; Brezis et al. 1986).

In models of toxic injury renal blood flow is often, but not consistently, decreased and volume expansion and vasodilatation do not cause a rise in GFR (Brezis et al. 1986). In ARF induced by uranyl nitrate, infusion of the vasodilatory PGE_1 restored blood flow but had no effect on GFR (Hostetter and Brenner 1988). In another study ACE inhibition restored Kf to normal without improving GFR (Hostetter and Brenner 1988).

Glycerol-induced ARF is associated with myoglobinuria and a major reduction in RBF. This model is enhanced by prior dehydration and some protection is afforded by previous chronic volume contraction (Hostetter and Brenner 1988).

Maintenance of Reduced GFR in Established Renal Failure

Vascular Pathology

In ATN following ischaemia the mechanism of continued reduction in renal blood flow after correction of systemic pressure and volume ("no reflow" phenomenon) is unknown. In renal sections, the dark zone at the outer medulla seen in ATN is due to intense vascular congestion. Using colloidal carbon or silicon rubber casts, obstruction of the vasculature in the deep cortex and outer medulla is consistently found in experimental models.

It has been suggested that endothelial swelling prevents recovery. However, endothelial swelling is patchy and transient (Kashgarian et al. 1976), with the exception in the cortico-medullary area were it is consistent and persists (Frega et al. 1976).

Finally, in these models, vascular pathology in resistance vessels in the form of focal and segmental arteriolar necrosis is seen. This is probably a consequence of the initial severe vasospasm, but may contribute to any continuing reduction in blood flow (Kashgarian et al. 1976; Adams et al. 1980; Matthys et al. 1983).

Haemodynamic Considerations

In experimental ATN, loss of renal autoregulation occurs (Adams et al. 1980; Matthys et al. 1983). This may have two consequences: first, there may not be the expected compensatory vasodilatation following the initial ischaemia, and second, the kidney will not be protected from any subsequent decreases in perfusion pressure. This may partly explain the observation in man that active tubular necrosis continues for some days after the initial insult.

Recent studies from Schrier and his colleagues have shown that following the induction of ATN there is a loss of endothelium-dependent vasodilatation within the kidney (Conger et al. 1988). This may also explain the paradoxical vasoconstriction in response to a decrease in perfusion pressure and the increased sensitivity to renal nerve stimulation which occur in ARF (Conger et al. 1988).

Following ischaemia, there is a rise in adenosine content in the kidney and adenosine may act as a potent mediator of vasoconstriction. Hypoxaemia in neonates and newborn rabbits is associated with a fall in GFR and RBF and this may be abolished by low doses of theophylline, an antagonist of adenosine (Gouyon and Guignard 1988).

Following ARF, glomeruli, examined in vitro, are refractory to vasoconstrictors including angiotension II, arginine vasopressin and noradrenaline (Wilkes et al. 1981; Ikuma et al. 1988).

Finally, locally produced vasoconstrictors such as thromboxane and leukotrienes may add a further insult to a compromised microcirculation.

Tubular Obstruction

The role of tubular obstruction in the maintenance of oliguria has provoked much debate for many years. It plays a role in some animal models, although there is less evidence for this in man (Myers and Moran 1986).

Tubular cell injury, probably, has an effect by compressing capillaries as a result of the cell swelling and interstitial oedema (Brezis et al. 1986; Frega et al. 1976). Sufficient cell swelling to contribute to "no-reflow" does not occur until anoxia has persisted for some 30–40 minutes. Following injury, cell volume regulation is inhibited and tubular epithelial cells swell. They become more permeable to sodium, and there is a rise in intracellular calcium. The medullary circulation is drained by the very thin-walled ascending vasa rectae, which are at particular risk of obstruction due to the proximity of the damaged ascending limb of Henle (Kriz 1982).

Endothelial Injury

Is Endothelial Injury or Intravascular Coagulation Involved?

There are several ways in which one might expect endothelial injury to play a role.

First, ischaemia may damage the capillary endothelium. This may cause endothelial swelling and capillary obstruction. However, as discussed above, there is very little evidence for this except in the medullary vessels (Kashgarian et al. 1976; Frega et al. 1976).

Second, endothelial damage may cause platelet aggregation and thrombosis to occur. It is possible that this may also occur in the glomerular as well as the tubular circulation. Unfortunately, platelets can only be identified by electron microscopy and if they are involved they are likely to have degranulated and be unrecognizable. Similarly fibrin may be very difficult to identify as the fibrinolytic capacity of the endothelium is so large that fibrin persists only when the system is overwhelmed. However, Clarkson et al. (1970) consistently found, by electron-microscopic examination of renal biopsies obtained during the oliguric phase, conspicuous intraglomerular deposition of fibrin and platelets consistent with intraglomerular capillary thrombosis. Moreover, there was often swelling of the glomerular endothelium or subendothelial deposits. These changes were found in ARF of various causes.

In attempting to address the question of the role of endothelial injury Mason et al. (1987) found that neither aspirin nor heparin were able to modify medullary vascular obstruction. However, both pathological and functional aspects of this injury were prevented by either raising perfusion pressure or lowering blood haematocrit (Mason et al. 1987).

Third, sepsis may trigger off localized intravascular coagulation leading to occlusion of the capillary microcirculation and secondary endothelial damage (Wardle 1974). Models of endotoxic shock can produce renal failure and thrombosis in the renal microcirculation. Infusion of endotoxin into baboons causes ATN with endothelial cell injury which is more prominent in peritubular than glomerular vessels (Richman et al. 1980).

In septicaemia and septic shock, however, there is little information regarding the renal microcirculation in either man or experimental models. In a study of 47 cases of disseminated intravascular coagulation (DIC) (seen out of 115 000 consecutive hospital admissions) 19 patients developed ARF, of whom 13 had an associated sepsis. All 19 had autopsies and none had evidence of microvascular thrombosis (Mant and King 1979).

In a model of septicaemia in sheep, the development of ARF was related to the severity of septicaemia but histological examination showed only mild tubular changes and no evidence of thrombosis (Cumming et al. 1988).

Fourth, it has been suggested that alterations in the morphology of glomerular endothelium, in particular a reduction in the size and number of fenestrations, may play a role in the reduction of GFR and Kf (Brezis et al. 1986; Gross and Anderson 1985). Significant changes have been reported in a number of models; but some of these changes may be artefactual, since very careful studies in other models have shown no abnormalities (Bulger et al. 1983).

Summary

As the pathogenesis of experimental ATN is unravelled the potential mechanisms and mediators multiply and the possibility of therapeutic intervention appears more remote. However, in man there are several circumstances in which ARF is associated with little or no tubular necrosis, such as cyclosporin nephrotoxicity and hepato-renal syndrome, and it seems certain that reduction in GFR must depend entirely on altered glomerular haemodynamics. The latter are regulated, above all, by the tone in afferent and efferent arterioles and in the mesangial cells. The effects of volume contraction and expansion in man, and new experimental models in which inhibition of several unrelated haemodynamic systems summate to cause ARF, again point to the primacy of haemodynamic events, at least in the induction of ARF. With the recent description of potent endothelium-derived vasoconstrictor and vasodilator factors clearer understanding may be imminent, with the possibility of practical therapeutic remedies.

References

Adams PL, Adams FF, Bell PD, Navar LG (1980) Impaired renal blood flow autoregulation in ischemic acute renal failure. Kidney Int 18: 68–76

Ausiello DA, Kreisberg JI, Roy C, Karinovsky MJ (1980) Contraction of cultured rat glomerular cells of apparent mesangial origin after stimulation with angiotensin II and arginine vasopressin. J Clin Invest 65: 754–760

Ballerman BJ, Levenson DJ, Brenner BM (1986) Renin, angiotensin, kinins, prostaglandins, and leukotrienes. In: Brenner BM, Rector FC (eds) The kidney, 3rd edn. WB Saunders, Philadelphia, pp 281–340

Blantz RC, Pelayo JC (1984) A functional role for the tubuloglomerular feedback mechanism. Kidney Int 25: 739–746

Brenner BM, Zatz R, Ichikawa I (1986a) The renal circulations. In: Brenner BM, Rector FC (eds) The kidney, 3rd edn. WB Saunders, Philadelphia, pp 93–123

Brenner BM, Dworkin LD, Ichikawa I (1986b) Glomerular Ultra filtration. In: Brenner BM, Rector FC (eds) The kidney, 3rd edn. WB Saunders, Philadelphia, pp. 124–144

Brezis M, Rosen S, Silva P, Epstein FH (1984a) Selective vulnerability of the thick ascending limb to anoxia in the isolated perfused rat kidney. J Clin Invest 73: 182–190

Brezis M, Rosen S, Silva P, Epstein FH (1984b) Renal ischaemia: a new perspective. Kidney Int 26: 375–383

Brezis M, Rosen S, Epstein FH (1986) Acute renal failure. In: Brenner BM, Rector FC (eds) The kidney, 3rd edn. WB Saunders, Philadelphia, pp 735–799

Bulger RE, Eknoyan G, Purcell DJ, Dobyan DC (1983) Endothelial characteristics of glomerular capillaries in normal, mercuric chloride-induced and gentamicin-induced acute renal failure in the rat. J Clin Invest 72: 128–141

Clarkson AR, MacDonald MK, Fuster V et al. (1970) Glomerular coagulation in acute ischaemic renal failure. Q J Med 39: 585

Conger JD, Robinette JB, Schrier RW (1988) Smooth muscle calcium and endothelium-derived relaxing factor in the abnormal vascular responses of acute renal failure. J Clin Invest 82: 532–537

Cumming AD, Driedger AA, McDonald JWD, Lindsay RM, Solez K, Linton AL (1988) Vasoactive hormones in the renal response to systemic sepsis. Am J Kidney Dis 11: 23–32

Edwards RM (1985) Response of isolated renal arterioles to acetylcholine, dopamine, and bradykinin. Am J Physiol 248: F183–F189

Frega NS, DiBona DR, Guertler B, Leaf A (1976) Ischaemic renal injury. Kidney Int 10: S17–S25

Furchgott RF, Zawadski JV (1980) The obligatory role of endothelial cells in the relaxation of arterial smooth muscle by acetylcholine. Nature 288: 373–376

Gouyon J-B, Guignard J-P (1988) Theophylline prevents the hypoxemia-induced renal hemodynamic changes in rabbits. Kidney Int 33: 1078–1083

Griffith TM, Edwards DH, Lewis MJ, Newby AC, Henderson AH (1984) The nature of endothelium-derived vascular relaxant factor. Nature 308: 645–647

Griffith TM, Edwards DH, Davies R Ll, Harrison TJ, Evans KT (1987) EDRF coordinates the behaviour of vascular resistance vessels. Nature 329: 442–445

Gross PA, Anderson RJ (1985) Acute renal failure and toxic nephropathy. In: Klahr S, Massry SG (eds) Contemporary nephrology. Plenum, New York, p 447

Heller J (1987) Effect of vasoactive mediators on renal haemodynamics. Nephrol Dial Transplant 2: 197–204

Heyman SN, Brezis M, Reubinoff CA et al. (1988) Acute renal failure with selective medullary injury in the rat. J Clin Invest 82: 401–412

Hostetter TM, Brenner BM (1988) Renal circulatory and nephron function in experimental acute renal failure. In: Brenner BM, Lazarus JM (eds) Acute renal failure, 2nd edn. Churchill Livingstone, London, pp 67–89

Ikuma K, Honda N, Yonemura K, Ahishi K, Hishida A, Nagase M (1988) Glomerular refractoriness to contractile stimuli in rabbits recovering from ischemic acute renal failure. Nephron 48: 306–309

Kashgarian M, Siegel NJ, Ries AL, DiMeola HJ, Hayslett JP (1976) Hemodynamic aspects in development and recovery phases of experimental postischemic acute renal failure. Kidney Int 10:S160–S168

Knox FG, Granger JP (1985) Renal hemodynamics and sodium chloride excretion. In: Klahr S, Massry SG (eds) Contemporary nephrology. Plenum, New York, pp 61–90

Kreisberg JI, Venkatachalam MA (1988) Morphological factors in acute renal failure. In: Brenner BM, Lazarus JM (eds) Acute renal failure, 2nd edn. Churchill Livingstone, London, pp 45–65

Kreisberg JI, Ventkatachalam MA, Troyer D (1985) Contractile properties of cultured glomerular mesangial cells. Am J Physiol 249: F457–F463

Kriz W (1982) Structural organization of renal medullary circulation. Nephron 31: 290–295

Lamas S, Olivera A, Obregon L, et al. (1988a) Cyclosporin A-induced contraction of isolated human and rat glomeruli and cultured rat mesangial cells. Nephrol Dial Transplant 3: 487(abstr)

Lamas S, Olivera A, Puyol DR, Lopez JM (1988b) Adenosine-induced rat mesangial cell contraction: an effect mediated by the A1 receptor type. Nephrol Dial Transplant 3: 487(abstr)

Levinsky NG (1977) Pathophysiology of acute renal failure. New Engl J Med 296: 1453–1458

Mant MJ, King EG (1979) Severe, acute disseminated intravascular coagulation. Am J Med 67: 557–563

Mason J, Torhorst J, Welsch J (1984) Role of the medullary perfusion defect in the pathogenesis of ischaemic renal failure. Kidney Int 26: 283–293

Mason J, Welsch J, Torhorst J (1987) The contribution of vascular obstruction to the functional defect that follows renal ischaemia. Kidney Int 31: 65–71

Matthys E, Patton MK, Osgood RW, Venkatachalam MA, Stein JH (1983) Alterations in vascular function and morphology in acute ischaemic renal failure. Kidney Int 23: 717–724

Mene P, Dunn MJ (1986) Modulation of mesangial cell contraction by arachidonate metabolites. Trans Assoc Am Physicians 99: 125–131

Mene P, Dubyak GR, Dunn MJ (1988) Actions and second messengers of thromboxane A2 and prostaglandins in cultured rat mesangial cells. In: Davison AM (ed) Nephrology (Proc Xth Int Congress Nephrol). Bailliere Tindall, London, pp 98–106

Myers BD, Moran SM (1986) Hemodynamically mediated acute renal failure. N Engl J Med 314: 97–105

Neuwirth R, Singhal P, Satriano JA, Braquet P, Schlondorff D (1987) Effect of platelet activating factor antagonists on cultured rat mesangial cells. J Pharmacol Exp Ther 243: 409–414

Palmer RMJ, Ferrige AG, Moncada S (1987) Nitric oxide release accounts for the biological activity of endothelium-derived relaxing factor. Nature 327: 524–526

Radomski MW, Palmer RMJ, Moncada S (1987a) Endogenous nitric oxide inhibits human platelet adhesion to vascular endothelium. Lancet II: 1057–1058

Radomski MW, Palmer RMJ, Moncada S (1987b) The anti-aggregating properties of vascular endothelium: interactions between prostacyclin and nitric oxide. Br J Pharmacol 92: 639–646

Rapoport RM, Draznin MB, Murad F (1983) Endothelium-dependent relaxation in rat aorta may be mediated through cyclic GMP-dependent protein phosphorylation. Nature 306: 174–176

Richman AV, Gerber LI, Balis JU (1980) Peritubular capillaries: a major target site of endotoxin-induced vascular injury in the primate kidney. Lab Invest 43: 327–332

Schmidt HHHW, Klein MM, Niroomand F, Bohme E (1988) Is arginine a physiological precursor of endothelium-derived nitric oxide? Eur J Pharmacol 148: 293–295

Simonson MS, Dunn MJ (1986) Leukotriene C4 and D4 contract rat glomerular mesangial cells. Kidney Int 30: 524–531

Vanhoutte PM (1988) The endothelium – modulator of vascular smooth-muscle tone. N Engl J Med 319: 512–513

Vari RC, Natarajan LA, Whitescarver SA, Jackson BA, Ott CE (1988) Induction, prevention and mechanisms of contrast media-induced acute renal failure. Kidney Int 33: 699–707

Wardle EN (1974) Fibrin in renal disease: functional considerations. Clin Nephrol 2: 85–92

Wilkes BM, Caldicott WJH, Schulman G, Hollenberg NK (1981) Loss of the glomerular contractile response to angiotensin in rats following myohemoglobinuric acute renal failure. Circ Res 49: 1190–1195

Williams RH, Thomas CE, Navar LG, Evan AP (1981) Hemodynamic and single nephron function during the maintenance phase of ischemic acute renal failure in the dog. Kidney Int 19: 503–515

Wolfert AI, Laveri LA, Reilly KM, Oken KR, Oken DE (1987) Glomerular hemodynamics in mercury-induced acute renal failure. Kidney Int 32: 246–255

Yanagisawa M, Kurihara H, Kimura S, et al. (1988) A novel potent vasoconstrictor peptide produced by vascular endothelial cells. Nature 332: 411–415

Discussion

The discussion centred on the various observations in the literature which suggest that mesangial contraction may occur in vitro and whilst this may well change the surface area for glomerular filtration, this need not necessarily change glomerular blood flow. All participants agreed that the studies of mesangial cells in culture were convincing – they contracted in response to a variety of substances and relaxed in response to others. Nevertheless, this may not be a generalized phenomenon with all mesangial cells responding in the same way. Dr Myers emphasized that whilst mesangial contraction might be a real phenomenon in vitro, it remained to be seen exactly what role it had to play in changes in Kf and glomerular blood flow in patients with acute renal failure. All agreed that further studies of the role of the mesangium in the pathogenesis of acute renal failure were required and considerable interest centred on the effects of the new vasoactive compounds EDRF and endothelin which might also play an important part in the redistribution of blood flow within the kidney.

Chapter 9

Role of the Medulla in Acute Renal Failure

F. H. Epstein, M. Brezis and S. Rosen

The mammalian kidney poses an interesting paradox with regard to the adequacy of its oxygen supply. The flow of blood to the kidney is high in relation to its weight, and renal arteriovenous oxygen difference is low. The high renal blood flow is commonly viewed as designed to maximize flow-dependent clearance of wastes, and it is often assumed that the supply of oxygen does not normally limit the ability of the kidney to do work. A generous flow of blood should also protect the kidney from potential ischaemic insults, by giving it a larger margin of security than other organs and making it the least likely organ in the body to be damaged by compromised blood flow. Nevertheless, the kidney is remarkably susceptible to hypoperfusion, ischaemic acute renal failure being one of the most frequent complications of hypotension or hypovolaemia, and exceeding by a significant margin the incidence of injury to brain, myocardium or liver in the same clinical setting. The explanation for this paradox lies in the remarkable inhomogeneity of blood flow and oxygen supply within the kidney. Selective regional hypoxia is potentially, therefore, an important cause of localized injury during renal hypoperfusion (Brezis et al. 1984a).

Gradients of Oxygen Supply Within Mammalian Kidney

Gradients of oxygen availability within the renal parenchyma have been appreciated for many years. More than 20 years ago, Aukland and Krog (1960) demonstrated that the pO_2 of the medulla was strikingly lower than renal arterial pO_2. Some 10 years later Leichtweiss et al. (1969; Baumgartl et al. 1972) confirmed and extended this idea, demonstrating that the medullary pO_2, measured with microelectrodes sensitive to oxygen, was consistently in the region of 10 mmHg in the kidney of the dog and of the rat, both *in situ* and during isolated perfusion of the kidneys. Oxygenation of renal tissue in the cortex of the kidney was also shown to be heterogeneous. The sharp corticomedullary gradient of oxygen is most easily explained by the organization of vessels in the medulla, which allows countercurrent diffusion of oxygen between the arterial and venous branches of the hairpin loops of the vasa recta. The demonstration that large variations in respired oxygen concentrations hardly affect medullary pO_2 (Baumgartl et al. 1972), and the illustration of A-V shunting within the kidney of oxygen and of krypton (Levy and Imperial 1961; Longley et al. 1958) have made the countercurrent exchange of oxygen within the medulla a plausible explanation of the low medullary pO_2.

What was not clear from the direct observations by Leichtweiss was whether the tissue pO_2 values that he determined, low as they were, were sufficiently low to influence the redox state of kidney cell mitochondria and therefore possibly alter the rate and manner of oxygen utilization in local areas of the kidney. A gradient in oxygen pressure must exist to enable oxygen to diffuse across the distances from capillary to cell border and from cell border to mitochondria. The "critical pO_2" at which oxygen concentration in the medium limits the rate of oxygen consumption therefore depends on the rate of oxygen consumption and on where the pO_2 is measured. It is higher for intact separated cells than for isolated mitochondria because the diffusion distance for oxygen is longer and the diffusivity of oxygen is reduced in high protein solutions (Goldstick et al. 1975). For similar reasons the critical pO_2 is higher still in intact perfused organs. Thus, while the K_m for oxygen in mitochondria is normally equivalent to 1–2 mmHg (Chance 1957), the critical pO_2 of a suspension of separated renal tubules was estimated to be in the neighbourhood of 10 mmHg by Balaban et al. (1980). The critical pO_2 of isolated whole perfused kidneys was estimated to be between 6 and 28 mmHg with a maximum abundance at 8 mmHg by using microelectrode pO_2 probes (Leichtweiss et al. 1969). Thus there is a possibility that substantial numbers of cells, particularly in the renal medulla, might normally operate in an atmosphere of partial anoxia in which mitochondrial cytochromes would be partially or completely reduced.

Redox State of Mitochondrial Cytochromes Within the Kidney

Direct observations using the techniques of optical spectroscopy, have confirmed these predictions (Epstein et al. 1982). Cytochrome aa_3 (cytochrome C oxidase), the terminal electron carrier of the mitochondrial chain, is almost completely oxidized at normal oxygen tensions and, in mitochondria and separated cells, it exists largely in the oxidized state (Chance 1957; Balaban et al. 1980). In a variety of cells it has been shown that cytochrome aa_3 does not become significantly reduced until the level of oxygen delivery to the tissue has become insufficient to maintain maximal oxidative metabolism in at least a portion of the tissue. For this reason cytochrome aa_3 is well suited for the monitoring of tissue oxygenation in whole organs through the application of the dual-wavelength principle to whole organ absorbance and reflectance spectrophotometry. In experiments on isolated perfused rat kidneys, approximately 30%–45% of cytochrome aa_3 in the whole perfused kidney was found to be in the reduced state (Epstein et al. 1982). These rather surprising findings were consistent with analogous experiments done in vivo in exposed kidneys of anaesthetized rats using the technique of reflectance spectrophotometry (Balaban and Silvia 1981). Experiments designed to reduce oxidative metabolism in proximal tubules and hence improve oxygenation in the cortex were without effect in altering the redox state. In contrast, the loop diuretics bumetanide and frusemide, which have their major locus of action in the medullary thick ascending limb, invariably produced partial oxidation of cytochrome aa_3 (Epstein et al. 1982).

These findings suggest that a substantial number of cells in the intact perfused kidney normally operate at or close to the brink of anoxia. It seems likely that these are predominantly in the renal medulla, probably in the thick ascending limb of Henle's loop, since they are affected by changes in transport work induced by the loop diuretics. The phenomenon is most likely not merely an artifact in the isolated perfused kidney inasmuch as cytochrome aa_3 was also found to be partially reduced in rat kidneys studied in vivo (Balaban and Silvia 1981). Furthermore, the studies by Leichtweiss et al. (1969) with oxygen microelectrodes suggest that the perfused kidney is better oxygenated than are kidneys *in situ* perfused with the animal's own blood at atmospheric pressures of oxygen. That oxygen supplied to the kidney may be marginally adequate rather than superabundant is also suggested by studies showing that hypoxia produces diuresis by decreasing tubular transport (Selkurt 1953).

The reduction in cytochrome aa_3 detected on absorbance spectrophotometry may represent the result of spatial oscillations in the redox state, whereby individual cells would fluctuate in their degree of cytochrome reduction but the total amount of reduced cytochrome would remain relatively constant. This possibility is suggested by some evidence that in the kidney, as in brain and muscle, there are rhythmic fluctuations in microvascular flow (Eggert and Weiss 1980).

An implication of these results is that a delicate and sensitive mechanism must exist to regulate local blood flow in response to metabolic demand. Derangement of this mechanism is likely to predispose to ischaemic necrosis. If the thick ascending limb were particularly susceptible to anoxic interference with active transport, it would be easy for relatively minor degrees of global renal ischaemia to initiate glomerular vasoconstriction via the tubuloglomerular feedback mechanism and thus contribute to the functional impairment of acute renal failure.

Selective Anoxic Injury to Medullary Thick Ascending Limb

It is the cells of the thick limb of the renal medulla, therefore, immersed in a hypoxic milieu and requiring energy to carry out a substantial fraction of active reabsorptive transport, that must in a sense pay a price for the ability of mammalian kidneys to concentrate the urine via countercurrent exchange. The morphological consequence of this special susceptibility is easily observed. During isolated perfusion of the rat kidney with cell-free albumin–Ringer's medium, the medullary thick ascending limb appears selectively vulnerable to anoxic injury (Brezis et al. 1984b). A specific lesion is consistently observed, occurring within minutes and confined to this nephron segment, that progresses from mitochondrial swelling to nuclear pyknosis and complete cellular disruption. The lesion involves about 50% of the thick ascending limbs under normal circumstances, and is most prominent in those tubules removed from vascular bundles and near the inner medulla, areas most likely to be anoxic according to expected gradients of pO_2. Hypoxic perfusion markedly exaggerates the lesion and extends it to all medullary thick limbs (Brezis et al. 1984e). Oxygen-enriched perfusion using rat erythrocytes or haemoglobin prevents the lesion (Brezis et al. 1984b). These findings strengthen the hypothesis that the medullary thick ascending limb is exquisitely susceptible to anoxic damage because of a low oxygen supply imposed by the medullary countercurrent exchange system and the high rate of metabolism mandated by active reabsorption of sodium chloride.

It is of some pathophysiological significance, we feel, that in the medulla of all mammalian kidneys, including the human, the relation between thick limbs and vascular bundles follows a definite pattern (Kriz and Kaissling 1985). Short-looped nephrons, which originate in the superficial cortex, have their thick limbs located at a distance from the vascular bundles while long-looped nephrons, originating in the deeper regions of the kidney, have their thick limbs adjacent to the vascular bundles. This means that with medullary hypoxia, it will be the thick limbs of the short-looped nephrons that will suffer the most. If ischaemic damage to the thick limb reduces single nephron glomerular filtration rate via a tubuloglomerular feedback mechanism, then when renal circulation is menaced, blood flow and glomerular filtration to the most superficial portions of the renal cortex would decline first. Juxtamedullary circulation would be maintained until medullary hypoxia became more severe. This is, of course, exactly what has been observed in patients and animals with reductions in renal blood flow.

Relation of Anoxic Injury to Transport

Of particular interest is that inhibition of cell transport activity with frusemide or ouabain, or by the abolition of glomerular filtration, using a hyperoncotic non-filtering mode, can protect the medullary thick limb and consistently prevents injury to this segment of the nephron in the isolated perfused kidney (Brezis et al. 1984c). Severe and extensive anoxic damage produced in this model by perfusion with cyanide or by a hypoxic medium (pO_2 less than 40 mmHg) is also remarkably attenuated by reduction of active transport produced by ouabain or frusemide (Brezis et al. 1984c). Furthermore, perfusion with a polyene antibiotic such as amphotericin or nystatin, which increases membrane permeability and stimulates the sodium pump, reproduces extensive anoxic-like injury to the medullary thick ascending limbs (Brezis et al. 1984d). This damage is prevented if active ion transport is inhibited by ouabain. These experiments with amphotericin suggest that other forms of cellular injury produced by agents that increase membrane permeability – for example, the attack complex of complement, or the increased cell permeability produced by lysolecithins – might also be modulated by active transport in an hypoxic environment.

These results suggest the concept that oxygen deficiency is related to its demand. The outer medulla apparently exhibits a sort of anginal syndrome in which the degree of cellular anoxia depends on the demand for oxygen as well as its supply. This principle may have important implications for the understanding of ischaemic damage to the medulla, since complete cessation of blood flow, so frequently used as a model of ischaemic renal injury, necessarily abolishes glomerular filtration and thus tends to protect the medullary thick limb and prevent the full expression of injury to this segment that would have been produced by hypoperfusion. This is presumably the basis of attenuation of ischaemic injury by frusemide and ouabain.

Role of ATP Depletion in Ischaemic Injury in the Medullary Thick Ascending Limb (mTAL)

A natural supposition is that in this model, anoxic and transport-dependent injury is the result of depletion of cellular stores of ATP. Further experiments in our laboratory, however, have thrown doubt on that presumption. In the isolated perfused rat kidney, perfusion with rotenone or antimycin, which interrupt mitochondrial electron flow proximal to cytochrome b, appears to ameliorate rather than worsen the anoxic lesion in medullary thick ascending limb cells, while further reducing, rather than increasing, the content of ATP in medullary tissue. A similar paradoxical sparing of cell injury is produced by certain inhibitors of intermediary metabolism like deoxyglucose or fluoroacetate. These results raise the question whether, at least in this portion of the nephron, hypoxic damage may not be mediated by some function of mitochondrial electron flow or redox state, rather than by depletion of ATP. It is conceivable, for example, that the formation of certain free radicals would be enhanced by factors (like cell work) that accelerate the tendency for mitochondrial electron transport in the presence of an anoxic block. Diminution of cell work or blockade of electron transport early in the mitochondrial chain would be protective by decreasing the formation of these free radicals.

Implications of Medullary Hypoxia for the Genesis of Acute Renal Failure

In the perspective of the precarious balance of oxygen demand and supply in the outer medulla, the reduction of cortical blood flow during hypotension may be viewed as designed to protect medullary cells from ischaemic injury, both directly by increasing the relative proportion of oxygen delivery to the medulla and indirectly by decreasing oxygen demand for solute reabsorption as glomerular filtration rate drops. When this regulatory mechanism fails and medullary ischaemia occurs, solute reaching the macula densa will activate tubuloglomerular feedback (Thurau and Boylan 1976). The ensuing profound decrease in glomerular filtration rate might be viewed as designed to decrease further the needs for solute reabsorption and oxygen demand in a last ditch effort to protect the ischaemic medullary thick ascending limb from further damage (Brezis et al. 1984a). It is pertinent that decreased concentrating ability, implying impaired function of the mTAL, is not only the most consistent defect encountered in acute renal failure, but is also a very early sign of impending renal failure in advanced prerenal azotaemia secondary to hypotension or to a decrease in cardiac output.

Endogenous Inhibitors of Transport

The close dependence of experimental ischaemic injury on active transport suggests that endogenous inhibitors of transport might play an important physiological role in modulating the susceptibility of the medulla to anoxic injury. Possible candidates for this role are adenosine and perhaps other purine metabolites, and derivatives of arachidonic acid.

Adenosine has been suggested as a possible endogenous modulator of ischaemic injury in brain and heart. The hydrolysis of ATP in excess of its synthesis is thought to lead to a rise in the intracellular concentration of AMP, which is hydrolysed to adenosine by 5'-nucleotidase. In low concentrations, adenosine activates inhibitory receptors which reduce the activity of adenylate cyclase and diminish the burden of cell work in excitable and secretory tissues. It is, therefore, of great interest that we have recently found that adenosine, at concentrations of 10^{-8}–10^{-5} mol l^{-1}, diminishes substantially the rate of transport-associated respiration in a homogeneous preparation of isolated cells of the thick ascending limb of rabbit medulla.

In preliminary experiments by Steven Hebert, a single isolated thick ascending limb of the mouse was perfused, and active transport was monitored electrically. When phenylisopropyladenosine was added to the basolateral surface of the tubule, an immediate and reversible reduction in active transport was produced. There are, therefore, receptors for adenosine in the thick ascending limb, and an adenosine analogue reduces transport in this nephron segment. In isolated perfused kidneys we have now been able to show that the same analogue dramatically reduces anoxic injury to medullary thick ascending limb when it is added to the perfusate. Furthermore, this protection is reversed by adding 8-phenyltheophylline, a competitive adenosine antagonist. These experiments suggest that adenosine, a normal byproduct of ATP breakdown during ischaemia, may serve a protective function in the medulla by down-regulating transport in the thick ascending limb so that these cells do not literally die of overwork.

Adenosine undoubtedly plays additional roles in the pathophysiology of acute renal failure. Though it reduces blood flow to the kidney cortex (Spielman et al. 1987) it is a powerful vasodilator of vasa recta flow (Miyamoto et al. 1988). Furthermore, adenosine and its analogues markedly enhance tubuloglomerular feedback (Schnermann 1988; Soejima and Schnermann 1988; Franco et al. 1988). Liberation of adenosine during ischaemia, therefore, might do three things designed to protect the mTAL cell from injury: (a) increase the supply of oxygen by improving vasa recta flow; (b) decrease the work of transport in thick limbs;

(c) further decrease the necessity for active transport by depressing glomerular filtration rate via an exaggerated tubuloglomerular feedback. The last effect would, of course, contribute paradoxically to the evolution of acute renal failure. Evidence in favour of this hypothesis can be adduced from the beneficial effect of theophylline, an adenosine antagonist, in ameliorating certain forms of experimental acute renal failure (Lin et al. 1988).

Prostaglandin E_2 and other arachidonic acid derivatives are known to be produced by cells of the medullary thick ascending limb. Prostaglandin E_2 is a potent vasodilator and also inhibits active transport in the thick limb. When added to the medium bathing isolated thick ascending limb cells prostaglandin E_2 has a profound effect on decreasing transport-associated oxygen consumption. Very recently, we have been able to show that enhancing the endogenous production of PGE_2 by rat kidneys also confers protection from the ischaemic injury seen in the isolated perfused kidney. In rats fed on safflower oil, containing the arachidonic acid precursor linoleic acid, urinary excretion of PGE_2 was approximately twice that of control rats fed on fish oil which does not contain this arachidonic acid precursor. The percentage of thick ascending limbs in the medulla that were damaged after 60 minutes of perfusion was greatly reduced by safflower oil. Damage seen in the medulla was only half as extensive as in the controls fed on fish oil, which produced a much lower renal prostaglandin excretion. These experiments suggest a kind of conversation between inner medulla and outer medulla whereby protective prostaglandins manufactured in the papilla, or inner medulla, may be carried by vasa recta blood to their neighbours in the outer medulla to spare thick ascending limb cells from ischaemic damage.

It might be predicted that indomethacin and other cyclooxygenase inhibitors would exaggerate the lesions of hypoxia seen in the isolated perfused kidney. This is indeed the case. The addition of indomethacin to the perfusion medium greatly increases the extent and severity of cell injury seen in the renal medulla, presumably because the restriction of transport work imposed by endogenous prostaglandins is removed. We believe that this effect, demonstrable in perfused kidneys, is primarily responsible for the lesion of analgesic nephropathy, seen in patients addicted to daily ingestion of large amounts of pain-relieving medications and characterized by interstitial fibrosis that is especially marked in the renal medulla, progressing to papillary necrosis. It may also be responsible in part for the predilection to acute renal failure conferred by non-steroidal anti-inflammatory drugs.

Arachidonic acid derivatives that are not prostaglandins may also modulate ischaemic injury by altering transport. Some of these unsaturated fatty acid derivatives are synthesized in large amounts by medullary thick ascending limb cells and act as specific inhibitors of Na,K-ATPase (Schwartzman et al 1985). Products of the cytochrome P-450 monooxygenase pathway, in particular the epoxyeicosatetraenoic acids (EETs), are especially potent in inhibiting transport. Preliminary experiments in our own laboratory have shown that during prolonged incubation, medullary thick limb cells release an endogenous inhibitor of transport-related respiration into the surrounding fluid. Formation of the endogenous inhibitor is blocked by lipoxygenase inhibitors and is exaggerated by the inclusion of arachidonic acid in the incubation medium. These are examples of a general phenomenon by which endogenous substances serve to condition and modulate cellular work in this critical region of the nephron.

Medullary Ischaemia and Acute Renal Failure in Animals and Man

An important question is whether medullary ischaemia, so easily demonstrated in the perfused kidney, has any relevance to the phenomenon of acute renal failure as observed in man and produced in experimental animals. It should be emphasized that there are marked differences between most experimental models of renal failure produced in animals and the morphological picture seen in human patients with acute renal failure. In most experimental animal models, usually produced by complete interruption of blood flow to the kidney followed by a variable period of reflow, there is extensive and severe damage to cortical portions of proximal tubules. In man, on the other hand, it is now appreciated that proximal convoluted tubular damage is extremely scanty and focal, if indeed it is present at all. One reason for these differences may be that experimental renal failure in animals is usually a *universal* response to *severe* ischaemia. Human renal failure, on the other hand, occurs in a setting of shock in which renal blood flow is usually not completely interrupted; it is therefore a very *occasional* response to *incomplete* ischaemia. In animals, the attractiveness of a simply designed experiment has led most investigators to administer a single but powerful insult. On the other hand, most cases arising in the clinic have at least two predisposing factors and frequently more.

Brezis and his collaborators have recently developed a model of acute renal failure in intact rats in which selective damage to the renal medulla appears in fact to produce a syndrome that resembles human acute renal failure (Heyman et al. 1988). Produced in rats kept on a salt-free diet, given indomethacin, and with renal reserve reduced by uninephrectomy, it resembles the human form of acute renal failure in that it is the resultant of several predisposing factors. As with many of our patients, these initial events set the stage for renal failure produced by intravenous sodium iothalamate. The radiocontrast agent produces extensive cellular necrosis confined to the medulla and to cells lining the medullary thick ascending limb. Serum creatinine rises progressively, and the elevation in serum creatinine is directly proportional to the percentage of medullary thick ascending limbs showing necrosis in a careful morphometric examination of the kidneys. Interestingly, similar damage can be demonstrated when radiocontrast agents are administered to isolated perfused rat kidneys, and the damage can be reduced or eliminated by inhibiting active transport with ouabain. We do not yet know what particular property of the radiocontrast medium is necessary to produce this result. It should be emphasized again that in this model necrosis is limited selectively to cells lining the medullary thick limb.

Medullary Injury and Human Acute Renal Failure

The evidence for predominant involvement of the renal medulla in human acute renal failure is admittedly indirect and incomplete. One reason for this is that renal biopsies of patients with acute renal failure are usually limited (intentionally) to the renal cortex; furthermore, bloc fixation of autopsy material does not yield the histological detail necessary to perceive the earliest morphological signs of ischaemic injury in affected cells. Severe necrotic changes have been reported, however, in the straight portion of the proximal tubule (S_3) which extends into the outer medulla, as well as in thick ascending limbs, as mentioned below. Certainly a hallmark of the clinical syndrome of acute renal failure is early and severe impairment of concentrating ability, pre-eminently the function of the thick ascending limb and the medulla. The universal finding, especially after urine flow is re-established, of urinary casts composed of Tamm–Horsfall protein, suggests that it is the thick ascending limb of the nephron, where this glycoprotein is exclusively located, that bears the brunt of damage.

Perhaps the most telling evidence that human acute renal failure involves the medulla is to be found in the first meticulous accounts of the disorder that date back to World War II (Bywaters and Beall 1941; Dunn et al. 1941; Bywaters and Dible 1942). These papers uniformly emphasize the predominant involvement of the renal medulla, focusing particularly on the medullary thick ascending limb (hence the appellation, "lower nephron nephrosis") (Lucke 1946). Fig. 9.1 illustrates a microdissected nephron (Oliver et al. 1951), illustrating the necrotic rent in the medullary thick limb in a kidney removed at autopsy from a victim of crush injury in the London bombings of World War II, who died in acute renal failure.

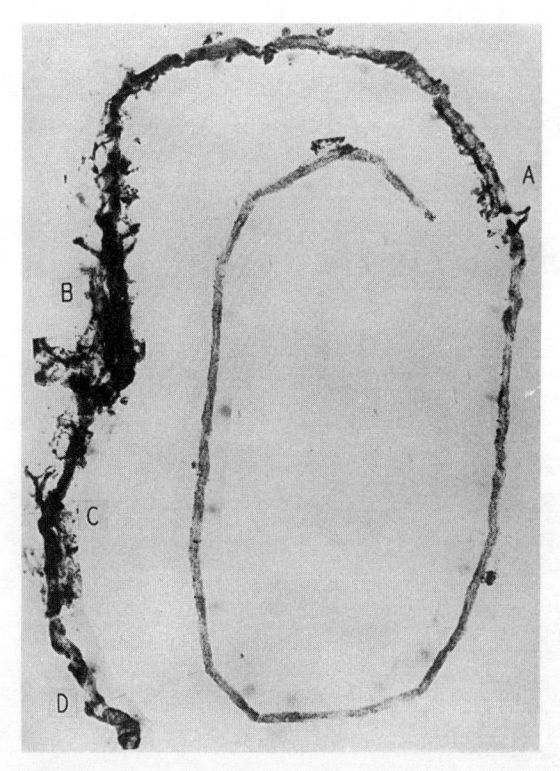

Fig. 9.1. Dissected nephron from case of Dunn et al. (1941), a young woman who died on the ninth day of oliguria following crush injury. A shows disruption of the medullary thick ascending tubule at a point of necrosis. At B the tubule is distended with a black pigment cast and there is fragmentation of the tubule wall. (Reprinted from Oliver et al. (1951)).

Summary

The price we pay for the efficient countercurrent system that permits us to concentrate our urine is that certain key portions of the nephron located in the medulla (e.g. the straight portion of the proximal tubule and the medullary thick ascending limb) always operate on the edge of anoxia. They are, therefore, exquisitely vulnerable to a decrease in the supply of oxygen without a commensurate reduction in transport work. Early in the course of ischaemia a decrease in thick ascending limb function leads to loss of concentrating ability and to a decrease in glomerular filtration secondary to tubuloglomerular feedback. Glomerular constriction first involves the cortical nephrons since their thick limbs are at greatest risk of anoxia, being located farthest from the vasa recta. As medullary anoxia becomes more widespread, all nephrons participate, contributing to the syndrome of acute renal failure. It seems possible that the renal toxicity of certain drugs and even the mechanism of immune injury might also be related to their impact on cellular work in the presence of limited oxygen supply. Because of the uniquely low ambient partial pressure of oxygen in the renal medulla it seems likely that a variety of, as yet undiscovered, mechanisms has evolved that permit the medullary cells to function on the verge of anoxia while protecting them from irreversible ischaemic injury. Interference with these primitive protective mechanisms is likely to predispose to the development of acute renal failure.

Acknowledgements. This work was aided by USPHS Grant No. DK18078 and a grant from the US–Israel Binational Science Foundation.

References

Aukland K, Krog J (1960) Renal oxygen tension. Nature 188:671
Balaban RS, Silvia AL (1981) Spectrophotometric monitoring of O_2 delivery to the exposed rat kidney. Am J Physiol 241: F257–F262
Balaban RS, Soltoff SP, Storey JM, Mandel LJ (1980) Improved renal cortical tubule suspension: spectrophotometric study of O_2 delivery. Am J Physiol 238: F50–F59
Baumgartl H, Leichtweiss HP, Lubbers DW, Weiss CH, Huland H (1972) The oxygen supply of the dog kidney: measurements of intrarenal pO_2. Microvasc Res 4: 247–257
Brezis M, Rosen S, Silva P, Epstein FH (1984a) Renal ischemia: a new perspective. Kidney Int 26: 375–383
Brezis M, Rosen S, Silva P, Epstein FH (1984b) Selective vulnerability of the thick ascending limb to anoxia in the isolated perfused rat kidney. J Clin Invest 73: 182–190
Brezis M, Rosen S, Silva P, Epstein FH (1984c) Transport activity modifies thick ascending limb damage in isolated perfused kidney. Kidney Int 25: 65–72
Brezis M, Rosen S, Silva P, Spokes K, Epstein FH (1984d) Polyene toxicity in renal medulla: injury mediated by transport activity. Science 224: 66–68
Brezis M, Rosen S, Silva P, Spokes K, Epstein FH (1984e) Transport-dependent anoxic cell injury in the isolated perfused rat kidney. Am J Pathol 116: 327–341
Bywaters EGL, Beal D (1941) Crush injuries with impairment of renal function. Br Med J i: 427–423
Bywaters EGL, Dible JH (1942) The renal lesion in traumatic anuria. J Pathol Bacteriol 54: 111–120
Chance B (1957) Cellular oxygen requirements. Fed Proc 16: 671–680

Dunn JS, Gillespie M, Niven JSF (1941) Renal lesions in two cases of crush syndrome. Lancet II: 549–551
Eggert P, Weiss C (1980) Periodic microflow pattern measured with a new microflow probe within the rat kidney cortex. Pflugers Arch 383:223–227
Epstein FH, Balaban RS, Ross BD (1982) Redox state of cytochrome a, a_3 in isolated perfused rat kidney. Am J Physiol 243: F356–F363
Franco M, Bell PD, Navar LG (1988) Intratubular effect of adenosine A_1 analog on tubuloglomerular feedback (TGF) mechanism. Kidney Int 33: 263
Goldstick TK, Ciuryla VT, Zuckerman L (1975) Diffusion of oxygen in plasma and blood In: Groete J, Renear D, Thews G (eds) Oxygen transport to tissue vol II. Plenum, New York, pp 183–190
Heyman SN, Brezis M, Reubinoff CA, Greenfeld Z, Lechene C, Epstein FH, Rosen S (1988) Acute renal failure with selective medullary injury in the rat. J Clin Invest 82: 401–412
Kriz W, Kaissling B (1985) Structural organization of the mammalian kidney. In: Seldin DW, Giebisch G (eds) The kidney, physiology and pathophysiology. Raven Press, New York, pp 265–306
Leichtweiss HP, Lubbers DW, Weiss CH, Baumgartl H, Reschke W (1969) The oxygen supply of the rat kidney: measurement of intrarenal pO_2. Pflugers Arch 309: 328–349
Levy MN, Imperial ES (1961) Oxygen shunting in renal cortical and medullary capillaries. Am J Physiol 200: 159–162
Lin J-J, Churchill PC, Bidani AK (1988) Theophylline in rats during maintenance phase of postischemic acute renal failure. Kidney Int 33: 24–28
Longley JB, Lasser NA, Lilienfeld LS (1958) Tracer studies on renal medullary circulation. Fed Proc 17: 99 (abstract)
Lucke B (1946) Lower nephron nephrosis. The renal lesions of the crush syndrome of burns, transfusion and other conditions affecting the lower segments of the nephron. Milit Surg 99: 371–396
Miyamoto M, Larson TS, Robertson CP, Jamison RL (1988) Effect of intrarenal adenosine on renal function and vasa recta blood flow in the rat. Kidney Int 33: 276
Oliver J, MacDowell M, Tracy A (1951) The pathogenesis of acute renal failure associated with traumatic and toxic injury: renal ischemia, nephrotoxic damage and the ischemuric episode. J Clin Invest 30: 1307–1351
Schnermann J (1988) Effect of adenosine analogues on tubuloglomerular feedback responses. Am J Physiol 255: F33–F42
Schwartzmann M, Ferreri NR, Carroll MA, Sougu-Mize E, McGiff JC (1985) Renal cytochrome P-450-related arachidonate metabolite inhibits (Na^+-K^+) ATPase. Nature 314: 620–622
Selkurt EE (1953) Influence of hypoxia on renal circulation and on excretion of electrolytes and water. Am J Physiol 172: 700–708
Soejima H, Schnermann J (1988) The effect of adenosine analogues on tubuloglomerular feedback responses. Kidney Int 33: 413
Spielman WS, Arend LJ, Forrest JN Jr (1987) The renal and epithelial actions of adenosine. In: Gerlach E, Becker BF (eds) Topics and perspectives in adenosine research. Springer-Verlag, Berlin, Heidelberg, New York, pp 249–260
Thurau K, Boylan JW (1976) Acute renal success. The unexpected logic of oliguria in acute renal failure. Am J Med 61: 308–315

Discussion

Dr Steinhausen voiced some doubts over the distribution of the damage seen in the kidney, in the model presented by Dr Epstein. Dr Steinhausen maintained, for example, that an infusion of noradrenaline into the renal artery in various animal models will give a necrosis primarily in the proximal tubules. He doubted that the medullary thick ascending limb of the loop of Henle was always involved in hypoxic damage to the kidney. Dr Epstein agreed that one cannot move directly from the isolated perfused rat kidney to acute renal failure in human beings. He admitted that he was using a paraphysiological model. Nevertheless, this model demonstrated certain principles and the concept of hypoxia within the medulla of the kidney remained essential in an understanding of the pathogenesis of acute renal failure. Dr Ledingham asked how tubuloglomerular feedback, even amplified by the release of adenosine, could maintain oliguria for such prolonged periods as seen in human acute renal failure. Dr Epstein admitted that this was a difficult question, and whilst the initial oliguria might be related to tubular glomerular feedback, it was not clear what mechanism could account for prolonged oliguria. Dr Epstein concluded that it was very likely that the mediators of the prolonged reduction in GFR seen in acute renal failure have not yet been discovered, and might well be related to peptides derived from the damaged endothelial cells.

Chapter 10

Ischaemic Acute Renal Failure in an Intact Animal Model

P. J. Ratcliffe, Z. H. Endre, J. D. Tange and J. G. G. Ledingham

Most experimental studies of ischaemic acute renal failure have been devoted to defining the mechanism of loss of excretory function in the damaged kidney and relatively little consideration has been given to the pathophysiological mechanisms leading to the occurrence of ischaemia; yet clinical strategies for prevention of acute renal failure in the Intensive Care Unit might best be drawn from such an understanding. In respect of this we have drawn a parallel with myocardial ischaemia where knowledge of the pathophysiology of the coronary circulation has provided a rational basis for therapeutics. Similar research in nephrology has been hampered by the difficulty of detecting ischaemia in the intact kidney either clinically or experimentally, in contrast with the myocardium where chest pain or changes in the surface electrocardiogram provide markers of ischaemia and permit physiological evaluation and timing of therapeutic intervention. This chapter describes our experience with the use of ^{31}P nuclear magnetic resonance (^{31}P NMR) to detect renal ischaemia in a model of haemorrhagic shock in the rat.

Recently, interest has been focused on the pathophysiology of renal ischaemia by the suggestion that oxygen delivery may be barely sufficient in certain potentially susceptible areas of the kidney while whole organ oxygen delivery is high; ischaemic damage might then result from only a slight impairment of perfusion providing a possible explanation for the apparent susceptibility of the kidney to injury despite high resting renal blood flow and low arteriovenous oxygen extraction (Epstein et al. 1982; Brezis et al. 1984a). Alternatively susceptibility to renal ischaemia might have its basis in the reactivity of the arterial vessels supplying the kidney which could render the organ at risk of a major decrease in total renal perfusion when systemic haemodynamics are threatened (Trueta et al. 1947).

In support of the first suggestion, areas of impaired renal tissue oxygenation have been demonstrated by direct measurement of pO_2 (Aukland and Krog 1960; Leichtweiss et al. 1969), spectroscopic observation of the redox state of cytochrome aa_3 (Epstein et al. 1982; Balaban and Sylvia 1981), and surface fluorescence of flavin nucleotides (Franke et al. 1976). However, the precise relationship of these findings to the occurrence of damaging cellular ischaemia is unclear; for instance, the limiting pO_2 at which hypoxic cell damage ensues is not known. Nevertheless, recent morphological findings in the isolated perfused kidney have convincingly demonstrated the importance of regionally impaired intrarenal oxygen delivery in generating localized injury, at least in that preparation (Brezis et al. 1984b).

Alcorn et al. (1981) described the rapid development of selective damage affecting the thick ascending limb of Henle's loops in the inner stripe of the outer medulla, during perfusion with cell-free media. Brezis et al. (1984b,c) by manipulating oxygen delivery by varying the oxygen content of the perfusate showed that this lesion had an hypoxic component and suggested that this region was specifically predisposed to hypoxic injury. The isolated perfused kidney, however, differs in a number of important ways from the kidney in vivo; for instance the oxygen is carried as oxyhaemoglobin rather than in solution. Predisposition of the cell-free perfused kidney to medullary thick ascending loop (mTAL) damage may be dependent on increased shunt diffusion in the renal medulla when oxygen is delivered entirely in a physically dissolved form; a possibility supported by our findings that supplementation of the perfusate with erythrocytes to a haematocrit of 2%–4% strikingly alters the pattern of hypoxic damage so that the proximal tubule rather than the mTAL is now most susceptible to damage (Endre et al. 1988) (Figure 10.1). Thus, extrapolation from results obtained by controlled decreases in oxygen delivery to the perfused kidney to in vivo conditions is subject to some uncertainty. Since in vivo, controlled decreases in renal oxygen delivery are more difficult to achieve, analogous experiments have not been performed. A means of detecting damaging renal cellular hypoxia or ischaemia in vivo would be of great value in clarifying the pathophysiology of renal ischaemia.

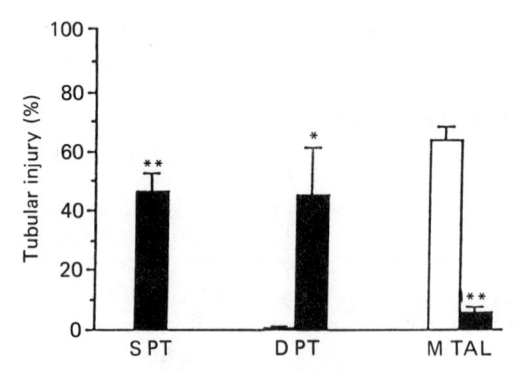

Fig. 10.1. Comparison of morphological damage at equivalent rates of total oxygen delivery (25–30 μmol min^{-1} per kidney) in erythrocyte perfused kidney (*black columns*) and cell-free perfused kidney (*open columns*) in three nephron segments: proximal tubules in the superficial cortex (*S PT*), proximal tubules in the deep cortex (*D PT*) and thick ascending limbs of Henle's loop in the inner stripe of the outer medulla (*M TAL*).

Detection of Renal Ischaemia by ^{31}P NMR

The first applications of ^{31}P NMR to intact kidney demonstrated that changes in the ^{31}P NMR spectrum consisting of accumulation of inorganic phosphate, tissue acidosis, and a reduction in ATP occurred early in ischaemic models of acute renal failure (Sehr et al. 1979; Chan et al. 1982). The precise importance of each of these changes in the molecular pathology of ischaemic cell injury has been much debated but remains unclear. In our recent work we have chosen to use reduction in ATP levels rather than phosphate accumulation or acidosis as a marker of cell ischaemia, principally because the latter are strongly influenced by vascular flow in the absence of energy provision. Thus, in pure hypoxic injury accumulation of protons and phosphate is only slight (Ratcliffe et al. 1988). Since ATP is the substrate for the majority of energy-requiring reactions and is the main product of oxidative metabolism, reduction of cellular levels of ATP in the face of diminished oxygen supply should indicate the occurrence of an important compromise in cellular metabolism. The importance of change of ATP concentrations in ischaemic injury has, however, been challenged. The level of ATP may not accurately reflect cellular energy status; phosphorylation potential (ATP)/(ADP) × (P_i) may be more important, but unfortunately the concentration of ADP is too low for direct measurement in kidney by current NMR techniques (Stubbs et al. 1984). Reduction of ATP by non-ischaemic means, for instance phosphate trapping by fructose (Shapiro et al. 1987), does not mimic ischaemic injury and other events, e.g. proton accumulation, calcium entry, membrane damage are clearly involved in cell injury (Farber et al. 1981; Cheung et al. 1982). After total interruption of renal blood flow profound ATP depletion occurs within minutes, yet structural damage and cell death evolve much more slowly (Vogt and Farber 1968). These considerations indicate that reduction of ATP *per se* is not the immediate cause of renal cell death but they do not exclude the possibility that reduction in ATP in the setting of ischaemia or hypoxia is a valid marker of the disturbance of cell metabolism, which if uncorrected, will lead to renal damage. How might this possibility be assessed?

One problem in correlating the extent of reduction in ATP with subsequent cell injury is that a finite period is required for the generation of microscopically visible structural change, so that for simple correlation a stable period of ATP depletion is required. This is not easily produced in vivo except by total interruption of blood flow, and cannot be achieved in the model of haemorrhagic hypotension to be described, where changes in ATP levels when they occur are characteristically sudden and unpredictable. In contrast, in the isolated perfused kidney a controlled decrease in oxygen delivery can be achieved by altering the oxygen content of the perfusate. In this model, we found that a single stepped decrease in oxygen delivery produced a single stepped reduction in ATP level to a new stable plateau which could be compared with the extent of subsequent morphological damage (Ratcliffe et al. 1988) (Fig. 10.2). A good correlation was found between the extent of ATP depletion and the total volume of injured cells (Fig. 10.3). The relationship is difficult to explain unless the overall reduction of ATP in whole kidney is taken to reflect severe depletion in those cells subsequently showing morphological injury, with the remainder undisturbed (an all-or-none phenomenon). The data therefore support the interpretation of ATP

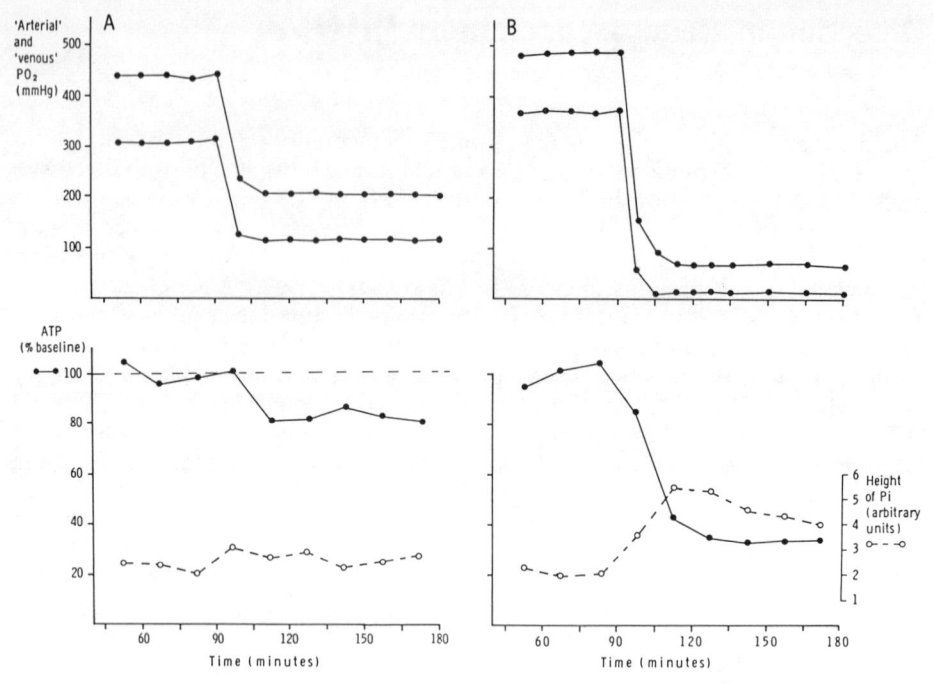

Fig. 10.2. Changes in the steady-state level of ATP and inorganic phosphate (P_i) in response to a single-stepped decrease in oxygen delivery achieved by altering the perfusate oxygen tension to the isolated perfused kidney. **A** Moderate hypoxia; **B** Severe hypoxia. Reproduced with permission from Ratcliffe et al. (1988).

depletion in the face of reduced oxygen delivery as a marker of incipient cell injury with the extent of ATP depletion reflecting the number of cells at risk.

Some further support is provided by experiments in the intact animal in which changes in renal ATP (accompanied by changes in P_i and acidosis) were correlated with renal function during and immediately after a defined 30-minute period of hypotension induced by rapid haemorrhage (Ratcliffe et al. 1986). The changes observed by ^{31}P NMR were highly correlated with post-hypotensive renal function. In animals which suffered no biochemical change during hypotension, retransfusion immediately restored normal renal function, whereas when metabolic changes were observed during hypotension, they were invariably associated with impaired renal function in the immediate post-hypotensive period. A typical experiment is illustrated in Fig. 10.4 where it can be seen that a short period of ATP depletion occurring abruptly towards the end of the post-hypotensive period was associated with decreased inulin clearance and increased fractional excretion of sodium after restoration of blood pressure by retransfusion. On the basis of these results we postulated that these changes in cellular energy status during hypotension distinguished prerenal failure from what may be the counterpart of early or incipient ATN.

In other experiments we have found a correlation between extensive ATP

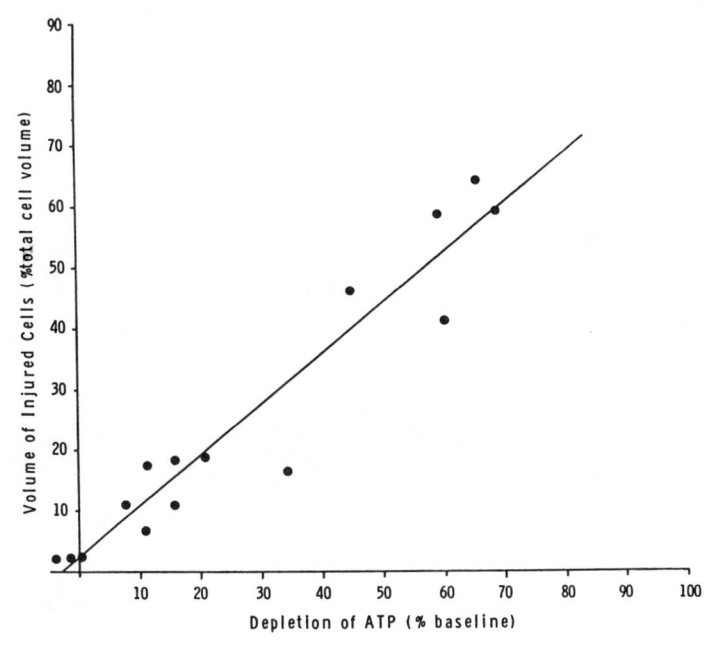

Fig. 10.3. The relationship between volume of injured cells (v) and reduction in whole kidney ATP (ΔATP) in the hypoxic perfused rat kidney. A linear regression has been fitted yielding the relationship $v = 0.83 (\pm 0.07) \Delta\text{ATP} + 2 (\pm 7)$ ($r = 0.956$). Reproduced with permission from Ratcliffe et al. (1988).

depletion during haemorrhagic hypotension and extensive cellular damage occurring principally in the renal cortex, although because of the uncontrollable nature of ATP depletion in this model, no comparison of graded change could be made.

Thus, reduction in the steady-state level of ATP appears to act as a marker of incipient renal injury. It is important to understand one major limitation to this statement; it only applies to settings of reduced oxygen delivery. First, as has been mentioned, reduction in ATP by other means does not produce cell injury. Second, although no change in ^{31}P NMR spectra were found by Chan et al. (1982) in non-ischaemic models of acute renal failure, ATP depletion may clearly occur as a secondary consequence of non-ischaemic cell injury (Endre et al. 1987), and third, after resumption of energy supply recovery of ATP will initially be incomplete. Although these considerations are important in relationship to the possible application of ^{31}P NMR in the diagnosis of renal ischaemia in man, they do not detract from the use of ^{31}P NMR in detecting the occurrence of damaging cellular ischaemia during a manoeuvre designed to reduce renal oxygen delivery. Thus in the cell-free isolated perfused kidney preparation, all levels of reduced oxygen delivery were associated with some reduction of ATP (Ratcliffe et al. 1988); a result in keeping with the suggestion (Epstein et al. 1982) that the preparation operates at the brink of hypoxia. A different result was obtained when renal perfusion pressure was reduced by hypotension in vivo.

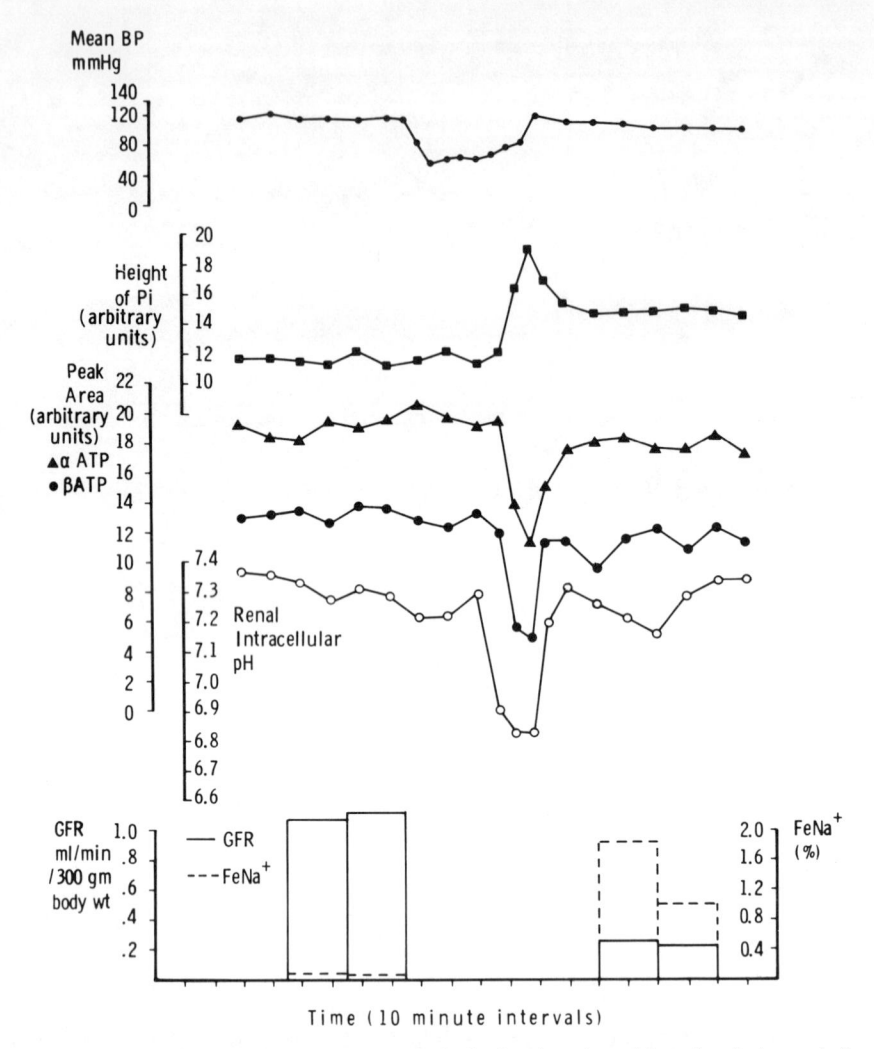

Fig. 10.4. Changes in blood pressure, metabolite levels and renal function during and after a period of approximately 30 minutes' haemorrhagic hypotension. Reproduced with permission from Ratcliffe et al. (1986).

Timing the Onset of Renal Ischaemia in vivo Using ^{31}P NMR

To examine the occurrence of renal ischaemia in vivo we have applied the ^{31}P NMR method to a model of progressive haemorrhagic hypotension. Under anaesthesia induced by sodium pentobarbital and maintained by halothane 1%–2% in a 3 : 1 mixture of nitrous oxide/oxygen male Wistar rats (300–340 g body wt) were bled under a variety of circumstances at a constant rate of 0.1 ml min^{-1} (Fig. 10.5). In this model it was possible to compare the ^{31}P NMR data timing the onset of cellular ischaemia with blood pressure, the volume of blood removed and

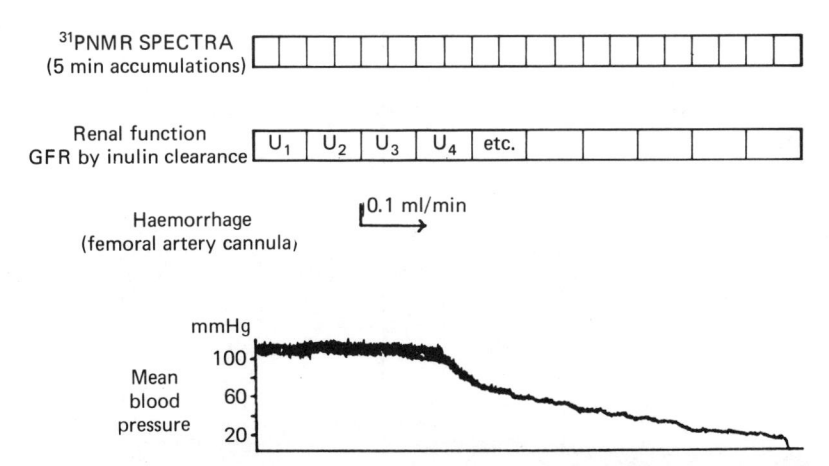

Fig. 10.5. Protocol for experiments designed to time the onset of changes in renal cellular energetics by ^{31}P NMR during the gradual induction of haemorrhagic hypotension.

GFR as assessed by inulin clearance (Ratcliffe et al. 1989). Several findings of potential importance in relation to the pathophysiology of renal ischaemia emerged.

First, there was no overall critical blood pressure or volume of blood removed which could be related to development of renal ischaemia. Several complicating manoeuvres were performed during haemorrhage which included the effect of concurrent myoglobin infusion, prior renal ischaemia, concurrent stimulation of the sciatic nerve, mannitol infusion, and uncomplicated haemorrhage in spontaneously hypertensive rats (SHR). Two situations, uncomplicated haemorrhage in SHR and concurrent stimulation of the sciatic nerve, led to NMR changes indicative of renal ischaemia occurring at significantly higher blood pressures and after significantly less blood had been withdrawn. In each of these cases the blood pressure at which NMR changes indicating ischaemia occurred were particularly variable, for instance, reduction in ATP by 25% occurred at a blood pressure varying from 42 to 140 mmHg in SHR (Fig. 10.6).

Second, all animals had become profoundly oliguric before alterations in the steady-state levels of ATP were detected. In some animals inulin clearance was measured under mannitol diuresis (Fig. 10.7) where it can be seen that at the lower mean blood pressure of approximately 60 mmHg, inulin clearance fell to unmeasurable levels associated with profound oliguria. Thus profound reduction in inulin clearance preceded the reduction in ATP. The implications of this preceding fall in GFR are important. It has long been established that a large proportion of total renal energy consumption is expended on tubular reabsorption and therefore varies with glomerular filtration (Cohen 1986). Thus it appears that under the circumstances pertaining in this experimental model, transport work and thus an important element to renal energy demand is decreased when or before a critical limitation of energy supply was induced. Such a response could be viewed as protective. The potential importance of tubular transport work rates in the genesis of renal injury has been elegantly demonstrated in the isolated perfused kidney where the hypoxic lesion in the mTAL can be ameliorated by inhibition of transport work (Brezis et al. 1984c,d). The decline in glomerular

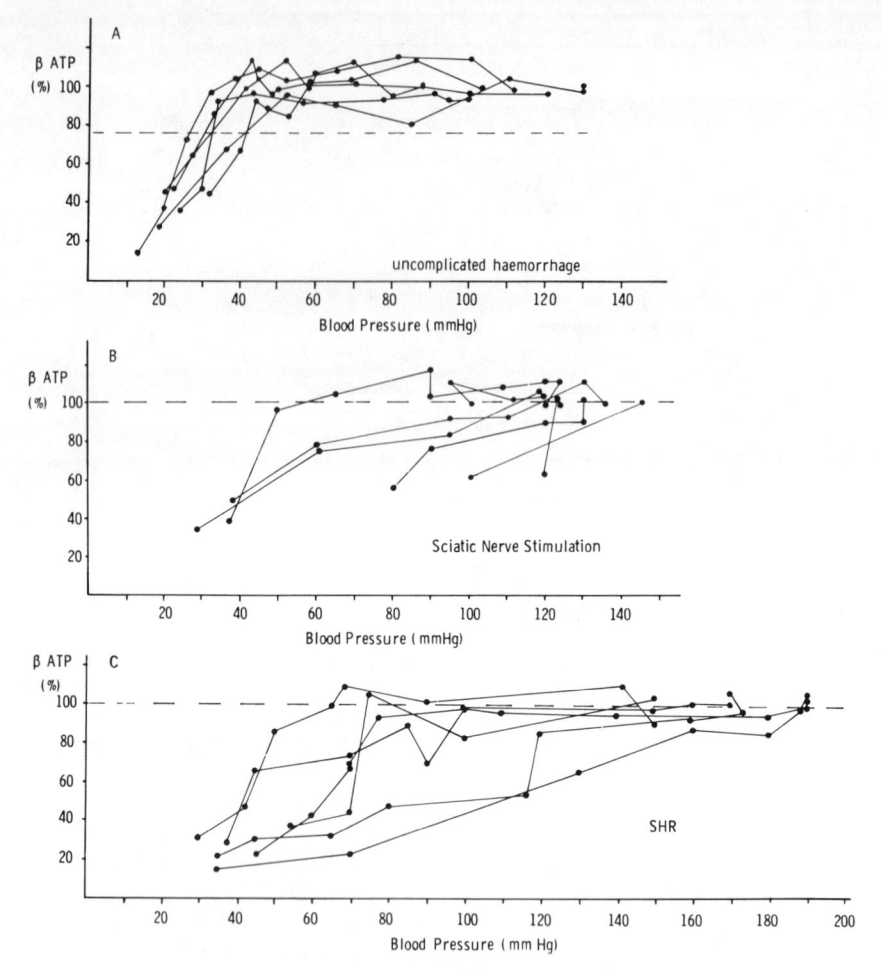

Fig. 10.6. Relationship between whole kidney ATP (% baseline) and mean systemic blood pressure during: **A** uncomplicated haemorrhage in Wistar rats; **B** haemorrhage and stimulation of the sciatic nerve in Wistar rats; **C** uncomplicated haemorrhage in spontaneously hypertensive rats.

filtration in these experiments prior to changes in ATP may well explain the inconsistent occurrence of damage to the mTAL in this (Ratcliffe et al. 1987) and some other models of haemorrhagic hypotension (Kreisberg et al. 1976; Dobyan et al. 1977), and further indicates the need for caution in extrapolating from the hypoxic isolated perfused kidney to in vivo.

Third, in most experiments, when changes in ^{31}P NMR spectra were observed they were marked. Thus a large decrease in whole kidney ATP generally occurred suddenly, presumably indicating that a critical limitation of energy supply had been reached concurrently in a large proportion of renal cells. An example from a spontaneously hypertensive animal is shown in Fig. 10.8, where it can be seen that this metabolic change took place when the fall in systemic blood pressure had reached a plateau. No measurements of blood flow and thus of oxygen delivery were possible in these experiments, but to achieve this level of

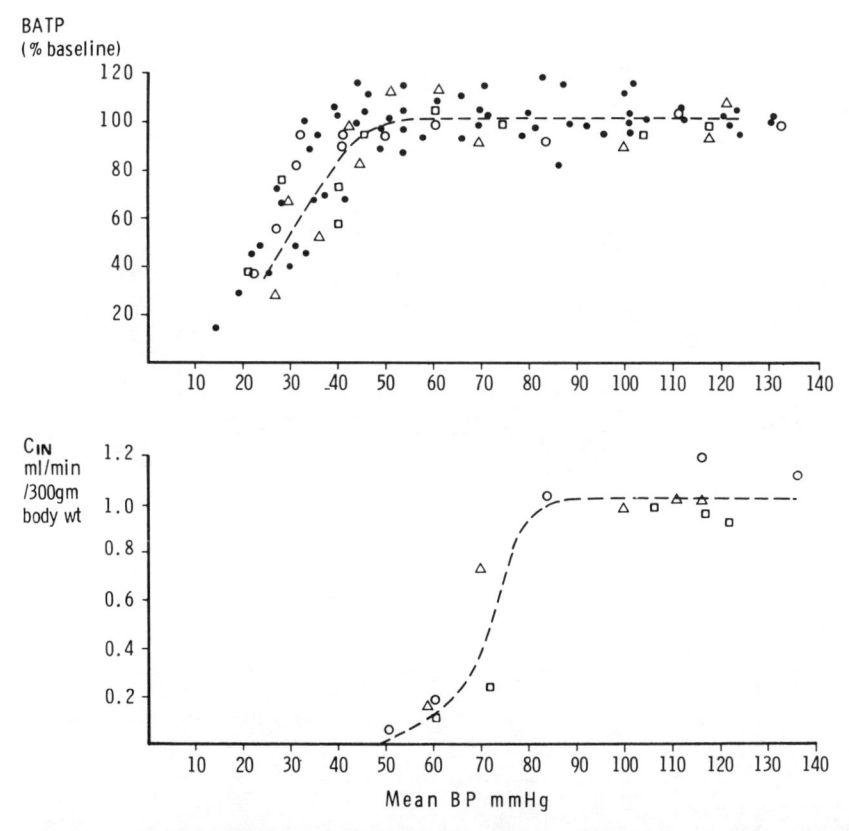

Fig. 10.7. Relationship between decline in whole kidney ATP during uncomplicated haemorrhage and decline in inulin clearance measured under mannitol diuresis. *Open symbols*, mannitol infusion, *filled symbols*, no mannitol infusion. The same experiments are illustrated in Fig. 10.6(A).

ATP reduction by hypoxia in the IPK a very profound reduction in oxygen delivery was required, suggesting that a very rapid decrease in renal blood flow occurred, probably dependent on renal vasoconstriction.

The hypothesis that renal vasoconstriction is of central importance in determining the occurrence of renal ischaemia is unproven, but it is supported by the pattern of metabolic change, its occurrence at very variable blood pressures, and by more ready occurrence in models in which enhanced tendency to renal vasoconstriction might be expected. Whilst such an increase in renal vascular resistance could be triggered by factors extrinsic to the kidney, mechanisms such as adenosine release, stimulation of tubuloglomerular feedback or renal chemoreceptors (Miller et al. 1978; Bell and Reddington 1983; Recordati et al. 1978) might also allow changes in tubular cell energetics to trigger renal vasoconstriction, thus reinforcing renal ischaemia and accounting for the very large and rapid decline in whole kidney ATP.

In summary, we have presented evidence supporting the validity of reductions in the steady-state level of ATP measured by ^{31}P NMR in the intact kidney as a marker of renal cell ischaemia. We have illustrated this technique with reference to a model of progressive haemorrhagic hypotension in the rat. The results of

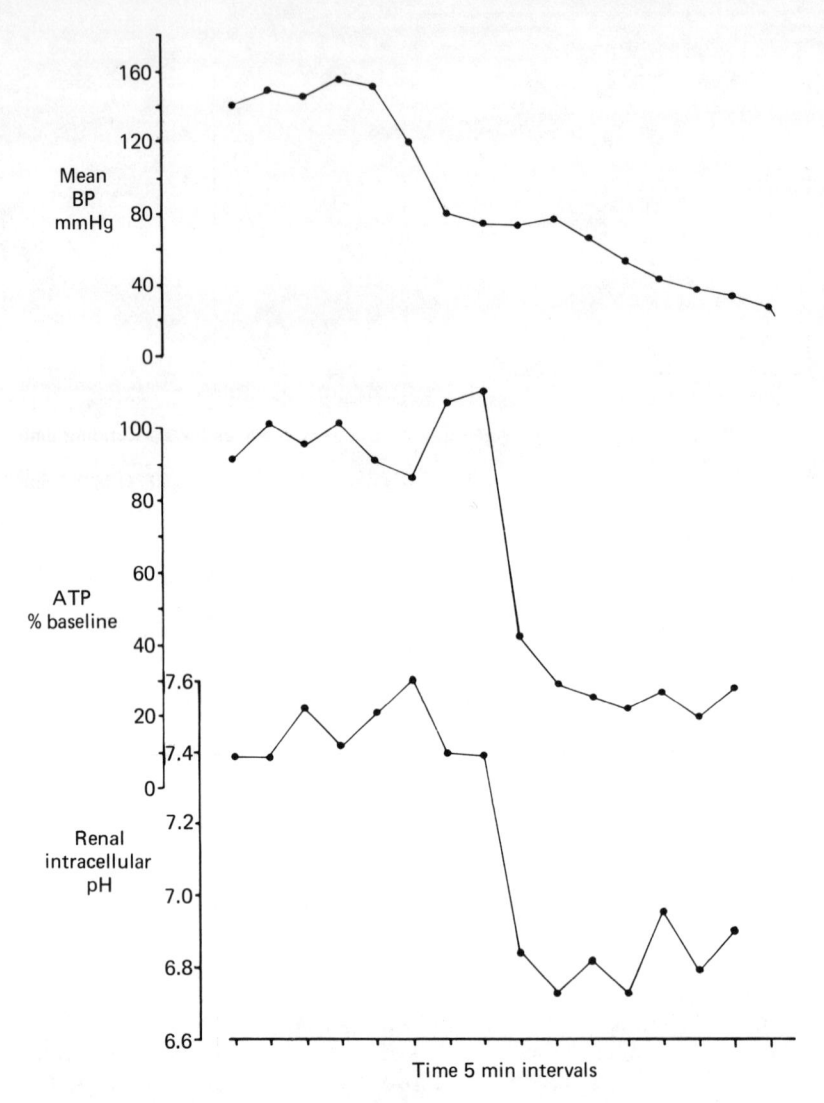

Fig. 10.8. Time course of change in blood pressure, whole kidney ATP and renal intracellular pH during haemorrhage in a spontaneously hypertensive rat.

these experiments demonstrate that renal ischaemia is not an inevitable consequence of reduced perfusion pressure and suggests that excessive and sometimes inappropriate renal vasoconstriction may be of central importance. Further work aimed at defining the factors responsible for excessive renal vasoconstriction is likely to be a fruitful approach to the prevention of acute renal failure in the ITU.

Acknowledgements. This work was supported by the MRC (UK). The authors are grateful to Professor G. K. Radda for advice and for provision of the NMR facilities.

References

Alcorn D, Emslie KR, Ross BD, Ryan GB, Tange JD (1981) Selective distal nephron damage during isolated kidney perfusion. Kidney Int 19: 638–647

Aukland K, Krog J (1960) Renal oxygen tension. Nature 188: 671

Balaban RS, Sylvia AL (1981) Spectrophotometric monitoring of O_2 delivery to the exposed rat kidney. Am J Physiol 241: F257–F262

Bell PD, Reddington M (1983) Intracellular calcium in the transmission of tubuloglomerular feedback signals. Am J Physiol 245: 295–302

Brezis M, Rosen S, Silva P, Epstein FH (1984a) Renal ischaemia: A new perspective. Kidney Int 26: 375–383

Brezis M, Rosen S, Silva P, Epstein FH (1984b) Selective vulnerability of the medullary thick ascending limb to anoxia in the isolated perfused rat kidney. J Clin Invest 73: 182–190

Brezis M, Rosen S, Spokes K, Silva P, Epstein FH (1984c) Transport dependent anoxic cell injury in the isolated perfused rat kidney. Am J Pathol 116: 327–341

Brezis M, Rosen S, Silva P, Epstein FH (1984d) Transport activity modifies thick ascending limb damage in the isolated perfused kidney. Kidney Int 25: 65–72

Chan L, Ledingham JGG, Dixon JA, Thulborn KR, Waterton JC, Radda GK, Ross BD (1982) Acute renal failure: a proposed mechanism based upon ^{31}P nuclear magnetic resonance studies in the rat. In: Eliahou HE (ed.) Acute renal failure. John Libbey, London, pp 35–41

Cheung JY, Bonventre JV, Malis CD, Leaf A (1982) Calcium and ischemic injury. N Engl J Med 314: 1670–1676

Cohen JJ (1986) Relationship between energy requirements for Na^+ reabsorption and other renal functions. Kidney Int 29: 32–40

Dobyan DC, Nagle RB, Bulger RE (1977) Acute tubular necrosis in the rat kidney following sustained hypotension. Lab Invest 37: 411–422

Endre ZH, Ratcliffe PJ, Nicholls LG, Ledingham JGG, Tange JD, Radda GK (1987) ^{31}Phosphorus NMR studies of mercuric chloride nephrotoxicity in the in vitro perfused rat kidney. In: Boeh PH, Lock EA (eds) Nephrotoxicity: extrapolation from in vitro to in vivo and animals to man. Plenum Press, London, pp 503–508

Endre ZH, Ratcliffe PJ, Tange JD, Ferguson DJP, Radda GK, Ledingham JGG (1988) Erythrocytes alter the pattern of renal hypoxic injury: predominance of proximal tubular injury with moderate hypoxia. Clin Sci (in press)

Epstein FH, Balaban RS, Ross BD (1982) Redox state of cytochrome aa_3 in isolated perfused rat kidney. Am J Physiol 243: F356–F363

Farber JL, Chien KR, Mittnacht S (1981) The pathogenesis of irreversible cell injury in ischemia. Am J Pathol 102: 271–281

Franke H, Barlow CH, Chance B (1976) Oxygen delivery in perfused rat kidney: NADH fluorescence and renal functional state. Am J Physiol 231: 1081–1089

Kreisberg JI, Bulger RE, Trump BF, Nagle RB (1976) Effects of transient hypotension on the structure and function of rat kidney. Virchows Arch [Cell Pathol] 22: 121–133

Leichtweiss H-P, Lubbers DW, Weiss Ch, Baumgartl H, Reschke W (1969) The oxygen supply of rat kidney: Measurement of intrarenal pO_2. Pflugers Arch 309: 328–349

Miller WL, Thomas RA, Berne RM, Rubio R (1978) Adenosine production in the ischemic kidney. Circ Res 43: 390–397

Ratcliffe PJ, Moonen CTW, Holloway PAH, Ledingham JGG (1986) Acute renal failure in haemorrhagic hypotension: Cellular energetics and renal function. Kidney Int 30: 355–360

Ratcliffe PJ, Endre ZH, Tange JD, Ledingham JGG, Radda GK (1987) Renal energetics and cellular injury in haemorrhagic hypotension. Tenth International Congress of Nephrology (abstract)

Ratcliffe PJ, Endre ZH, Scheinman SJ, Tange JD, Ledingham JGG, Radda GK (1988) ^{31}P nuclear magnetic resonance study of steady-state adenosine 5′-triphosphate levels during graded hypoxia in the isolated perfused rat kidney. Clin Sci 74: 437–448

Ratcliffe PJ, Moonen CTW, Ledingham JGG, Radda GK (1989) Timing of the onset of changes in renal energetics in relation to blood pressure and glomerular filtration in haemorrhagic hypotension in the rat. Nephron 51: 225–232

Recordati GM, Moss NG, Waselkov L (1978) Renal chemoreceptors in the rat. Circ Res 43: 534–543

Sehr PA, Bore PJ, Papatheofanis J, Radda GK (1979) Non-destructive measurement of metabolites and tissue pH in the kidney by ^{31}P Nuclear Magnetic Resonance. Br J Exp Pathol 60: 632–641

Shapiro JI, Chan L, Cheung C, Itabashi A, Rossi NF, Schrier RW (1987) Effect of adenosine triphosphate depletion in the isolated perfused rat kidney. Miner Electrolyte Metab 13: 415–421
Stubbs M, Freeman DM, Ross BD (1984) Formation of NMR-invisible ADP during renal ischaemia in rats. Biochem J 224: 241–246
Trueta J, Barclay AE, Daniel DPM, Franklin KJ, Prichard MML (1947) Studies of the renal circulation. Blackwell, Oxford
Vogt MT, Farber E (1968) On the molecular pathology of ischemic renal cell death. Am J Pathol 53: 1–26

Discussion

At the opening of the discussion Dr Ratcliffe described in more detail his technique of using NMR to assess energy levels within renal tubular cells. As he explained in his summary of the technique, a certain number of assumptions have to be made concerning the field generated by the magnets and that the results obtained reflect the physiological condition of the whole kidney since the whole organ fits inside the coil.

Dr Bihari reflected on the concept that hypoxia might have some other effects on cellular function which could occur before the inhibition of oxidative phosphorylation. Thus a number of extramitochondrial oxygen-requiring reactions might well be inhibited at partial pressures of oxygen which have no effect on the rate of ATP production. Certainly this does seem to be the case in the brain in which neurotransmitter synthesis is inhibited long before there is a reduction in ATP production. Similarly, the various eicosanoids derived from the cyclo-oxygenase and lipoxygenase enzymes might well be related to the oxygen tension of the cell in which these compounds were being elaborated. The cyclo-oxygenase enzyme requires oxygen as well as arachidonate as substrate and is inhibited (with a Michaelis–Menten constant of 25 µM O_2 (pO_2, 16 mmHg) at concentrations of oxygen which have little effect on the lipoxygenase enzyme (K_m 16 µM O_2; pO_2 9 mmHg). Dr Ratcliffe agreed that it was possible that other mechanisms could modulate the signal of hypoxia and account for some of the disturbances in cellular function. He also concurred with Dr Epstein that it was difficult to extrapolate from the isolated, perfused rat kidney in vivo, especially when it was perfused with a perfusate with a pO_2 of 400 mmHg; whilst the model gave some insight into the response of the kidney to hypoxia it was not without its limitations. Dr Lopez-Novoa emphasized that whilst the level of ATP in renal tubular cells might be normal in various conditions the turnover of the compound might be increased. This rate of turnover might be the important variable in the assessment of the effects of a hypoxic milieu. A number of participants expressed concern at the use of ATP alone as a marker of ischaemic damage to the kidney. Dr Ledingham agreed that without some sort of correlation between morphology, function, and energetics coupled together with renal blood flow, it was difficult to establish a change in the ATP level within the cell as a mechanism leading directly towards the cell damage associated with acute renal failure.

Chapter 11

Eicosanoids and Acute Renal Failure

A. Schieppati and G. Remuzzi

Introduction

Many theories have been proposed over the last decades to explain the reduced glomerular filtration rate (GFR) in acute renal failure (ARF). However, the precise pathogenetic mechanisms of this syndrome are still largely undefined. Several animal models of ARF have been employed over the years and different experimental conditions in the same animal model have been studied, in the attempt to dissect the components of the pathogenetic mechanisms. Traditionally, the causes of ARF can be divided in the two broad categories of ischaemic and nephrotoxic type. Ischaemic injury to the kidney may occur in the clinical setting as a consequence of volume depletion, septic shock, cardiovascular failure, major trauma. A particular and interesting condition of postischaemic ARF is represented by cadaver renal transplantation, which occurs when the warm or the cold ischaemia are too prolonged. Experimental models of ischaemic injury are obtained by glycerol injection, intrarenal infusion of vasoconstrictor agents, such as noradrenaline, and vascular clamp of the renal arteries. Nephrotoxic ARF is today largely due to iatrogenic causes, in association with aminoglycoside antibiotics, X-ray contrast media, non-steroidal anti-inflammatory drugs, cis-platinum, and, more recently, the novel immunosuppressive agent cyclosporin A. All these agents have been used in laboratory animals to reproduce the ARF, in addition to the traditional models of nephrotoxic ARF (mercuric chloride, uranyl nitrate).

Four main pathogenetic factors, potentially involved in the induction and maintenance phase of ARF, have been proposed (for excellent reviews see Hostetter et al. 1983; Schrier and Conger 1986):

1. Leakage of the filtered tubular fluid into the interstitial space, due to the disruption of the normal lining of tubular epithelial cells

2. Tubular obstruction due to the presence of cast and cellular debris in the tubular lumen
3. Haemodynamic alterations of renal circulation (reduction of renal blood flow (RBF))
4. Permeability changes at the glomerular level

The first two mechanisms relate to the effects on tubular cell functions induced by the ischaemic or nephrotoxic insult. The other two mechanisms affect the renal haemodynamic functions and may be influenced by neural and hormonal factors. In the last two decades, research from several laboratories has attempted to identify all the potential mediators of the described pathogenetic mechanisms. Among these mediators much attention has been paid to the arachidonic acid metabolites. The purpose of this chapter is to review the available information that implicates the eicosanoids in the pathogenesis of ARF.

Eicosanoids and ARF

Arachidonic Acid Metabolism in the Kidney

During the last decade great interest has developed in the area of arachidonic acid (AA) metabolism in the kidney and a large body of evidence has emerged to indicate that eicosanoids play an important role in renal physiological and pathological processes (Schlondorff and Ardillou 1986; Stork et al. 1986).

The metabolic fate of AA is illustrated in Fig. 11.1. AA is a 20-carbon free fatty acid, and is usually esterified in the 2 position of phospholipids (phosphatidylinositol, phosphatidylethanolamine and phosphatidylserine). It is present in all cellular membranes of different organs (Lands 1979); a negligible amount of the fatty acid is in a free form (Lands 1979).

AA is released from these stores by the action of calcium-dependent phospholipases (Lands 1979), and subsequently converted into its metabolites through two different metabolic pathways. The cyclooxygenase pathway leads to the formation of prostaglandins (PGs) and thromboxanes (TX); the lipoxygenase pathway converts AA into the hydroxyacid compounds and leukotrienes. Cyclic endoperoxides are unstable intermediates of cyclooxygenase metabolism and are obligatory steps in AA metabolism in all tissues; the subsequent conversion of these compounds into the final metabolic products (prostaglandins and thromboxane) may vary greatly among different tissues or even among different structures of the same organ (Sun et al. 1981). Differences in the pattern of PG formation depend on several factors, such as the enzyme/substrate ratio, cofactor requirement and hormonal stimulation.

AA is metabolized through the lipoxygenase pathway, and converted into hydroperoxides and leukotrienes (Samuelson 1981). It has been shown that the renal medulla synthesizes 12-HETE and 15-HETE (Winokur and Morrison 1981); rat and human glomeruli seem to possess the synthetic potential for these lipoxygenase products (Jim et al. 1982; Sraer et al. 1983). Finally, AA may be metabolized by several oxidases (Ellin et al. 1972, Zenser et al. 1978), which have

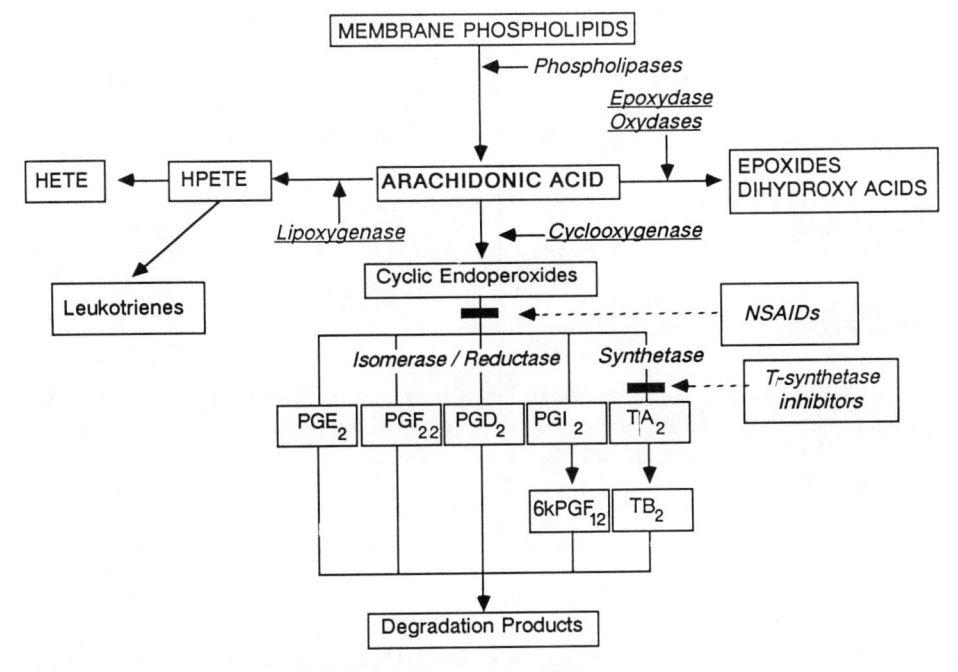

Fig. 11.1. Arachidonic acid metabolism in mammalian cells.

also been identified in the kidney. Recently, AA products, not derived from cyclooxygenase or lipoxygenase, have been identified in the thick ascending limb of the loop of Henle (Ferreri et al. 1984; Schwartzman et al. 1985), and their activity may be important in sodium and water transport in this and other portions of the nephron.

The kidney, especially the renal medulla, is a considerable source of eicosanoid synthesis. Cyclooxygenase has been localized in the renal tissue by an indirect immunofluorescence technique (Smith and Bell 1978). Positive staining has been found in the cortex associated with the endothelial cells of arteries and arterioles, and with the epithelial cells of Bowman's capsule, but not with capillaries and proximal tubules, loop of Henle and distal convoluted tubules (Smith and Bell 1978). In the medulla strong positive immunofluorescence has been found in collecting tubules and interstitial cells (Smith and Bell 1978).

Synthesis of PGs in the kidney has been studied by several techniques, using homogenates or microsomes of renal tissues from different animal species, including man (Sun et al. 1981). Isolated fragments of the nephron (glomeruli, proximal, distal and collecting tubules) (Folkert and Schlondorff 1979; Kirschenbaum et al. 1982; Schlondorff et al. 1985b; Sraer et al. 1979) and renal cell cultures have been employed (Bohman 1977; Dunn et al. 1976; Petrulis et al. 1981; Schlondorff et al. 1985a). Finally, attention has been focused on the pattern of urinary PG excretion, aiming to differentiate the systemic versus the renal origin of the various compounds (Frolich et al. 1975; Fitzgerald et al. 1983; Patrono and Pugliese 1980).

Table 11.1 reports the main renal sites of prostaglandin synthesis and their most important physiological actions.

Table 11.1. Sites of synthesis and actions of prostaglandins in the kidney

Localization	Prostanoid	Action
Arterioles	PGI_2	Vasodilation, ↑ RBF
Glomerulus	PGI_2, PGE_2	Vasodilation, maintain GFR
	TXA_2	↑ Mesangial contraction, ↓ GFR
Collecting tubule	PGE_2, $PGF_{2\alpha}$	Modulate Na and water excretion
Juxtaglomerular apparatus	PGI_2, PGE_2	↑ Renin release
Medullary interstitial cells	PGE_2	Vasodilation, promotes natriuresis and diuresis

Renal Actions of Prostaglandins

Evidence has been accumulated to indicate that PGs play an important role in the maintenance of renal homeostatis in different animal species; the results justify the interest in the study of renal PGs in the pathophysiology of ARF. The actions of PGs on renal functions include control of renal blood flow (RBF) and glomerular filtration rate, regulation of renin release, modulation of the urine concentrating mechanism and regulation of NaCl reabsorption (Schlondorff and Ardillou 1986). PGs and TXA_2 may participate in regulation of RBF in different regions of the kidney. PGE_2 and PGI_2 have a vasodilatory effect on the renal vascular bed (Jackson et al. 1982), whereas TXA_2 is a potent vasoconstrictor and it has been shown to contract isolated glomeruli (Scharschmidt et al. 1983). These mediators are involved in a complex interplay with other vasoactive substances in the kidney since it has been shown that vasopressin (Walker et al. 1978), angiotensin II (Aiken and Vane 1981; Needleman et al. 1979; Schwartzman et al. 1981), bradykinin (Needleman et al. 1979; Schwartzman et al. 1981) and catecholamines (Needleman et al. 1974) can all stimulate PG synthesis (Fig. 11.2). Glomerular filtration rate may be influenced by PGs and TXA_2 by several mechanisms. The glomerular filtration determinants may be altered by regulating the contraction of the mesangial cells (Scharschmidt et al. 1983). PGs may exert a regulatory effect on glomerular haemodynamics by affecting the afferent and efferent arteriolar tone (Schor et al. 1981). The tubuloglomerular feedback is also influenced by AA metabolites (Schnerman et al. 1984).

Several studies have investigated the role of the renin–angiotensin system (RAS) in ARF. It has been postulated that activation of the RAS may have a central role in affecting renal haemodynamics (reviewed by Hollemberg et al. 1983). Since it has been demonstrated that PGE_2 and PGI_2 enhance plasma renin activity in vivo and in vitro (Gerber et al. 1981; Heinrich 1981) and that angiotensin II is a potent stimulator of PG synthesis in the kidney (Aiken and Vane 1981; Needleman et al. 1979; Schwartzman et al. 1981), it may be postulated that an interaction between the two systems takes place in ARF.

Much less is known about the role of leukotrienes (LTs) in normal physiology and in pathological conditions in the kidney. The sulphopeptide leukotrienes LTC_4 and LTD_4 have been shown to increase renal vascular resistance in intact animals (Badr et al. 1984), and in the isolated perfused kidney (Rosenthal and Pace-Asciak 1983). In vitro they contract isolated glomeruli (Dunn and Simonson 1985) which have been shown to possess LT binding sites (Ballerman et al. 1985).

In hydronephrotic kidneys, an increase in lipoxygenase activity has been demonstrated, although it still remains unclear whether these products originate

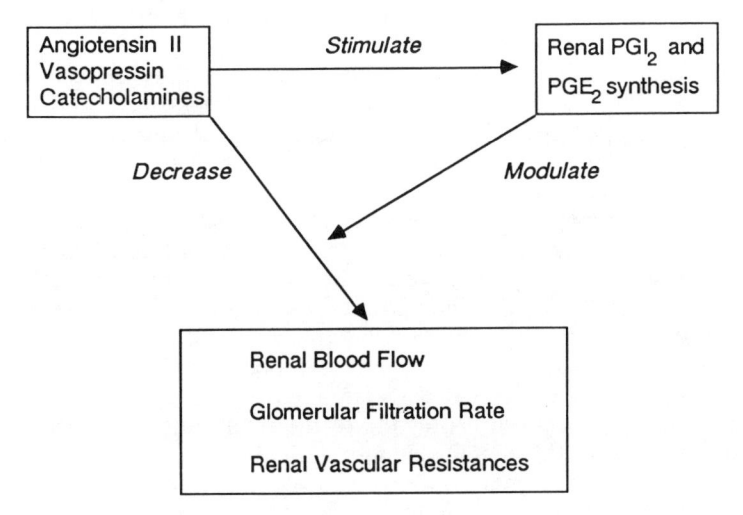

Fig. 11.2. Hypothetical scheme of interaction between hormones and renal prostaglandin system.

from renal tissues or from the invading inflammatory cells (Nishikawa et al. 1977; Okegawa et al. 1983).

It appears that the physiological role of eicosanoids in the kidney is complex; moreover different AA metabolites may exert opposite actions at the same anatomical sites. It seems reasonable, therefore, to postulate that these compounds may be involved in the complex sequence of events that take place in the various phases of ARF.

Role of Prostaglandins and Thromboxane in Acute Renal Failure

Ischaemic ARF

Torres et al. (1975) found that in experimental ARF, obtained by glycerol injection, the whole kidney PGE_2 synthesis was enhanced. The administration of indomethacin prevented the increase of PGE_2 and aggravated the incidence and severity of ARF. A similar finding was also reported by Papanicolau et al. (1975) who showed that indomethacin abolished the protective effect of saline loading in glycerol-treated animals. The role of PGs in the haemodynamic alterations occurring in the glycerol-induced ARF has also been investigated by several other groups. Benabe et al. (1980) demonstrated that isolated perfused kidney from rabbits, previously treated by subcutaneous injection of glycerol, released a vasoconstrictor agent, that was identified as TXA_2 by GC/MS. Sraer et al. (1981) demonstrated that the possible source of this compound could be the glomerulus. They studied PG synthesis in vitro by isolated glomeruli from rats with glycerol-induced ARF, and found that at 24 hours after glycerol PGE_2, $PGF_{2\alpha}$ and TXA_2 synthesis were greater than in glomeruli from control animals; this activity was enhanced by stimulation with AA. The effect on increased PG synthesis in glycerol-induced ARF was prevented by pretreatment with captopril, indicating a possible interaction on glomerular PG synthesis by angiotensin II or bradykinin, which are affected in opposite ways by captopril.

Plasma PG levels were measured in rats with ARF secondary to renal ischaemia (Lelcuk et al. 1985). The surgical operation itself significantly stimulated PG synthesis in sham-operated animals; however, after 45 minutes of renal ischaemia a further marked increase in plasma TXB_2 levels was measured, whereas plasma levels of 6-keto-$PGF_{1\alpha}$ the stable metabolite of PGI_2 decreased. When a cyclooxygenase inhibitor, ibuprofen, was administered prior to induction of ischaemia, the rise in TXB_2 levels was abolished. Pretreatment with OKY 046, an imidazole derivative which has been proved to be a selective thromboxane synthetase inhibitor, completely changed the pattern of plasma PGs in ischaemic animals: TXB_2 was significantly reduced and 6-keto-$PGF_{1\alpha}$ increased over baseline values. The re-orientation of PG synthesis, obtained by selective thromboxane synthetase inhibition (described also in other tissues (Fischer et al. 1983)) was associated with a significant protection of the renal function: serum creatinine levels were similiar to those in the sham-operated group. Histological sections of renal tissue revealed a normal to mildly damaged tubular epithelium in animals pretreated with OKY 046, but not in those who received ibuprofen. The authors, therefore, propose that the ratio PGI_2/TXA_2 may be critical in moderating the injury in renal ischaemia, possibly leading, when tipped in favour of thromboxane synthesis, to vasoconstriction and uncontrolled platelet aggregation in the glomerular capillaries (Fig. 11.3).

Papanicolau et al. (1987) measured renal function parameters and urinary prostaglandin excretion in glycerol-induced acute renal failure in rats. They observed a significantly increased urinary excretion of PGE_2, 6-keto-$PGF_{1\alpha}$ and TXB_2, in association with a significant decrease in creatinine clearance, and fractional excretion of sodium (FE_{Na}). Selective inhibition of TXB_2 partially prevented the decrease in creatinine clearance; FE_{Na} was actually increased, indicating an inhibition of sodium reabsorption. The authors propose that TXA_2 may exert a potent antidiuretic action in acute renal failure, and be pivotal in the developing phases of ARF. It should be mentioned, however, that in this (Watson et al. 1986) and other experimental models (Vanholder et al. 1987) of

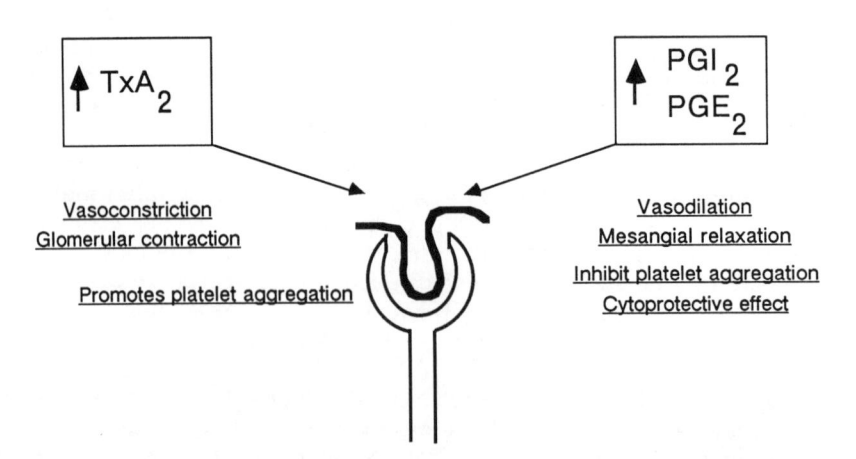

Fig. 11.3. Possible opposite effects of eicosanoids in the pathogenesis of ARF.

acute renal failure, other groups could not demonstrate any beneficial effect on renal function by selective inhibition of thromboxane synthetase, arguing against a major role for thromboxane in ARF.

Several studies have also addressed the question as to whether vasodilatory prostaglandins play a protective role in different models of ARF. Mauk et al. (1977) studied the effect of PGE_2 infusion in two models of ARF in dogs, i.e. uranyl nitrate administration and intrarenal infusion of norepinephrine – a nephrotoxic and an ischaemic model of ARF. The results of this study indicated a significant protective effect only in the ischaemic model. In a different model of renal ischaemia, obtained by clamping the renal artery in dogs, Tobimatsu et al (1985) infused PGE_1 after 1 or 2 hours of ischaemia. They showed a significant protection on renal function as renal cortical blood flow was restored towards normal values in PGE_1-treated animals as compared to controls. In postoperative days serum creatinine levels increased from basal values of 1.0 ± 0.1 mg dl^{-1} to 2.1 ± 0.3 mg dl^{-1} in treated animals whereas in controls serum creatinine reached a peak of 11.4 mg dl^{-1}. Several groups have also investigated the effect of another more potent vasodilatory PG, PGI_2, in renal ischaemia and a positive protective effect has been consistently reported (Haisch et al. 1983; Lifschitz and Barnes 1984; Mundy et al. 1980). Recently Finn et al. (1987) have addressed the question of whether or not prostacyclin attenuates the severity of ischaemia through a haemodynamic effect. PGI_2 was infused prior to and after 45 minutes of renal ischaemia in rats and several parameters of renal and systemic haemodynamics were measured. Immediately after the end of the ischaemic period, reflow of blood in rats receiving PGI_2 was delayed as compared to animal receiving glycine buffer alone; RBF returned to only $76 \pm 19\%$ of initial values in treated animals, as compared to $90 \pm 12\%$ in untreated rats. In the following hours renal function improved to a greater extent in PGI_2 rats than in control animals, although there was no significant difference in RBF between the two groups. Renal histology showed that PGI_2 had a significant protective effect on tubular epithelium, as revealed by less-evident cellular necrosis. In this study the beneficial effects of PGI_2 on renal function after ischaemia could not be attributed to its vasodilatory properties, and other mechanisms have to be postulated. Prostacyclin has been shown to exert a cytoprotective effect in several tissues, such as gastric mucosa (Miller and Jacobson 1979), hepatic cells (Sikujara et al. 1983), myocardium (Lefer et al. 1978), and pancreas (Gabryelewicz et al. 1983). The mechanisms of these cytoprotective properties are not yet understood: they may be related to interactions with free-radical anions (Thiemerman et al. 1984; Zsoldos et al. 1984), or to the stimulation of adenosine triphosphate and other cyclic nucleotides (Mozsik et al. 1983).

Endotoxin-induced ARF

ARF is a frequent complication of systemic sepsis, but the pathogenetic mechanisms are still poorly understood. Renal haemodynamic changes (Churchill et al. 1987) and intravascular coagulation (Koffler and Paronetto 1966) are believed to play a major role in the pathogenesis of acute renal dysfunction. In experimental animals intravenous injection of endotoxin promotes glomerular capillary thrombosis and bilateral cortical necrosis (Beller and Graeff 1967). However, severe reduction of the GFR after endotoxin administration could be demonstrated even in the absence of fibrin deposition (Conger et al. 1981). These data suggest that the observed renal haemodynamic changes in the course of septic shock may be due to factors other than the activation of the haemostatic cascade, and PGs are a likely candidate for this role. Endotoxin stimulates white blood cells to release AA and its metabolites (Bottoms et al. 1985). Elevated plasma TXB_2 levels have been measured in rats following endotoxin infusion (Cook et al. 1980). A pathogenetic role for the AA metabolite in septic shock was suggested by the evidence that the inhibition TXA_2 synthesis, by imidazole or indomethacin, or TXA_2 activity, by a TXA_2 antagonist – 1,3-azoprostanoic acid – was associated with a significant decrease in the mortality rate in rats given endotoxin (Cook et al. 1980).

TXA_2 has been also shown to be a potent vasoconstrictor of the pulmonary vascular bed in goats given endotoxin (Winn et al. 1983); its inhibition by a selective inhibitor, dazoxiben, ameliorated the pulmonary circulation. On the other hand, in a different animal model, prostacyclin infusion showed a protective effect against endotoxic shock, by increasing cardiac index and systemic blood pressure, restoring urinary output, and protecting against intravascular coagulation (Krausz et al. 1981).

Badr et al. (1987) studied renal haemodynamics and renal prostaglandin synthesis in rats injected with *E. coli* purified endotoxin. A rapid decrease in RBF and GFR was observed; 50 min after endotoxin injection, renal cortical generation of TXB_2, PGE_2 and 6-keto-$PGF_{1\alpha}$ was significantly increased over basal values. When animals were pretreated with a thromboxane inhibitor, dazoxiben, there was a substantial preservation of RBF and GFR. The authors also investigated the possible role of leukotrienes (LTs) in this particular model of ARF; they showed that the LT antagonist FPL-55712 partially prevented the decrease in RBF, which was completely restored 70 min after endotoxin administration. However, the observed fall in GFR was only partially attenuated. Taken together the results of all these studies suggest that AA metabolites may play a major role in the pathogenesis of endotoxin-induced renal failure and that the pharmacological manipulation may provide a useful therapeutic approach.

Cyclosporin A Nephrotoxicity

The introduction of cyclosporin A (CyA) in the treatment of allograft rejection has improved organ survival in heart, kidney, and liver transplantation (European Multicentre Trial Group 1983; Oyer et al. 1981; Starzl et al. 1981). However, acute and chronic CyA nephrotoxicity immediately appeared as one of the most common and important side effects of this drug (Bennett and Pulliam 1983). Studies have indicated that in the pathogenesis of CyA nephrotoxicity haemodynamic factors are involved. Murray et al. (1985) studied the effects of acute CyA infusion in conscious rats, and found that RBF was significantly decreased and RVR augmented in CyA-treated animals. Plasma renin activity (PRA) and urinary excretion of 6-keto-$PGF_{1\alpha}$ were both increased by CyA, but whereas cyclooxygenase inhibition worsened renal haemodynamics, the inhibition of angiotensin-converting enzyme did not prevent the decrease in RBF, suggesting that the observed vasoconstriction was not mediated by angiotensin II. Perico et al. (1986) have examined the relationship between the reduction of

GFR and the alteration in renal AA metabolism after short-term administration of CyA. They found that glomerular synthesis and urinary excretion of TXB_2 increased during CyA treatment and that this increase precedes the rise in serum creatinine and the fall in GFR. They also confirmed the finding that PRA was enhanced by CyA, but in this study renal PGI_2 and PGE_2 synthesis remained unchanged. The authors therefore suggest that the observed decrease in GFR in CyA nephrotoxicity may result from the potentiation of the action of angiotensin II and TXA_2 on mesangial cell contractility not counter-regulated by a parallel increase in glomerular PGE_2 and PGI_2.

Non-steroidal Anti-inflammatory Drug Nephrotoxicity

NSAIDs have become one of the most often prescribed (and self-prescribed) categories of drugs, because they are indicated for such diverse clinical conditions as rheumatoid arthritis, headache, gout and dysmenorrhoea. Reports on their adverse effects on renal functions have been growing in recent years and several clinical syndromes associated with the use of these compounds have been described (reviewed by Heinrich 1988). It has been proposed that adverse renal effects of NSAIDs are strictly related to the inhibition of renal PG synthesis, and evidence has accumulated to support this hypothesis (Patrono and Dunn 1987).

Two patterns of acute reduction of renal function are recognized: ARF due to haemodynamic mechanisms and acute interstitial nephritis. Sodium and water retention and a tendency toward hyperkalaemia have also been associated with the use of NSAIDs. It must be pointed out, however, that in normal circumstances NSAIDs do not alter renal functions significantly. This is demonstrated by the discrepancy between the enormous number of subjects exposed to these compounds, and the relatively small number of patients who develop renal complications attributable to NSAIDs. On the other hand, experimental work has shown (and we have illustrated several examples) that under particular circumstances, when vasoconstrictor hormones are activated, renal function may become dependent on an intact PG system. In these situations PG blockade by NSAIDs may be detrimental.

The haemodynamic type of ARF is considered the most common form of acute renal impairment due to NSAIDs (Table 11.2); it has been frequently reported in association with indomethacin, probably because this drug has been on the market for several years and is popular among doctors and patients (Gary et al.

Table 11.2. Characteristics of haemodynamic form of NSAID-induced ARF

True incidence not clearly established
Onset after few days of exposure to the offending drug
Clinical picture characterized by oliguria, azotaemia, hyperkalaemia, urinalysis usually not significant
Predisposing conditions: congestive heart failure, pre-existing nephropathies, chronic renal failure, cirrhosis, dehydration, advanced age
Seldom requires dialytic treatment
Usually reversible upon drug withdrawal

1980; Richardson and Alderfer 1963; Tan et al. 1979b; Walshe and Venuto 1979). The clinical spectrum of NSAID-associated ARF is characterized by initial oliguria, which ensues only a few days after the taking of the drug. Serum creatinine rises rapidly, but after discontinuation of the compound, rapidly returns toward normal values. Corwin and Bonventre (1984) reported 27 episodes of NSAID-associated ARF: in the study population serum creatinine increased in men from a value of 1.6 ± 0.1 mg dl^{-1} to a maximum value of 3.3 ± 0.3mg dl^{-1} with a return to 1.7 ± 0.1 mg dl^{-1} after withdrawal of the offending drug. The same group reported that six patients showed severe hyperkalaemia in spite of mild renal insufficiency, and one patient had a cardiac arrest secondary to hyperkalaemia. This finding may be explained by a state of hyporeninaemic hypoaldosteronism due to PG inhibition (Tan et al. 1979a). Urinalysis is often unremarkable in this clinical condition; urinary sodium fractional excretion may not be useful as in other forms of oliguric ARF. Dialysis is seldom required: in Corwin's report no patient required dialysis; in a clinical survey by Garella and Matarese (1984), only 3 of 27 patients with NSAID-induced ARF required dialysis, and two of them had underlying renal insufficiency; in a report by Adams et al. (1986) the proportion of patients who needed dialysis was somewhat higher (2 out of 7 patients). Analysis of reported cases reveals that predisposing factors or pathological conditions are often present in patients who developed NSAID-induced ARF. They include: (a) congestive heart failure; (b) nephrotic syndrome; (c) chronic renal failure; (d) liver cirrhosis; (e) dehydration; (f) old age; (g) previous diuretic use. Many of these clinical conditions are associated with an increased urinary PG excretion. It may be speculated that in these conditions the activation of the renal PG system may act as a defence mechanism to maintain renal functions; disruption of this mechanism by NSAIDs further impairs renal haemodynamics.

Interstitial nephritis is characterized by a slower onset and a progressive renal insufficiency, which may not be promptly reversible upon drug withdrawal (Abrham and Keane 1984). The clinical picture is often that of a nephrotic syndrome, with oedema and significant proteinuria. At variance with the haemodynamic form of ARF, NSAID-induced interstitial nephritis does not appear to be associated with predisposing factors. Renal histology shows a picture of interstitial oedema and infiltration of blood-borne cells (monocytes, eosinophils). Sometimes steroids are helpful in treating this clinical condition. The pathogenetic mechanisms involved are still obscure. The chronic inhibition of cyclooxygenase enzyme may be important: a shunt of the AA metabolism toward the lipoxygenase pathway, leading to an increased leukotriene synthesis, has been proposed as a possible mechanism (Torres 1982).

It has been reported that up to 25% of patients receiving NSAIDs for arthritis developed a sodium-retaining state; if water retention is exaggerated in respect to sodium retention hyponatraemia may result (Walshe and Venuto 1979). The mechanisms involved in sodium retention states associated with the use of NSAIDs have been excellently reviewed by several authors (Clive and Stoff 1984; Dunn 1983, 1984). Hyperkalaemia has also been reported in patients taking NSAIDs (Zimram et al. 1985); age over 65 years and pre-existing chronic renal insufficiency are a predisposing factor. It has been proposed that the inhibition of the renin–angiotensin–aldosterone system by NSAIDs is responsible for the tendency to hyperkalaemia in patients using these drugs (Tan et al. 1979a).

Conclusions

This brief review has attempted to highlight the possible roles of the renal prostaglandin system in ARF. Experimental data and clinical observations have suggested that in ischaemic and nephrotoxic forms of ARF, AA metabolism is actively stimulated and that complex interactions between vasodilatory PGs and vasoconstrictor TXA_2 take place. Moreover AA metabolites modulate or cooperate with other mediators (angiotensin II, bradykinins, catecholamines) in regulating renal circulation. More recently, other mediators have gained the attentions of several investigators; interactions of PGs/TXA_2 with free-radical species, calcium ions, platelet-activating factor are of potentially great interest.

Recent data (Badr 1987) also indicate that lipoxygenase products may be involved in the pathogenesis of some forms of ARF; further experimental work in this area is likely to lead to new insight on the role of these eicosanoids in ARF.

The cytoprotective effect of PGI_2, which has been demonstrated in several tissues, is potentially relevant in determining the observed preservation of renal function in animals treated with prostacyclin.

Pharmacological manipulation of the AA metabolism, with selective inhibitors of detrimental products, may hold forth the promise of a new beneficial therapeutic approach in some forms of ARF.

References

Abrham PA, Keane WF (1984) Glomerular and interstitial disease induced by nonsteroidal anti-inflammatory drugs. Am J Nephrol 4: 1

Adams DH, Howie AJ, Michel J, McConkey B, Bacon PA, Adu D (1986) Non-steroidal anti-inflammatory drugs and renal failure. Lancet I: 57

Aiken JW, Vane JR (1981) Intrarenal prostaglandin attenuates the renal vasoconstrictor activity of angiotensin. J Pharmacol Exp Ther 184: 678

Badr KF, Baylis C, Pfeffer JM, Pfeffer MA, Soberman RJ, Lewis RA, Austen KF, Corey EJ, Brenner BM (1984) Renal and systemic hemodynamic responses to intravenous infusion of leukotriene C4 in the rat. Circ Res 54: 492

Badr FK, Kelley VE, Rennke HG, Brenner BM (1987) Roles for thromboxane A_2 and leukotrienes in endotoxin-induced acute renal failure. Kidney Int 30: 474

Ballerman BJ, Lewis RA, Corey EJ, Austen KF, Brenner BM (1985) Identification and characterization of leukotriene C4 receptors in isolated rat renal glomeruli. Circ Res 56: 324

Beller FK, Graeff H (1967) Deposition of glomerular fibrin in the rabbit after infusion with endotoxin. Nature 215: 295

Benabe JE, Klahr S, Hoffman MK, Morrison AR (1980) Production of thromboxane A_2 by the kidney in glycerol-induced acute renal failure in the rabbit. Prostaglandins 19: 333

Bennet WM, Pulliam JP (1983) Cyclosporine nephrotoxicity. Ann Intern Med 99: 851

Bohman SO (1977) Demonstration of prostaglandin synthesis in collecting duct cells and other cell types of the rabbit renal medulla. Prostaglandins 14: 729

Bottoms GD, Johnson ME, Lamar CH, Fessler JF, Turek JJ (1985) Endotoxin-induced eicosanoid production by equine vascular endothelial cells and neutrophils. Circ Shock 15: 155

Churchill PC, Bidani AK, Schwartz MM (1987) Renal effects of endotoxin in the male rat. Am J Physiol 253: F244

Clive DM, Stoff JS (1984) Renal syndromes associated with nonsteroidal anti-inflammatory drugs. N Engl J Med 310: 563

Conger JD, Falk SA, Guggenheim SJ (1981) Glomerular dynamics and morphologic changes in the generalized Shwartzman reaction in post partum rats. J Clin Invest 67: 1334

Cook JA, Wise WC, Halushka PV (1980) Elevated thromboxane levels in rat during endotoxic shock. J Clin Invest 65: 227

Corwin HL, Bonventre JV (1984) Renal insufficiency associated with nonsteroidal anti-inflammatory agents. Am J Kidney Dis 4: 147

Dunn MJ (1983) Renal prostaglandins. In: Dunn MJ (ed) Renal endocrinology. Williams and Wilkins, Baltimore, p 1

Dunn MJ (1984) Nonsteroidal anti-inflammatory drugs and renal failure. Ann Rev Med 35: 411

Dunn MJ, Simonson (1985) The effects of leukotriene C45 (LTC) on rat glomerular mesangial cells in culture. Kidney Int 27: 256 (abstract)

Dunn MJ, Staley RS, Harrison M (1976) Characterization of prostaglandin production in tissue culture of rat renal medullary cells. Prostaglandins 12: 37

Ellin A, Jakbson SV, Schenkman JB, Orrenus S (1972) Cytochrome P450K of rat kidney microsomes, its involvement in fatty acid W- and (W-1)-hydroxylation. Arch Biochem Biophys 150: 64

European Multicentre Trial Group (1983) Cyclosporin in cadaveric renal transplantation: One-year follow-up of a multicentre trial. Lancet II: 986

Ferreri NR, Schwartzman M, Ebrahan NG, Chender DN, McGiff JC (1984) Arachidonic acid metabolism in a cell suspension isolated from rabbit renal outer medulla. J Pharmacol Exp Ther 231: 441

Finn WF, Hak LJ, Grossman SH (1987) Protective effect of prostacyclin in postischemic acute renal failure in the rat. Kidney Int 32: 479

Fischer S, Struppler M, Bohlig B, Bernutz C, Wober W, Weber PC (1983) The influence of selective thromboxane synthetase inhibition with a novel imidazole derivative UK-38,485 on prostanoid formation in man. Circulation 68: 821

FitzGerald GA, Pedersen AK, Patrono C (1983) Analysis of prostacyclin and thromboxane biosynthesis in cardiovascular disease. Circulation 67: 1174

Folkert VW, Schlondorff D (1979) Prostaglandin synthesis in isolated glomeruli. Prostaglandins 17: 79

Frolich JC, Wilson TW, Sweetman BJ, Smigel M, Bies AS, Carr K, Watson JY, Oates JA (1975) Urinary prostaglandins: identification and origin. J Clin Invest 55: 763

Gabryelewicz A, Dlugosz J, Brzozowsky J, Musiatowicz B, Sidun-Kurylowicz Z, Wereszczynska U, Triebling A (1983) Prostacyclin: effect on pancreatic lysosomes in acute experimental pancreatitis in dogs. Mt Sinai J Med 50: 218

Garella S, Matarese RA (1984) Renal effects of prostaglandins and clinical adverse effects of non-steroidal anti-inflammatory drugs. Medicine, 63: 165

Gary NE, Dodelson R, Eisinger RP (1980) Indomethacin associated acute renal failure. Am J Med 69: 135

Gerber JG, Olson RD, Nies AS (1981) Interrelationship between prostaglandins and renin release. Kidney Int 19: 816

Haisch CE, Deepe RM, Hall WR, Park HK, Larkin EW, Thomas FT (1983) Protective effects of prostacyclin in acute renal ischemia. Surg Forum 34: 13

Heinrich WL (1981) The role of prostaglandins in renin secretion. Kidney Int 19: 822

Heinrich WL (1988) Nephrotoxicity of nonsteroidal antiinflammatory agents. In: Schrier RW, Gottschalk CW (eds) Diseases of the kidney. Little, Brown, Boston/Toronto, p 1319

Hollemberg NK, Wilkes BM, Schulman G (1983) The renin–angiotensin system in acute renal failure. In: Brenner BM, Lazarus JM (eds) Acute renal failure. WB Saunders, Philadelphia, p 137

Hostetter TH, Wilkes BM, Brenner BM (1983) Renal circulatory and nephron function in experimental acute renal failure. In: Brenner BM, Lazarus JM (eds) Acute renal failure. WB Saunders, Philadelphia, p 99

Jackson EK, Heidemann HT, Branch RA, Gerkens JF (1982) Low dose intrarenal infusion of PGE_2, PGI_2 and 6-keto-PGE_1 vasodilate the in vivo rat kidney. Circ Res 51: 67

Jim K, Hassid A, Sun F, Dunn MJ (1982) Lipoxygenase activity in rat kidney glomeruli, glomerular epithelial cells and cortical tubules. J Biol Chem 257: 10294

Kirschenbaum MA, Lowe AG, Trizna W, Fine LG (1982) Regulation of vasopressin action by prostaglandin. Evidence for prostaglandin synthesis in the rabbit cortical collecting tubule. J Clin Invest 70: 1193

Koffler O, Paronetto F (1966) Fibrinogen deposition in acute renal failure. Am J Pathol 49: 383

Krausz MM, Utsunomiya T, Feuerstein G, Wolfe JHN, Shepro D, Hecthman HB (1981) Prostacyclin reversal of lethal endotoxemia in dogs. J Clin Invest 67: 1118

Lands WEM (1979) The biosynthesis and metabolism of prostaglandins. Ann Rev Physiol 41: 633

Lefer AM, Ogletree ML, Smith JB, Silver MJ, Nicolau KC, Barnette WE, Gasic GP (1978) Prostacyclin: A potentially valuable agent for preserving myocardial tissue in acute myocardial ischemia. Science 200: 52

Lelcuk S, Alexander F, Kobzik L, Valeri CR, Shepro D, Hectman HB (1985) Prostacyclin and thromboxane A_2 moderate postischemic renal failure. Surgery 98: 207

Lifschitz MD, Barnes JL (1984) Prostaglandin I_2 attenuates ischemic acute renal failure in the rat. Am J Physiol 247: F714

Mauk RH, Patak RV, Fadem SZ, Lifschitz MD, Stein JH (1977) Effect of prostaglandin E administration in a nephrotoxic and a vasoconstrictor model of acute renal failure. Kidney Int 12: 122

Miller TA, Jacobson ED (1979) Gastrointestinal cytoprotection by prostaglandins. Gut 20: 75

Mozsik G, Moron F, Fiegler M, Javor T, Nagy L, Patty I, Ternok F (1983) Interrelationships between the membrane-bound ATP-dependent energy system, gastric mucosal damage produced by NaOH, hypertonic NaC1, HC1 and alcohol, and prostacyclin-induced gastric cytoprotection in rats. Prostaglandins Leukotrienes Med 12: 423

Mundy AR, Bewick M, Moncada S, Vane JR (1980) Experimental assessment of prostacyclin in the harvesting of kidneys for transplantation. Transplantation 30: 251

Murray BM, Paller MS, Ferris TF (1985) Effect of cyclosporine administration on renal hemodynamics in conscious rats. Kidney Int 28: 767

Needleman P, Douglas JR, Jakschik B, Stoeklein PB, Johnson EM (1974) Release of renal prostaglandin by catecholamines, relationship to renal endocrine function. J Pharmacol Exp Ther 188: 453

Needleman P, Wyche A, Bronson SD, Holmberg S, Morrison AR (1979) Specific regulation of peptide-induced renal prostaglandin synthesis. J Biol Chem 254: 9772

Nishikawa K, Morrison A, Needleman P (1977) Exaggerated prostaglandin biosynthesis and its influence on renal resistance in isolated hydronephrotic rabbit kidney. J Clin Invest 59: 1143

Okegawa T, Sonas PE, DeSchryver K, Kawasaky A, Needleman P (1983) Metabolic and cellular alterations underlying the exaggerated renal prostaglandin and thromboxane synthesis in ureter obstruction in rabbits. J Clin Invest 71: 81

Oyer PE, Stinson EB, Jamieson SW (1981) Cyclosporine in cardiac transplantations: a 2 1/2 year follow-up. Transplant Proc 15(Suppl 1): 2546

Papanicolau N, Gallard P, Bariety J, Milliez P (1975) The effect of indomethacin and prostaglandin (PGE_2) on renal failure due to glycerol in saline-loaded rats. Clin Sci Mol Med 49: 507

Papanicolau N, Hatzaintoniou C, Dontas A, Gkikas EL, Paris M, Gkikas G, Bariety J (1987) Is thromboxane a potent antinatriuretic factor and is it involved in the development of acute renal failure? Nephron 45: 277

Patrono C, Dunn MJ (1987) The clinical significance of inhibition of renal prostaglandin synthesis. Kidney Int 32: 1

Patrono C, Pugliese F (1980) The involvement of arachidonic acid metabolism in the control of renin release. J Endocrinol Invest 3: 193

Perico N, Zoja C, Benigni A, Ghilardi F, Gualandris L, Remuzzi G (1986) Effect of short-term cyclosporine administration in rats on renin–angiotensin and thromboxane A_2: possible relevance to the reduction in glomerular filtration rate. J Pharmacol Exp Ther 239: 229

Petrulis AS, Aikawa M, Dunn MJ (1981) Prostaglandins and thromboxane synthesis by rat glomerular epithelial cells. Kidney Int 20: 469

Richardson JH, Alderfer HH (1963) Acute renal failure caused by phenylbutazone. N Engl J Med 268: 809

Rosenthal A, Pace-Asciak CR (1983) Potent vasoconstriction of the isolated perfused rat kidney by leukotrienes C4 and D4. Can J Pharmacol 61: 325

Samuelson B (1981) Leukotrienes, mediators of immediate hypersensitivity reactions and inflammation. Science 220: 568

Scharschmidt LS, Lianos E, Dunn MJ (1983) Arachidonate metabolites and the control of glomerular function. Fed Proc 42: 3058

Schlondorff D, Ardillou R (1986) Prostaglandins and other arachidonic metabolites in the kidney. Kidney Int 29: 108

Schlondorff D, Perez J, Satriano JA (1985a) Differential stimulation of PGE_2 synthesis in mesangial cells by angiotensin and A23187. Am J Physiol 248: C119

Schlondorff D, Satriano JA, Schwartz GJ (1985b) Synthesis of prostaglandin E_2 in different segments of isolated collecting tubules from adult and neonatal rabbits. Am J Physiol 248: F134

Schnerman J, Briggs JP, Weber PC (1984) Tubuloglomerular feedback, prostaglandins and angiotensin in the autoregulation of glomerular filtration rate. Kidney Int 25: 53

Schor N, Ichikawa I, Brenner BM (1981) Mechanisms of action of various hormones and vasoactive substances on glomerular ultrafiltration in the rat. Kidney Int 20: 442

Schrier RW, Conger JD (1986) Acute renal failure: pathogenesis, diagnosis, and management. In: Schrier RW (ed) Renal and electrolyte disorders. Little, Brown, Boston/Toronto, p 423

Schwartzman M, Lieberman E, Raz A (1981) Bradykinin and angiotensin II activation of arachidonic acid deacylation and PGE_2 formation in rabbit kidney. Hormone-sensitive versus hormone-insensitive lipid pools of arachidonic acid. J Biol Chem 256: 2329

Schwartzman M, Ferreri NR, Carrol MA, Songu Mize E, McGiff JC (1985) Renal cytochrome P450-related arachidonate metabolite inhibits $(Na^+-K^+)ATPase$. Nature 314: 620

Sikujara O, Monden M, Toyoshima K, Okamura J, Kosaki G (1983) Cytoprotective effect of prostaglandin I_2 on ischemia-induced hepatic cell injury. Transplantation 36: 238

Smith WL, Bell TG (1978) Immunohistochemical localization of the prostaglandin-forming cyclooxygenase in renal cortex. Am J Physiol 235: F451

Sraer J, Sraer JD, Chansel D, Russo-Marie F, Kouznetzova B, Ardillou R (1979) Prostaglandins synthesis by isolated rat renal glomeruli. Mol Cell Endocrinol 16: 29

Sraer JD, Moulonguet-Doleris L, Delarue F, Sraer J, Ardillou R (1981) Prostaglandin synthesis by glomeruli isolated from rats with glycerol-induced acute renal failure. Circ Res 49: 775

Sraer J, Rigaud M, Bens M, Rabinovitch H, Ardaillou R (1983) Metabolism of arachidonic acid via the lipoxygenase pathway in human and murine glomeruli. J Biol Chem 258: 4325

Starzl TE, Klintmalm GB, Porter KA, Itwatsuki S, Schroder GPJ (1981) Liver transplantation with the use of cyclosporine A and prednisone. N Engl J Med 305: 266

Stork JE, Rahman MA, Dunn MJ (1986) Eicosanoids in experimental and human renal disease. Am J Med 80 (suppl 1A): 34

Sun FF, Taylor BM, McGiff JC, Wong PK (1981) Metabolism of prostaglandins in the kidney. Kidney Int 19: 760

Tan SY, Shapiro R, Franco R, Stockard H, Murlow PJ (1979a) Indomethacin-induced prostaglandin inhibition with hyperkalemia: a reversible cause of hyporeninemic hypoaldosteronism. Ann Int Med 90: 783

Tan SY, Shapiro R, Kish MA (1979b) Reversible acute renal failure induced by indomethacin. JAMA 241: 2732

Thiemerman C, Steinhagen-Thiessen E, Schros K (1984) Inhibition of oxygen-centered free-radical formation by stable prostacyclin-mimetic iloprost (ZK 36 374) in acute myocardial ischemia. J Cardiovasc Pharmacol 6: 365

Tobimatsu M, Konomi K, Saito S, Tsumagari T (1985) Protective effect of prostaglandin E_1 on ischemia-induced acute renal failure in dogs. Surgery 98: 45

Torres VE (1982) Present and future of the nonsteroidal anti-inflammatory drugs in nephrology. Mayo Clin Proc 57: 389

Torres VE, Strong CG, Romero JC, Wilson DW (1975) Indomethacin enhancement of glycerol-induced acute renal failure in rabbits. Kidney Int 7: 170

Vanholder R, Laekman G, Herman A, Lameirie N (1987) Influence of vasoactive substances on early toxic acute renal failure in the dog. Nephrol Dial Transplant 2: 332

Walker LA, Whorton AR, Smigel M, France R, Frolich JC (1978) Antidiuretic hormone increases renal prostaglandin synthesis in vivo. Am J Physiol 235: F180

Walshe JJ, Venuto RC (1979) Acute oliguric renal failure induced by indomethacin: possible mechanisms. Ann Intern Med 92: 47

Watson AJ, Stout RL, Adkinson NF, Solez K, Whelton A (1986) Selective inhibition of thromboxane synthesis in glycerol-induced acute renal failure. Am J Kidney Dis 8: 26

Winn R, Harlan J, Nadir B, Harker L, Hildebrandt J (1983) Thromboxane A_2 mediates lung vasoconstriction but not permeability after endotoxin. J Clin Invest 72: 911

Winokur TS, Morrison AR (1981) Regional synthesis of monohydroxy eicosanoids by the kidney. J Biol Chem 256: 10221

Zenser TV, Mattammal MB, Davis BB (1978) Differential distribution of the mixed-function oxidase activities in rabbit kidneys. J Pharmacol Exp Ther 207: 719

Zimram A, Kramer R, Plaskin M, Hershko C (1985) Incidence of hyperkalemia induced by indomethacin in a hospital population. Br Med J 291: 107

Zsoldos T, Czegledi B, Tigyi A, Javor T, Mozsik GY (1984) Interrelationship between the development of the gastric cytoprotective effects of prostacyclin, atropine, cimetidine and the gastric mucosal superoxide dismutase activity in rats. Acta Physiol Hung 64: 325

Discussion

Professor Cameron initiated the discussion by asking about the cytoprotective effects of prostacyclin. He mentioned that PGE_2 had been shown by Dr Epstein to reduce oxygen consumption; apparently prostacyclin did not have this effect in the thick, ascending limb of the loop of Henle in the rabbit. Dr Neild suggested that a similar situation to that observed with the use of non-steroidal anti-inflammatory drugs probably occurred in patients who develop cyclosporin nephrotoxicity. The production of vasodilatory prostaglandins by the kidney so as to modulate the effect of various vasoconstrictors seemed to be a very important mechanism in preserving renal blood flow. Dr Parsons raised the issue of from where these eicosanoid compounds were originating. He thought that it was conceivable that some of the metabolites measured were coming into the kidney from elsewhere. Dr Schieppati noted that the issue of the origin of urinary prostaglandin metabolites was somewhat controversial. Dr Remuzzi confirmed that many of these prostaglandin metabolites measured in urine were probably of an extrarenal origin. In the case of cyclosporin nephrotoxicity, it was extremely likely that much of the thromboxane B_2 detected in the urine was indeed coming from infiltrating platelets and macrophages. Dr Parsons mentioned that in his experience the development of acute renal failure in patients who were thrombocytopenic and neutropenic and who often developed sepsis and hypovolaemia, was rare. This was supported by some animal work that suggested that dogs made aplastic were more resistant to the development of acute renal failure associated with a noradrenaline infusion and sepsis. Dr Schrier thought that it was impossible to interpret measurements of urinary metabolites of the various eicosanoids without reference to the state of activation of the renin–angiotensin system. He mentioned a number of studies in compensated cirrhotic patients which had related urinary excretion of 6-oxo-$PGF_{1\alpha}$ and PGE in relation to the systemic concentration of angiotensin II. It appeared that the effects of indomethacin were much more pronounced in those cirrhotics with activation of the renin–angiotensin system. There was general agreement about this observation and all participants thought that further studies on the concentration of urinary metabolites of prostaglandins must be related to the systemic concentration of various renal vasoconstrictors.

Chapter 12

Disturbances in Renal Function Associated with Hepatic Dysfunction

J. M. López-Novoa

Introduction

Patients with chronic liver disease, especially those with cirrhosis, often show a progressive impairment of renal function that results in renal sodium retention leading to ascites and peripheral oedema formation. Only in the later stages of the disease, and often after one or several episodes of bleeding accompanied by haemodynamic and hepatic decompensation, does true renal failure develop. This so-called hepatorenal syndrome is usually irreversible and often leads to the patient's death (Epstein 1988). Despite extensive studies dealing with the pathophysiology of the impairment in renal sodium handling, the mechanisms mediating this abnormality remain incompletely defined. This brief review will focus on the efferent mechanisms responsible for sodium retention.

It is important to note the difficulty of analysing the data available, because most of the clinical studies have been performed on patients with advanced cirrhosis of different aetiologies and different levels of impairment of liver function. Since cirrhosis seems to be a disease in which hepatic impairment is progressive, it is likely that the relative contributions of the different mechanisms leading to sodium retention vary with the evolution of the disease.

Several experimental animal models which attempt to imitate human disease have been developed. Amongst these the most popular are the dimethylnitrosamine-induced cirrhosis in dogs (Levy 1977a,b), phenobarbital/carbon tetrachloride-induced cirrhosis in rats (López-Novoa 1988) and bile duct ligation in dogs and rats (Gliedman et al. 1970). These experimental models are helpful in the analysis of the sequential changes observed during the different stages of the liver disease.

Mechanisms of Sodium Retention in Cirrhosis

Decreased GFR vs Increased Tubular Reabsorption

Initial attempts to explain the abnormalities of renal sodium handling in cirrhosis focused on the decrements in glomerular filtration rate (GFR) that frequently occur in patients with advanced liver disease. However, although severe reductions in GFR and plasma sodium may result in a decreased filtered sodium load, it is unlikely that this alone could be the mechanism of sodium retention, because cirrhotic animals do not show decreased sodium excretion until the GFR is only a small percentage of the normal value (Bricker and Donavitch 1983). In addition, sodium retention may occur in the presence of normal or even elevated GFR, as demonstrated in cirrhotic patients (Klinger et al. 1970) or in experimental models of liver disease (Levy 1977a; López-Novoa 1988; López-Novoa et al. 1980). In fact, when renal function was assessed during the period in which rats developed ascites, increased sodium retention was associated with increases rather than with decreases in GFR (López-Novoa et al. 1980). This observation implies that tubular sodium reabsorption is increased. Micropuncture studies have revealed that this increase in tubular reabsorption occurs both in the proximal and in the distal tubule (López-Novoa et al. 1977, 1984), as seems to occur in cirrhotic patients and in other experimental models of cirrhosis (Chaimovitz et al. 1972; Bank and Aynedjian 1975; Levy 1977b; Chiandussi et al. 1978; Epstein et al. 1982). The mechanisms responsible for the augmentation in sodium reabsorption at these sites have not been clearly elucidated, but some of the possible explanations will be reviewed.

Following extracellular volume expansion, the inability of cirrhotic rats to increase adequately their sodium excretion (López-Novoa and Martinez-Maldonado 1982) seems to be due, at least in part, to changes in tubular reabsorption. Thus, extracellular volume expansion induced in control rats produced a marked decrease in proximal tubular water and sodium reabsorption (López-Novoa et al. 1984). This decrease was lower in rats with cirrhosis of the liver. A similar phenomenon has been observed with distal tubular reabsorption (López-Novoa et al. 1984). In addition, another mechanism which might be involved in the lack of diuretic and natriuretic responses to extracellular volume (ECV) expansion in cirrhotic rats relates to changes in intrarenal blood flow. In control animals, ECV expansion induces a redistribution of blood flow and GFR toward the outer nephrons (Baines 1973; López-Novoa et al. 1984). This redistribution has not been observed in rats with experimental cirrhosis (López-Novoa et al. 1984).

Peritubular Physical Forces

It has been postulated that in patients with cirrhosis as well as in experimental models of the disease an increase in renal vascular resistance may alter peritubular capillary physical forces, thus leading to increased tubular reabsorption (Epstein et al. 1976; Yarger 1976).

Renin–Angiotensin–Aldosterone Axis

Increased renin secretion, with subsequent increases in angiotensin II concentration may also be involved in the impairment of sodium excretion in cirrhosis. Although most of the studies report increased plasma renin activity in patients with cirrhosis and ascites, a careful analysis of the data reveals that, when patients are selected on the basis of the lack of previous history of manifest hepatic decompensation, bleeding or diuretic treatment, their renin activity is not increased from normal values (Epstein 1983a). In cirrhotic rats, plasma renin concentration (PRC) was not significantly different from control animals in any of the experimental protocols performed in our laboratory. When non-ascitic cirrhotic animals were subjected to acute extracellular volume expansion, PRC decreases by a percentage similar to that observed in control animals (López-Novoa et al. 1984), thus demonstrating intact regulation of renin release. Murray and Paller (1985) reported a threefold increase in plasma renin activity in non-ascitic, cirrhotic rats. We have no clear explanation for this discrepancy from our data, but as our rats have a very low sodium intake, this might induce a moderate activation of the renin–angiotensin system in both control and cirrhotic animals, masking possible differences between the groups.

There is also some evidence implicating aldosterone as an important factor in the increased distal sodium reabsorption in cirrhosis (Epstein 1983b). Plasma aldosterone concentrations are normal in cirrhotic patients without ascites, and increase in most patients with ascites (Arroyo et al. 1979; Wilkinson et al. 1979). Spironolactone, a specific aldosterone inhibitor is effective in inducing a diuresis in cirrhotic patients (Eggert 1970). Other investigators, however, have shown that the plasma aldosterone concentration is normal in a substantial number of cirrhotic patients with ascites (Wernze et al. 1978), and that sodium retention may persist in these patients despite the lowering of plasma aldosterone concentrations to normal levels (Rosoff et al. 1975; Epstein et al. 1977).

Studies performed in our laboratory on cirrhotic, sodium-retaining animals before ascites formation have revealed that plasma aldosterone is similar in control and in cirrhotic rats. Similar data were reported by Murray and Paller (1985). However, urinary aldosterone excretion was higher in cirrhotic than in control rats both in our study (López-Novoa et al. 1984) and in that of Murray and Paller (1985). Similar results concerning urinary aldosterone excretion were reported by Jimenez et al. (1985) in cirrhotic, sodium-retaining animals before the appearance of ascites, the differences between control and cirrhotic rats being substantially greater when ascites was evident. The same authors found that urinary aldosterone excretion showed a close correlation with sodium excretion, and that treatment with spironolactone prevented sodium retention and ascites accumulation in cirrhotic rats (Jimenez et al. 1985). However, we have found that bilateral adrenalectomy does not correct the inability of cirrhotic animals to increase adequately urinary sodium excretion in response to sodium loading (López-Novoa et al. 1978).

From these data it can be deduced that, although aldosterone seems to be an important modulator of sodium excretion in patients with advanced cirrhosis, it may merely constitute a permissive factor rather than act as the primary determinant of the sodium retention in cirrhosis.

Sympathetic Nervous System Activation and Increase of Plasma Catecholamines

Sympathetic activation can play a major role in tubular sodium reabsorption, indirectly through changes in renal and systemic haemodynamics and glomerular filtration rate, and by direct stimulation of proximal tubular sodium reabsorption (Di Bona 1982). In addition, sympathetic stimulation may also activate the renin–angiotensin–aldosterone system, thus increasing distal reabsorption. In patients with decompensated liver cirrhosis, increased plasma levels of catecholamines are often found (Henriksen et al. 1984). These increased levels are due to an increased production rather than a decreased metabolic clearance (Ring-Larsen et al. 1982; Nichols et al. 1985), and they show a positive correlation with the inability to excrete sodium (Bichet et al. 1982). Ring-Larsen et al. (1982) have demonstrated the renal origin of at least a part of these catecholamines by measuring their concentration in the right renal vein, observing higher concentrations than in the renal artery.

Rats with cirrhosis of the liver without ascites or oedema demonstrate increased urinary catecholamine metabolite excretion with normal plasma levels (Rodriguez-Puyol et al. 1988). These data may be interpreted as showing an activation of the sympathetic nervous system with increased catecholamine release and turnover but not enough to increase plasma levels.

The mechanism of sympathetic nervous system activation in cirrhosis is not clear. In the final stages of cirrhosis it may be a consequence of the decreased effective blood volume, detected in stretch receptors that exist in the cardiopulmonary system (Thames 1977). In the early stages, it may reflect a hepatorenal reflex initiated by intrasinusoidal portal hypertension (Kostreva et al. 1980). It must be noted that Levy and Wexler (1987) have recently reported that hepatic denervation improves sodium excretion in dogs with chronic bile duct ligation.

Prostaglandins

To define the role of prostaglandins in the impairment of renal sodium handling in patients with cirrhosis, three kinds of experimental approach have been used. First, endogenous prostaglandins have been administered and haemodynamics and renal function assessed. Thus the administration of PGA_1 induces increases in RBF, GFR and sodium excretion in cirrhotic patients with ascites (Boyer et al. 1979). However, the relevance of these results is questionable since PGA_1 is not a physiological prostaglandin, and because inactivation of this substance occurs in its first passage through the lungs.

A second approach is the inhibition of endogenous production of prostaglandin. This inhibition induces a decrease in RBF, GFR, sodium excretion and free-water clearance, that can be reversed by the exogenous administration of prostaglandins (Boyer et al. 1979; Planas et al. 1983; Mirouze et al. 1983). Similar results have been obtained in dogs with bile duct ligation and sodium retention (Levy et al. 1983; Zambraski et al. 1984). The third approach has been to measure urinary excretion or plasma levels of prostaglandins. Early studies reported that urinary PGE excretion was increased in cirrhotic patients with ascites (Boyer et al. 1979; Zipser et al. 1979). Perez-Ayuso et al. (1984) reported increased PGE_2 excretion in patients with a normal GFR and a relatively conserved ability to excrete water, whereas decreased urinary PGE_2 excretion occurs in patients with decreased GFR and a marked impairment in water excretion. Head-out water immersion in patients with cirrhosis induces an increase in urinary PGE excretion and plasma 6-keto-$PGF_{1\alpha}$, the stable metabolite of the vasodilator prostacyclin, that coincides with an increase in sodium excretion (Epstein 1986). In non-ascitic cirrhotic rats, it has been observed that plasma concentration of 6-keto-$PGF_{1\alpha}$ are higher than in control rats, whereas plasma levels of the vasoconstrictor TXB_2 are lower than in control rats (Santos et al. 1988). These data may be related to the peripheral vasodilation that occurs in rats with cirrhosis (Fernandez-Muñoz et al. 1985). In addition, urinary excretion and isolated glomerulus production of PGE_2 are lower in cirrhotic than in control rats (Santos et al. 1988). Moreover, volume expansion induces a lower PGE_2 urinary excretion and glomerular production in cirrhotic than in control rats (Santos et al. 1988). Similar studies have been performed by Murray and Paller (1985), who demonstrated that cirrhotic and control rats have similar urinary excretions of PGE_2 and $PGF_{2\alpha}$. Thus, reduced renal PGE_2 synthesis could be involved in the sodium retention and the impaired natriuretic response to volume expansion shown by cirrhotic, non-ascitic rats. When cirrhosis decompensates, prostaglandins seem to be involved in the maintenance of RBF and GFR in the presence of vasoconstrictors such as noradrenaline and angiotensin II (Epstein 1986). In extreme cases, such as the hepatorenal syndrome, an imbalance between vasodilator and vasoconstrictor prostaglandins may be one of the causes of the marked impairment in renal function (Zipser et al. 1982).

Kallikrein–Kinin System

This system could also be involved in the sodium retention associated with cirrhosis because kinins seem to be physiological renal vasodilators, thus promoting sodium excretion. Analysis of the available information is complicated by the fact that the plasma kallikrein–kinin system and the renal kinin system are different. Plasma levels of prekallikrein and bradykinin have been found to be reduced in patients with cirrhosis and ascites (Wong et al. 1977). Urinary excretion measurements have given contradictory results. Some authors have reported increased urinary kallikrein excretion (Perez-Ayuso et al. 1984), whereas others have reported decreased urinary kallikrein excretion (Zipser et al. 1981), even in the presence of increased plasma levels of aldosterone and urinary PGE_2 excretion; this suggests decreased activity and abnormal regulation of the kinin system in cirrhosis. Rats with cirrhosis of the liver without ascites show normal urinary kallikrein excretion in basal conditions. However, after volume expansion non-sodium-retaining cirrhotic rats increase their urinary kallikrein excretion whereas sodium-retaining rats do not (Santos et al. 1988). Thus although the kallikrein–kinin system might be involved in the regulation of natriuresis in cirrhosis, the data are preliminary and contradictory thereby preventing definite conclusions.

Circulating Natriuretic Factors

During the past 20 years, considerable evidence has accumulated suggesting the involvement of a humoral natriuretic factor in the renal response to extracellular volume expansion (De Wardener and Clarkson 1985). Today, the existence of at least two circulating substances with such properties, the "classical" natriuretic factor of natriuretic hormone, and the more recently described atrial natriuretic peptide, has been confirmed.

Atrial Natriuretic Peptide

Atrial natriuretic peptide (ANP), a circulating hormone synthesized and released by the atrial cardiocytes in response to atrial distension, induces potent and transient diuretic and natriuretic effects, which seem to be mediated by both changes in glomerular filtration rate and a direct tubular action (Ballerman and Brenner 1985). ANP does not affect the sodium pump nor proximal tubular reabsorption (Ballerman and Brenner 1985). ANP also has a vasodilating action, mainly in the renal vascular bed (Garcia et al. 1985; Caramelo et al. 1986a), where it opposes the constricting actions of angiotensin II and noradrenaline (Kleinert et al. 1984).

Several groups have found that plasma levels of ANP are increased in patients with cirrhosis of the liver and ascites (Fernandez-Cruz et al. 1985; Ginés et al. 1988) but others have not confirmed this observation (Shenker et al. 1985; Arendt et al. 1986). In addition, we have demonstrated that head-out water immersion induces a further increase in ANP plasma levels in cirrhotics, as well as in control subjects (Fernandez-Cruz et al. 1987). Cirrhotic rats without ascites show increased levels of ANP, and these levels increase further after extracellular volume expansion by saline infusion (Olivera et al. 1988). Thus, a blunted secretion of ANP does not seem to be involved in the impaired sodium excretion of cirrhotic patients nor in the blunted natriuretic response to volume expansion.

High levels of ANP in patients with cirrhosis of the liver are not due to a decreased catabolic rate of the hormone but are more likely related to an increased cardiac production (Ginés et al. 1988). Natriuretic response to exogenous synthetic ANP has been reported to be decreased in patients and rats with cirrhosis when compared to that of normal subjects (Salerno et al. 1988; Olivera et al. 1988).

The Classical Humoral Natriuretic Factor

In response to extracellular volume expansion, mammals synthesize a circulating natriuretic factor with the capacity to decrease tubular sodium reabsorption and increase vascular reactivity (DeWardener and Clarkson 1985; Buckalew and Gruber 1984). The biological effect of this factor seems to be mediated by the Na,K-ATPase or sodium pump. This factor appears to be an endogenous digitalis-like substance released by the hypothalamus (Buckalew and Gruber 1984).

It has been reported that the chromatographic plasma fraction in which this factor appears, induces natriuresis when injected into rats and blocks transcellular sodium transport (natriuretic and antinatripheric effects, respectively) (Kramer 1975). This fraction obtained from cirrhotic patients does not alter either the short circuit current or the potential difference of isolated frog skin (Kramer 1975). Naccarato et al. (1981) have reported a decreased natriuretic effect of the urine from non-ascitic cirrhotic patients as compared with the effect of the urine from normal controls. In addition, Hernando et al. (unpublished observations) have demonstrated that the plasma obtained from volume-expanded control animals has the capacity to inhibit the ouabain-sensitive sodium transport in erythrocytes, whereas plasma obtained from cirrhotic rats does not have this effect. These data have been interpreted as demonstrating the presence in plasma from normal, volume-expanded rats of a natriuretic substance that is absent in plasma from cirrhotic animals with the same degree of volume expansion, and agree with the data of Naccarato et al. (1981).

Microsomes from cirrhotic rat kidneys show higher Na,K-ATPase activity than microsomes from control rats (Tejedor et al. 1988). When control microsomes are dialysed for 24 hours, Na,K-ATPase activity increases to levels similar to that of cirrhotic rats, and in the dialysate, a substance can be recovered that inhibits Na,K-ATPase (Tejedor et al. 1988). By contrast, dialysis of cirrhotic microsomes does not induce signficant changes in ATPase activity, and no ATPase-inhibitor substance can be recovered from the dialysate (Tejedor et al. 1988).

Although incomplete and preliminary, the available evidence strongly suggests that a defect in natriuretic factor secretion could play a major role in the decreased natriuresis as well as in the impaired natriuretic response to volume expansion shown by patients and animals with cirrhosis of the liver.

Antidiuretic Hormone (ADH)

Among the derangements of renal function frequently encountered in patients with cirrhosis, is an impairment in renal water excretion that results in an inability to excrete a water load. Hyponatraemia occurs in a substantial number of individuals with liver disease (Vaamonde 1983). Some of the strongest support for a role of ADH in these abnormalities has been obtained in rats with carbon tetrachloride-induced cirrhosis of the liver. In this animal model, impaired water excretion has been verified by basal hyponatraemia and an impaired excretion of a water load (López-Novoa et al. 1977; Linas et al. 1981). Impaired urinary dilution has also been observed in rats with chronic bile duct ligation, although hyponatraemia has not been reported in these animals (Better and Massry 1972; Better et al. 1980).

Vasopressin levels are increased in cirrhotic rats when compared with controls (Linas et al. 1981). In addition, cirrhotic Battleboro rats, a strain with genetic diabetes insipidus and undetectable levels of ADH, in spite of histological, biochemical and renal haemodynamics comparable with Sprague–Dawley rats, do not show impairments in water excretion. Thus, high levels of ADH seem to be responsible for the impairment in water handling. Linas et al (1981) suggest that increased ADH levels in cirrhotic rats are caused by a non-osmolar stimulus due to the abnormal systemic haemodynamics (Fernandez-Muñoz et al. 1985).

Platelet Activating Factor (PAF)

PAF is an alkylphosphoglyceride with haemodynamic and renal actions when infused in normal rats that are reminiscent of those encountered in cirrhotic animals: antinatriuresis, hypotension and increased vascular permeability (Sanchez-Crespo et al. 1982). This substance has been found to be increased in blood of patients with cirrhosis of the liver (Caramelo et al. 1987). Cirrhotic rats also show increased blood levels of PAF (Villamediana et al. 1986). In addition, when treated with BN-52021, a synthetic substance that specifically blocks the binding of PAF to its receptor, cardiac output, that is increased in cirrhotic animals, decreases to near normal values, whereas the effect of this PAF-antagonist in control animals in negligible (Villamediana et al. 1986).

Conclusion

In summary, renal sodium retention in patients with advanced liver disease can be explained by a number of different, interacting mechanisms, some of which are only poorly understood. The relative contribution of each of these mechanisms to sodium retention in the various stages of chronic liver disease remains to be defined.

References

Arendt RM, Gerbes AL, Ritter D, Stanmgl E, Bach P, Zaehringer J (1986) Atrial natriuretic factor in plasma of patients with arterial hypertension, heart failure or cirrhosis of the liver. J Hypertens 4 (suppl): S131–S135
Arroyo V, Bosch J, Mauri M et al. (1979) Renin, aldosterone and renal hemodynamics in cirrhotics with ascites. Eur J Clin Invest 9: 69–73
Baines AD (1973) Redistribution of nephron function in response to chronic and acute solute loads. Am J Physiol 224: 237–244
Ballerman BJ, Brenner BM (1985) Biologically active atrial peptides. J Clin Invest 76: 2041–2048
Bank N, Aynedjian HS (1975) A micropuncture study of renal salt and water retention in chronic bile duct obstruction. J Clin Invest 55: 994–1002
Better OS, Massry SH (1972) Effect of chronic bile duct ligation on renal handling of salt and water. J Clin Invest 51: 402–411
Better OS, Aisenbrey GA, Berl T, Anderson RJ, Handelman WA, Linas SL, Guggenheim SJ, Schrier RW (1980) Role of antidiuretic hormone in impaired urinary dilution associated with chronic bile-duct ligation. Clin Sci 58: 493–500
Bichet DG, Van Putten VJ, Schrier RW (1982) Potential role of increased sympathetic activity in impaired sodium and water excretion in cirrhosis. N Engl J Med 307: 1552–1557
Boyer TD, Zia P, Reynolds TB (1979) Effect of indomethacin and prostaglandin A_1 in renal function and plasma renin activity in alcoholic liver disease. Gastroenterology 77: 215–222
Bricker MS, Donavitch GM (1983) In: Epstein M (ed.) The kidney in liver disease. Elsevier Biomedical, New York, pp 13–24
Buckalew VM Jr, Gruber KA (1984) Natriuretic hormone. Annu Rev Physiol 46: 343–358
Cantin M, Genest J (1985) The heart and the atrial natriuretic factor. Endocr Rev 6: 107–127
Caramelo C, Fernandez-Cruz A, Villamediana LM, Sanz E, Rodriguez-Puyol D, Hernando L, López-Novoa JM (1986a) Systemic and regional hemodynamic effects of a synthetic atrial natriuretic factor in conscious rats. Clin Sci 71: 323–325
Caramelo C, Fernandez-Muñoz D, Santos JC, Blanchart A, Rodriguez-Puyol D, López-Novoa JM, Hernando L (1986b) Effect of volume expansion on hemodynamics, capillary permeability and renal function in conscious, cirrhotic rats. Hepatology 6: 129–134
Caramelo C, Fernandez-Gallardo S, Santos JC, Iñarrea P, Sanchez-Crespo M, López-Novoa JM, Hernando L (1987) Increased levels of PAF-acether in blood from patients with cirrhosis of the liver. Eur J Clin Invest 17: 7–11

Chaimovitz C, Szylman P, Alroy G, Better OS (1972) Mechanisms of increased renal tubular reabsorption in cirrhosis. Am J Med 52: 198–202

Chiandussi L, Bartoli E, Arras S, Chaimovitz C, Alon V, Better OS (1978) Pathogenesis of salt retention in dogs with chronic bile duct ligation. Clin Sci 62: 65–70

DeWardener HE, Clarkson EM (1985) The natriuretic hormone. Physiol Rev 65: 658–759

DiBona CF (1982) The function of renal nerves. Rev Physiol Biochem Pharmacol 94: 75–181

Eggert RC (1970) Spironolactone diuresis in patients with cirrhosis and ascites. Br Med J 4: 401–403

Epstein M (1983a) The renin–angiotensin system in liver disease. In: Epstein M (ed.) The kidney in liver disease, 2nd edn. Elsevier, New York, pp 353–376

Epstein M (1983b) Renal sodium handling in cirrhosis. In: Epstein M (ed.) The kidney in liver disease, 2nd edn, Elsevier. New York, pp 25–53

Epstein M (1986) Renal prostaglandins and the control of renal function in liver disease. Am J Med 80: 46–55

Epstein M (1988) The hepatorenal syndrome. In: Epstein M (ed.) The kidney in liver disease, 3rd edn. Baltimore, Williams and Wilkins, pp 89–118

Epstein M, Pins DS, Schneider N, Levinson R (1976) Determinants of deranged sodium and water homeostasis in decompensated cirrhosis. J Lab Clin Med 87: 822–839

Epstein M, Levinson R, Sancho J, Haber E, Re R (1977) Characterization of the renin–angiotensin system in decompensated cirrhosis. Circ Res 41: 818–829

Epstein M, Ramachandran M, De Nuncio AG (1982) Interrelationship of renal sodium and phosphate handling in cirrhosis. Miner Electrolyte Metab 7: 305–315

Fernandez-Cruz A, Marco J, Cuadrado LM, Gutkowska J, Rodriguez-Puyol D, Caramelo C, López-Novoa JM (1985) Plasma levels of atrial natriuretic factor in cirrhotic patients. Lancet II: 1439–1440

Fernandez-Cruz D, Rodriguez-Puyol D, Gutkowska J, López-Novoa JM (1987) Effect of head-out water immersion on plasma natriuretic peptide levels in cirrhotics with ascites. In: Brenner BM, Laragh JH (eds) Biologically active natriuretic peptides. Raven Press, New York

Fernandez-Muñoz D, Caramelo C, Santos JC, Blanchart A, Hernando L, López-Novoa JM (1985) Systemic and splanchnic hemodynamics in conscious rats with experimental cirrhosis without ascites. Am J Physiol 249: G236–G240

Garcia R, Thibault G, Cantin M, Genest J (1985) Effect of purified atrial natriuretic factor on rat and rabbit vascular strips and vascular beds. Am J Physiol 247: R34–R39

Ginés P, Jiménez W, Arroyo V, Navasa EM, Titó L, López C, Serra A, Bosch J, Sang G, Rivera F, Rodés J (1988) Atrial natriuretic factor in cirrhosis with ascites. Plasma levels, cardiac release and splanchnic extraction. Hepatology 8: 636–642

Gliedman ML, Carrol HJ, Popowitz L, Mullane JF (1970) An experimental hepatorenal syndrome. Surg Gynecol Obstet 131: 30–40

Henriksen JH, Ring-Larsen H, Christensen NJ (1984) Sympathetic nervous system in cirrhosis. A survey of the plasma catecholamine studies. J Hepatol 1: 55–65

Hernando N, Caramelo C, Tejedor A, Fernandez-Cruz A, López-Novoa JM (1985) Lack of effect of synthetic atrial natriuretic factor on rubidium uptake by human erythrocytes. Biochem Biophys Res Commun 130: 1066–1071

Jimenez W, Martinez-Pardo A, Arroyo V, Bruix J, Rimola A, Gaya J, Rivera F, Rodés J (1985) Temporal relationship between hyperaldosteronism, sodium retention and ascites formation in rats with experimental cirrhosis. Hepatology 5: 245–250

Kleinert HD, Maack T, Atlas SA, Januscewicz A, Sealey JE, Laragh JH (1984) Atrial natriuretic factor inhibits angiotensin-, norepinephrin- and potassium-induced vascular contractility. Hypertension 6: 143–147

Klinger EL, Vaamonde CA, Vaamonde LS et al. (1970) Renal function changes in cirrhosis of the liver. A prospective study. Arch Intern Med 125: 1010–1015

Kostreva DR, Castaner A, Kampine JP (1980) Reflex effects of hepatic baroreceptors on renal and cardiac sympathetic nerves activity. Am J Physiol 238: R390–R394

Kramer HJ (1975) Natriuretic hormone. Its possible role in fluid and electrolyte disturbances in chronic liver disease. Postgrad Med J 51: 532–540

Levy M (1977a) Sodium retention and ascites formation in dogs with experimental portal cirrhosis. Am J Physiol 233: F572–F588

Levy M (1977b) Sodium retention in dogs with cirrhosis and ascites: efferent mechanisms. Am J Physiol 233: F586–F592

Levy M, Wexler MJ (1987) Hepatic denervation alters first-phase urinary sodium excretion in dogs with cirrhosis. Am J Physiol 253: F664–F671

Levy M, Wexler MJ, Fechner C (1983) Renal perfusion in dogs with experimental hepatic cirrhosis. Role of prostaglandins. Am J Physiol 245: F521–F529

Linas SL, Anderson RJ, Guggenheim SJ, Robertson GL, Berl T (1981) Role of vasopressin in impaired water excretion in conscious rats with experimental cirrhosis. Kidney Int 20: 173–180

López-Novoa JM (1988) The CCl_4/phenobarbital model of cirrhosis of the liver in rats. In: Epstein M (ed.) The kidney in liver disease, 3rd edn. Williams and Wilkins, Baltimore, pp 309–327

López-Novoa JM, Martinez-Maldonado M (1982) Impaired renal response to splanchnic infusion of hypertonic saline in conscious cirrhotic rats. Am J Physiol 242: F390–F394

López-Novoa JM, Rengel MA, Rodicio JL, Hernando L (1977) A micropuncture study of salt and water retention in chronic experimental cirrhosis. Am J Physiol 232: F315–F318

López-Novoa JM, Rengel MA, Hernando L (1978) Sodium excretion after bilateral nephrectomy in rats with experimental cirrhosis. Experientia 34: 1613–1614

López-Novoa JM, Rengel MA, Hernando L (1980) Dynamic of ascites formation in rats with experimental cirrhosis. Am J Physiol 238: F353–F357

López-Novoa JM, Santos JC, Caramelo C, Fernandez-Muñoz D, Blanchart A, Hernando L (1984) Mechanisms of the impaired diuretic and natriuretic responses to a sustained and moderate saline infusion in rats with experimental cirrhosis. Hepatology 4: 419–423

Mirouze D, Zipser RD, Reynolds TB (1983) Effect of inhibitors of prostaglandin synthesis on induced diuresis in cirrhosis. Hepatology 3: 50–55

Murray BM, Paller MS (1985) Decreased pressor reactivity to angiotensin II in cirrhotic rats. Circ Res 57: 424–431

Naccarato RM, Messa P, D'Angelo A et al. (1981) Renal handling of sodium and water in early chronic liver disease. Gastroenterology 81: 205–210

Nicholls KM, Shaphiro MDS, VanPutten VJ et al. (1985) Elevated plasma norepinephrine concentrations in decompensated cirrhosis. Association with increased secretion rates, normal clearance rates and suppressibility of central blood volume expansion. Circ Res 56: 457–464

Olivera A, Gutkowska J, Rodriguez-Puyol D, Fernandez-Cruz A, López-Novoa JM (1988) Atrial natriuretic peptide in rats with experimental cirrhosis of the liver without ascites. Endocrinology 122: 840–847

Perez-Ayuso RM, Arroyo V, Camps J, Rimola A, Costa J, Gaya J, Rivera F, Rodés J (1984) Renal kallikrein excretion in cirrhotics with ascites: relationship with renal hemodynamics. Hepatology 4: 247–252

Planas R, Arroyo V, Rimola A, Perez-Ayuso RM, Rodes J (1983) Acetylsalicylic acid suppresses the renal hemodynamic effect and reduces the diuretic action of furosemide in cirrhosis with ascites. Gastroenterology 84: 247–252

Ring-Larsen H, Hesse B, Henriksen JH, Christiensen NJ (1982) Sympathetic nervous activity and renal and systemic hemodynamic in cirrhosis: plasma norepinephrine concentration, hepatic extraction and renal release. Hepatology 2: 304–310

Rodriguez-Puyol D, Alsasua A, Blanchart A, López-Novoa JM (1988) Plasma catecholamines and urinary excretion of its main metabolites in 3 models of portal hypertension. Clin Physiol Biochem 6: 2301–2309

Rosoff L Jr, Zia P, Reynolds T, Horton R (1975) Studies of renin and aldosterone in cirrhotic patients with ascites. Gastroenterology 69: 698–705

Salerno F, Badalamenti S, Incerti P, Capozza L, Mainardi L (1988) Renal response to atrial natriuretic peptide in patients with advanced cirrhosis. Hepatology 8: 21–26

Sanchez-Crespo M, Alonso F, Alvarez V, Iñarrea P, Egido J (1982) Vascular actions of synthetic PAF-acether in the rat. Evidence of a platelet-independent mechanism. Immunopharmacology 4: 173–185

Santos JC, Rodriguez-Puyol D, Blanchart A, Hernando L, López-Novoa JM (1988) Urinary excretion and glomerular synthesis of PGE_2 and $PGF_{2\alpha}$ in cirrhotic, non-ascitic rats. The effect of sodium overload. Nephron 49: 322–327

Shenker Y, Sider RS, Ostafin EA, Grekin RJ (1985) Plasma levels of atrial natriuretic factor in healthy subjects and in patients with edema. J Clin Invest 76: 1684–1687

Tejedor A, Conesa D, Hernando N, Hernando L, López-Novoa JM (1988) Absence of an endogenous regulatory factor of Na,K,ATPase activity during experimental cirrhosis in the rat. Biochem Cell Biol 66: 218–230

Thames MD (1977) Neural control of renal function. Contribution of the cardiopulmonary receptors to the control of the kidney. Fed Proc 37: 1209–1213

Vaamonde CA (1983) Renal water handling in liver disease. In: Epstein M (ed.) The kidney in liver disease, 2nd edn. Elsevier, New York, pp 55–86

Villamediana LM, Sanz E, Fernandez-Gallardo S, Caramelo C, Sanchez-Crespo M, Braquet P, López-Novoa JM (1986) Effects of the platelet-activating factor antagonist BN 52021 on the hemodynamics of rats with experimental cirrhosis of the liver. Life Sci 39: 201–205

Wernze H, Spech HI, Mullert G (1978) Studies on the activity of the renin–angiotensin–aldosterone system in patients with cirrhosis of the liver. Klin Wochenschr 56: 389–397

Wilkinson SP, Jowett JDH, Slater JDH, Arroyo V, Moodie H, Williams R (1979) Renal sodium retention in cirrhosis. Relationship to aldosterone and nephron site. Clin Sci 56: 169–177

Wong PY, Talamo RC, Williams GH (1977) Kallikrein–kinin and renin–angiotensin system in functional renal failure of cirrhosis of the liver. Gastroenterology 73: 1114–1118

Yarger WE (1976) A micropuncture study of salt retention associated to bile duct ligation. J Clin Invest 57: 408–418

Zambraski EJ, Chremos AN, Dunn MJ (1984) Comparisons of the effects of sulindac with other cyclooxygenase inhibitors on prostaglandin excretion and renal function in normal and chronic bile duct ligated dogs and swine. J Pharmacol Exp Ther 228: 560–566

Zipser RD, Hoefs JC, Speckart PF, Zia PK, Horton H (1979) Prostaglandins: modulators of renal function and pressor resistance in chronic liver disease. J Clin Endocrinol Metab 48: 895–900

Zipser RD, Kerlin P, Hoefs JC, Zia P, Barg A (1981) Renal kallikrein excretion in alcoholic cirrhosis. Am J Gastroenterol 75: 183–187

Zipser RD, Radvan G, Kronborg J, Duke R, Littel T (1982) Urinary thromboxane B_2 and prostaglandin E_2 in the hepatorenal syndrome: evidence for increased vasoconstrictor and decreased vasodilator factors. Gastroenterology 87: 1228–1232

Discussion

Dr Epstein drew attention to the interesting observation that levels of atrial natriuretic peptide seemed to be increased in patients with cirrhosis. He thought it was difficult to explain the mechanism of this unless the extensive arterio-venous communications which develop in hepatic cirrhosis were responsible for increased atrial filling. He wondered whether there was evidence for this in rats and asked about the haemodynamic state of the cirrhotic rat. Dr López-Novoa replied that in all his rats with cirrhosis and ascites there was an increase in cardiac output and a decrease in peripheral vascular resistance. Nevertheless, he had been unable to demonstrate any arterio-venous shunting as such with the technique of radioactive microspheres. Dr Bihari remarked that whilst flow may be increased in cirrhosis, cardiac filling pressures are usually reduced, reflecting peripheral pooling of blood in the vasodilated peripheral circulation. He thought it was difficult to explain the increase in atrial natriuretic factor on the basis of increased cardiac filling pressures which tend not to occur. Dr López-Novoa agreed and thought that sympathetic stimulation might be another mechanism responsible for atrial natriuretic peptide release. Dr Schrier made several observations. He thought that the fact that most cirrhotics become ascites free when treated with large doses of spironolactone (400 mg), over a period of 3–4 weeks, suggests that aldosterone does indeed play a rather important role in the sodium retention associated with cirrhosis. He was concerned about restraining the rats in the experiments reported, since this restraint alone will increase blood catecholamine and renin levels. He also observed that atrial natriuretic peptide levels are increased in pregnancy, another condition where the blood pressure is low, the cardiac output raised and the peripheral vascular resistance reduced. Dr Ledingham reported that the effects of atrial natriuretic peptide appeared to be pressure dependent. The natriuretic effect of a certain concentration of atrial natriuretic peptide was related to the perfusion pressure of the kidney and this had been demonstrated in the isolated perfused rat kidney model.

Chapter 13

A Review of Mediators and the Hepatorenal Syndrome

K. Moore, V. Parsons, P Ward and R. Williams

Introduction

A discussion of renal failure accompanying liver failure needs a thorough dissection of the situation where the renal failure is either due to common features predisposing to ARF on the one hand and shared diseases on the other. Neither of these clinical diagnoses qualify for the definition of hepatorenal syndrome (HRS) but there is no doubt overlap in many cases (see Fig. 13.1). Often it is by the correction of the former predisposing causes such as hypovolaemia, sepsis, cardiac output and all the shared diseases that a diagnosis of HRS can be made.

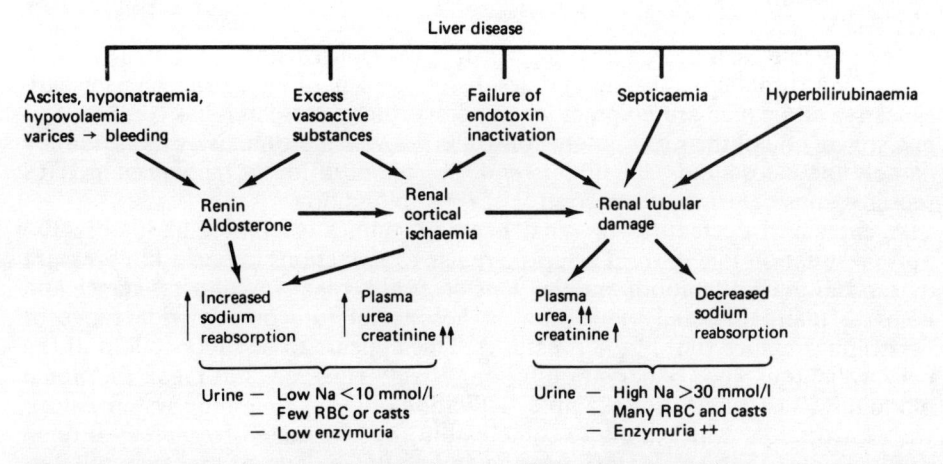

Fig. 13.1. Diagram to show relationship between HRS, acute renal failure and acute tubular necrosis.

With this narrowing down, what are the possible mechanisms of the renal dysfunction? There is good evidence to support the concept that the renal failure is functional in origin. The kidneys retain the ability to resorb sodium or concentrate the urine and pathological abnormalities are minimal. Transplantation of such kidneys into recipients with normal liver function leads to a return of renal function, and likewise liver transplantation into a recipient with HRS results in rapid renal recovery, suggesting that simple acute tubular necrosis (ATN) is not the dominant manifestation of the renal lesion (Koppel et al. 1969; Iwatsuki et al. 1973).

Liver failure alters the homeostatic environment for the kidney such that it ceases to provide effective glomerular filtration but retains tubular function. This is presumably due to substances which are not detoxified by the liver (e.g. endotoxins or vasoactive mediators) or failure by the liver to produce substances necessary for renal function. Whatever the mechanism, in subjects with liver failure, the renal vasculature is exquisitely sensitive to insults such as sepsis, volume depletion and perhaps endotoxaemia (Fig. 13.1).

Haemodynamic Changes in Hepatorenal Syndrome

Reduced renal blood flow in HRS has been demonstrated with several techniques, including PAH clearance, xenon washout and angiography (Ring-Larsen 1977; Wilkinson et al. 1974; Epstein et al. 1970). In some subjects it is associated with increased renal vascular resistance due to vasoconstriction, in which radiographic studies have demonstrated vasoconstriction of the primary branches of the renal artery, the interlobar arteries and the intrarenal (arcuate) vessels. This vasoconstriction is at least potentially reversible since the vessels become patent post mortem. Redistribution of blood flow from the cortical nephrons to the juxtamedullary nephrons causes a reduction of glomerular filtration rate (GFR).

The possible candidates for such reversible vasoconstriction are shown in Table 13.1. Unfortunately it is difficult to dissect which of these mechanisms are causative and which are epiphenomena. Nevertheless research has continued to investigate one of the most potent controllers of vasomotor activity in the kidney namely the eicosanoids. To understand the role of different mediators in HRS requires consideration of the control of renal blood flow.

A characteristic feature of renal haemodynamics is autoregulation. In the normal situation the afferent arteriole reacts to reductions in perfusion pressure by relaxation of its smooth muscle. This decreases renal vascular resistance and helps to maintain renal blood flow at a constant rate over a wide range of perfusion pressure (i.e. blood pressure). This appears to be independent of the nervous system since denervation has no effect. This does not mean that renal blood flow is constant. For example, activation of the sympathetic system causes vasoconstriction, which may, to some extent, be attenuated by increased renal production of the vasodilatory prostaglandins PG E_2 and prostacyclin (PGI_2). Reduction of renal blood flow activates the renin–angiotensin system with

Table 13.1. Vasoactive substances in hepatorenal syndrome

Angiotensin II	Constriction	Increased in HRS
Catecholamines	Constriction	Increased in HRS. Jaundice increases sensitivity
Vasopressin	Constriction	Increased in cirrhosis
Thromboxane	Constriction	Increased in decompensated liver disease. Mesangial cell contraction
Leukotrienes C_4 and D_4	Constriction	Increased in decompensated liver disease. Mesangial cell contraction
Bradykinin	Dilatation	Decreased in urine in HRS
Vasoactive polypeptide (VIP)	Dilatation	Increased in liver disease

concomitant efferent arteriolar vasoconstriction. This effect on the efferent arterioles not only decreases glomerular plasma flow but, by increasing glomerular pressure upstream, serves to increase the filtration fraction, i.e. that fraction of plasma arriving at the glomeruli that is actually filtered. This action helps to maintain the glomerular filtration rate (GFR). Angiotensin II (AT II) also stimulates renal production of PGE_2 and PGI_2, as well as promoting proximal tubular sodium resorption and aldosterone release from the adrenal cortex. Other factors may also have profound effects on both renal blood flow and glomerular microcirculatory haemodynamics. These include the kinin–kallikrein system, thromboxane A_2 (TXA_2) and the cysteinyl leukotrienes (LTC_4 and LTD_4). These factors, however, seem to have a pathophysiological role rather than one involved in day to day renal physiology. Thus, there is a complex interplay of various mediators with the action of some dominating under different circumstances (see Fig 13.2).

It is often assumed that the decrease in renal blood flow in hepatorenal syndrome is due to vasoconstriction. Studies demonstrating actual vasoconstriction rather than decreased blood flow have been few (Epstein et al. 1970).

The explanation for decreased renal blood flow lies in part in other haemodynamic changes that occur in liver disease. The fraction of cardiac output perfusing the kidneys (renal blood flow/cardiac output) depends on the ratio of renal vascular resistance to systemic vascular resistance. In hepatic decompensation there is both decreased systemic vascular resistance and increased cardiac output. The increased cardiac output fails adequately to compensate for the decreased systemic vascular resistance and consequently there is a modest fall in systemic pressure. Even if one assumes that there is no change in the calibre of the renal vessels, renal blood flow will fall since the cardiac output fails to compensate fully for the decreased systemic vascular resistance. This, together with the role of various vasoconstrictors which act to overcome the autoregulatory system, explains the fall in renal blood flow observed. However, the importance of decreased renal blood flow alone in the pathogenesis of hepatorenal syndrome has probably been overemphasized. Other factors may alter GFR independently of renal blood flow. For example the eicosanoids (TXA_2 and LTD_4) are also potent stimuli of mesangial cell contraction, and modulate the surface area available for glomerular filtration (Dunn et al. 1986).

An alternative explanation for decreased renal blood flow is that proposed by Alverstrand and Bergstrom (1984), who suggested that the liver normally produces a hormone (glomerulopressin) which maintains renal blood flow and

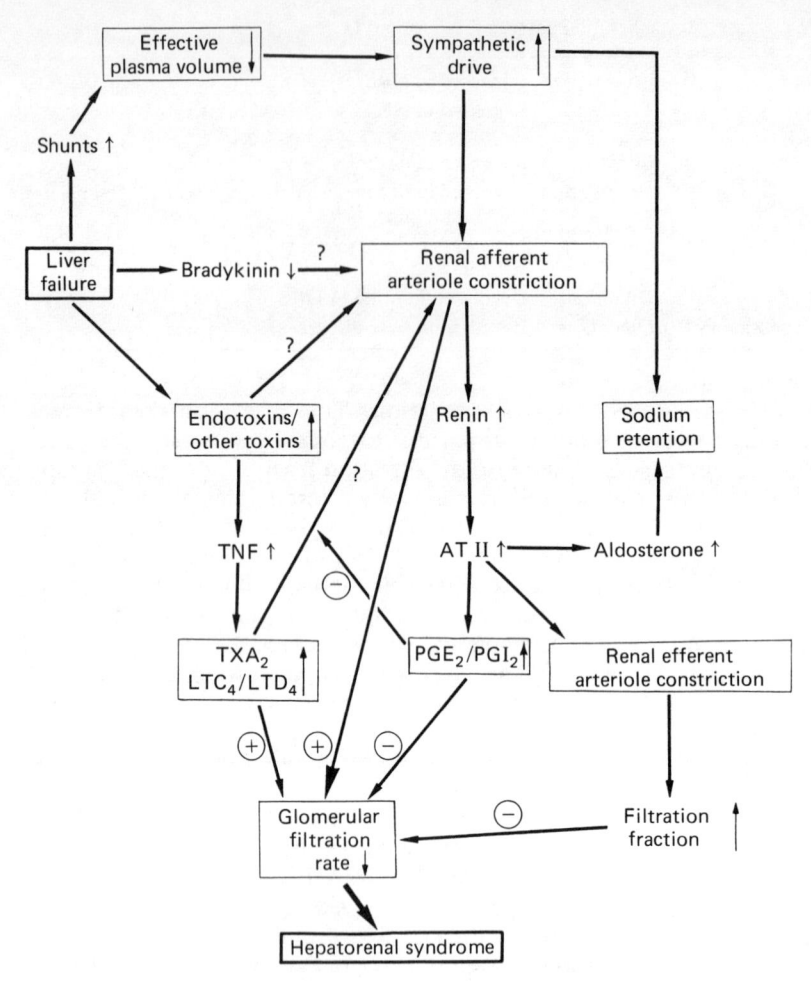

Fig. 13.2. An outline of proposed mechanisms involved in the pathogenesis of hepatorenal syndrome.

that a decrease in the level of glomerulopressin due to liver failure may be responsible for altered renal haemodynamics. To date there is no evidence in man to support this hypothesis.

The production of renal vasodilators is, however, likely to be important since cyclooxygenase inhibitors (e.g. indomethacin) cause a predictable decrease in glomerular filtration rate in cirrhotic subjects with ascites (Zipser 1979). This is thought to be secondary to inhibition of renal production of the vasodilatory prostanoids PGE_2 or PGI_2. Alternative but less-plausible explanations include diversion of arachidonic acid to the lipoxygenase pathway to form the cysteinyl leukotrienes (LTC_4 and LTD_4) themselves potent renal vasoconstrictors. Whatever the role for vasodilatory mediators, the observation that post-mortem angiograms show the renal vasculature to be naturally relaxed lead to the conclusion that the presence of a vasoconstrictor is necessary before the absence of a vasodilator becomes important.

Possible Mediators Involved in the Hepatorenal Syndrome

The Sympathetic Nervous System

Liver failure is associated with activation of the sympathetic nervous system. Recent studies have observed elevated levels of circulating catecholamines in peripheral blood of cirrhotic subjects with ascites or HRS (Arroyo et al. 1983). It is now generally believed that increased sympathetic activity is secondary to the systemic haemodynamic changes that occur in liver failure or end-stage cirrhosis. Indeed in HRS or ascites the peripheral noradrenaline level can be directly correlated with plasma renin activity (PRA). Further, α-adrenergic blockade does not improve renal blood flow or renal function (Epstein et al. 1970). A more recent novel approach, which seems to challenge this concept, has been selective blockade of the sympathetic supply at the level of L1 (i.e. that of the kidney) (Solis-Herruzo et al. 1987). This study observed an increase in glomerular filtration rate in some patients with HRS, suggesting that renal sympathetic stimulation may be a contributory factor decreasing renal blood flow and GFR in hepatorenal syndrome.

Angiotensin II

In view of its vasopressor activity it seemed an attractive hypothesis that AT II may be involved in altered intrarenal haemodynamics in HRS. Its formation is stimulated by the sympathetic nervous system which is activated in response to low effective plasma volume. However, AT II contracts the efferent arterioles rather than the afferent arterioles thus increasing the filtration fraction and maintaining GFR rather than the converse. There have been few studies measuring circulating levels of AT II since there are few specific antisera available for the assay, and it has a short half-life in peripheral blood making accurate collection and inhibition of in vitro metabolism difficult (Bernadi et al. 1982). To assess the role of AT II in vivo the effect of an AT II antagonist (saralasin) or enzyme inhibitor (captopril) on renal function in liver disease has been investigated (Pariente et al. 1985; Schroeder et al. 1976). Both of these approaches either had no effect or caused deterioration of renal function, presumably secondary to associated hypotension. There is little evidence to support a role of AT II in the pathogenesis of HRS. Indeed, there is good reason to believe that activation of the renin–angiotensin system is a physiological response designed to maintain glomerular filtration rate in the face of altered plasma volume and other vasoactive influences rather than an abnormal response resulting in renal failure.

Endotoxins

Endotoxins are derived from the cell wall of Gram-negative bacteria of which the active part is the lipid A component of the lipopolysaccharide moiety. Infusion of endotoxins into most animal species causes a reduction in both renal blood flow and GFR, and in man it has recently been shown to cause secretion of tumour necrosis factor (TNF) and interleukin-1 (IL-1) (Michie et al. 1988).

A correlation between the presence of endotoxaemia and the development of hepatorenal syndrome was first reported in 1974 (Wilkinson et al. 1974, 1976). Since then there have been a number of confirmatory and contradictory studies reflecting selection of patients for study, type of sample collected (platelet rich plasma or plasma) as well as differences in the assay (Gatta et al. 1981). Although still controversial, there appears to be a general consensus that endotoxaemia is more common in subjects with hepatorenal syndrome, compared with liver disease controls without renal failure. Whether this is important in the development of renal failure or merely a reflection of severity of liver disease *per se* is unknown.

Endotoxins are thought to mediate their effect via the formation and release of cytokines such as TNF or IL-1 from macrophages, and it is through these cytokines that endotoxins either act directly or release other mediators such as the eicosanoids (Hagmann et al. 1985). The effect of endotoxin on renal function and blood flow is believed to be mediated via thromboxane A_2 (TXA_2) and the cysteinyl leukotrienes (LTC_4 and LTD_4). Studies in vitro, however, demonstrate rapid tachyphylaxis such that subsequent stimulation of macrophages by endotoxin does not cause TNF formation and release (Gifford and Flick 1987). This is important since, if the effects of endotoxin are predominantly TNF mediated, one might expect tachyphylaxis in subjects with end-stage liver disease in whom there is chronic low-grade endotoxaemia rather than that mimicked by the injection of large boluses of endotoxins. The absence of endotoxin in the peripheral blood, however, does not necessarily exclude a toxin-mediated mechanism. Other toxins, e.g. staphylococcal toxin, may also be important, since these not only have potent biological effects, but, unlike endotoxin, do not cause tachyphylaxis in macrophages with respect to TNF production. It is interesting to speculate that chronic endotoxaemia primes the macrophage for response and acts synergistically with other toxins.

Eicosanoids

Prostaglandins and Thromboxane

Most recent interest has focused on the eicosanoids, in particular the vasoconstrictor TXA_2 and the vasodilatory prostanoids PGE_2 and PGI_2. Prostaglandins are derived from arachidonic acid which is released from phospholipids by the action of phospholipase A_2 or C. Arachidonic acid is converted by cyclooxygenase into PGG_2 and thence via other enzymes to a variety of prostanoids or thromboxane A_2. The half-lives of both TXA_2 and PGI_2 are very short. Systemically generated TXA_2 and PGI_2 are hydrolysed to TXB_2 and 6-keto-$PGF_{1\alpha}$ which themselves undergo further β-oxidation by the liver to the 2,3-dinor metabolites which are excreted in the urine. Relatively little urinary TXB_2 and 6-keto-$PGF_{1\alpha}$ is derived from systemic TXA_2 or PGI_2. Tracer studies infusing tritiated TXB_2 and 6-keto-$PGF_{1\alpha}$ and simultaneously measuring urinary excretion of endogenously formed TXB_2 and 6-keto-$PGF_{1\alpha}$ have convincingly demonstrated that these eicosanoids are present in peripheral blood at concentrations of <5 pg ml^{-1} (Fitzgerald et al. 1987; Zipser and Martin 1982). Most studies in liver disease and hepatorenal syndrome assume that urinary excretion of these metabolites reflects renal production of these eicosanoids. Since these eicosanoids are produced within the kidney, it is believed that the urinary excretion rate of these substances is not affected by renal failure.

Most patients developing HRS have severe jaundice and coagulopathy secondary to acute alcoholic hepatitis (with or without cirrhosis) or acute viral hepatitis. A second group of patients with end-stage cirrhosis and renal failure are relatively anicteric with only mild coagulopathy. It is this group who most frequently develop renal failure secondary to an identifiable event such as hypovolaemia (bleeding or overdiuresis) or sepsis, and who strictly speaking should be considered separately to HRS. Unfortunately many studies comparing "renal production" of TXB_2 and 6-keto-$PGF_{1\alpha}$ in subjects with liver disease fail to specify their means of excluding precipitating events, or use subjects in whom a diagnosis of HRS is made on the basis of mild renal impairment (creatinine just above normal) or a moderately reduced creatinine clearance. Second, most studies use stable cirrhotics or those with ascites as controls. The ideal control group for patients with HRS should be matched as closely as possible for hyperbilirubinaemia, coagulopathy and aetiology, and should be followed up to ensure that these subjects do not subsequently develop renal failure.

Zipser et al. (1983) first reported that the urinary excretion rate of PGE_2 was decreased in patients with HRS and suggested that deficiency of production of this renal vasodilator may be important in the changes in renal blood flow that accompany HRS. This group subsequently demonstrated that urinary TXB_2 concentration was highest in subjects with HRS compared with normals, cirrhotics, or subjects with alcoholic hepatitis, and suggested that a decrease in the ratio of PGE_2/TXB_2 was aetiologically important in the pathogenesis of HRS. It was reasoned that since urinary concentration of TXB_2 was unchanged in normals with or without fluid deprivation, i.e. the excretion rate fell with fluid deprivation, then the comparison of the concentration of this metabolite in these different groups was valid. This study also observed a higher urinary excretion rate of TXB_2 in HRS compared with normals but the data comparing the excretion rate for the other control groups (alcoholic hepatitis, cirrhosis with ascites or renal failure alone) was not given. Most studies have, however, compared the urinary excretion rate of these compounds as a reflection of renal production rate. These are summarized in Table 13.2.

To follow up the observation of increased production of TXB_2 in HRS, Zipser et al. (1984) also assessed the effects of dazoxiben (a thromboxane synthase inhibitor) in subjects with HRS. Unfortunately this had no effect on the subjects studied although many had advanced renal failure and inhibition of TXB_2 excretion was maximally reduced by only 50% in three patients. A more recent study in non-azotaemic cirrhotic subjects with ascites demonstrated an increase in glomerular filtration rate but not renal blood flow in subjects treated with a new and more effective thromboxane synthase inhibitor (OKY 046) (Gentilini and Laffi 1988). The potential benefits of thromboxane synthase inhibition may be masked to some extent by increased formation of PGD_2, which itself can interact with the thromboxane A_2 receptor.

Recently, immunostaining has been used to semiquantitate the capacity of the kidney to synthesize prostanoids (Govindarajan et al. 1987). Markedly diminished PG endoperoxide synthase staining activity was observed in patients with HRS, but PGI_2 synthase immunostaining activity was identical in cirrhotics,

Table 13.2. Eicosanoids in HRS

Author	Prostaglandin E_2		Thromboxane B_2		6-keto-$PGF_{1\alpha}$	
Zipser et al. (1983)	$ng\ h^{-1}$		$ng\ ml^{-1}$			
	↓	HRS	↑	HRS		
	N	Alc. hepatitis	N	Alc. hepatitis		
	↑	Ascites	N	Ascites		
Rimola et al. (1986)	$ng\ h^{-1}$		$ng\ h^{-1}$		$ng\ h^{-1}$	
	↑	Ascites	↑	Ascites	↑	Ascites
	N	HRS	N	HRS	↓	HRS
Guarner et al. (1986)	$pg\ min^{-1}$		$pg\ min^{-1}$		$pg\ min^{-1}$	
	↑	Cirrhosis	↑↑	Cirrhosis	↑↑	Cirrhosis
	↑	Ascites	↑↑	Ascites	↑↑	Ascites
	N	HRS	↑	HRS	N	HRS
Laffi et al. (1986a)	$ng\ h^{-1}$		$ng\ h^{-1}$		$ng\ h^{-1}$	
	N	Cirrhosis	N	Cirrhosis	N	Cirrhosis
	↑↑	Ascites	↑↑	Ascites	↑	Ascites
	↓	HRS	N	HRS	N	HRS

All results are related to normal (N) controls.

"normal subjects" and HRS. It was suggested that loss of PG endoperoxide synthase was responsible for the decreased PGE_2 excretion. It should be noted, however, that whereas PGI_2 synthase is primarily located in the renal cortex, PGE_2 is synthesized primarily in the renal medulla. Therefore, these findings might be expected to reduce medullary blood flow rather than cortical blood flow.

A further point that needs consideration is the effect of liver failure on capacity for β-oxidation of TXB_2 and 6-keto-$PGI_{1\alpha}$ to their dinor metabolites. If β-oxidation is reduced in liver failure or if TXB_2 or 6-keto-$PGF_{1\alpha}$ production exceed the β-oxidative capacity of the liver then there would be reduced metabolism of any systemically generated TXB_2 and 6-keto-prostaglandin $F_{1\alpha}$, which would be excreted in urine. Clearly, if this were the case one might expect equally high urinary excretion of these metabolites in an appropriately "sick" control group matched for liver dysfunction.

Serial Changes in Prostanoid Excretion During the Development of HRS

To assess the effect of renal failure on urinary excretion of TXB_2 and 6-keto-$PGF_{1\alpha}$, serial urine samples were collected from one patient with severe alcoholic hepatitis and who rapidly developed HRS. Urinary concentration and excretion rate of TXB_2 and 6-keto-$PGF_{1\alpha}$ and their dinor metabolites were measured by gas chromatography mass spectrometry (GCMS). The results are illustrated in Fig. 13.3. The excretion rates of TXB_2 and 6-keto-$PGF_{1\alpha}$ were both considerably elevated at an early stage of renal failure and decreased approximately in parallel to creatinine clearance with the onset of renal failure. The initial excretion rates of these compounds were considerably higher than any other reported values. If the stage of renal impairment is taken into account then our results do not differ from others when matched for renal impairment. The excretion rate of these metabolites was also measured in three subjects with severe hepatocellular dysfunction (alcoholic or viral hepatitis) (mean bilirubin 480 μM, mean prothrombin time 25 s) who did not develop progressive renal failure, and all of whom

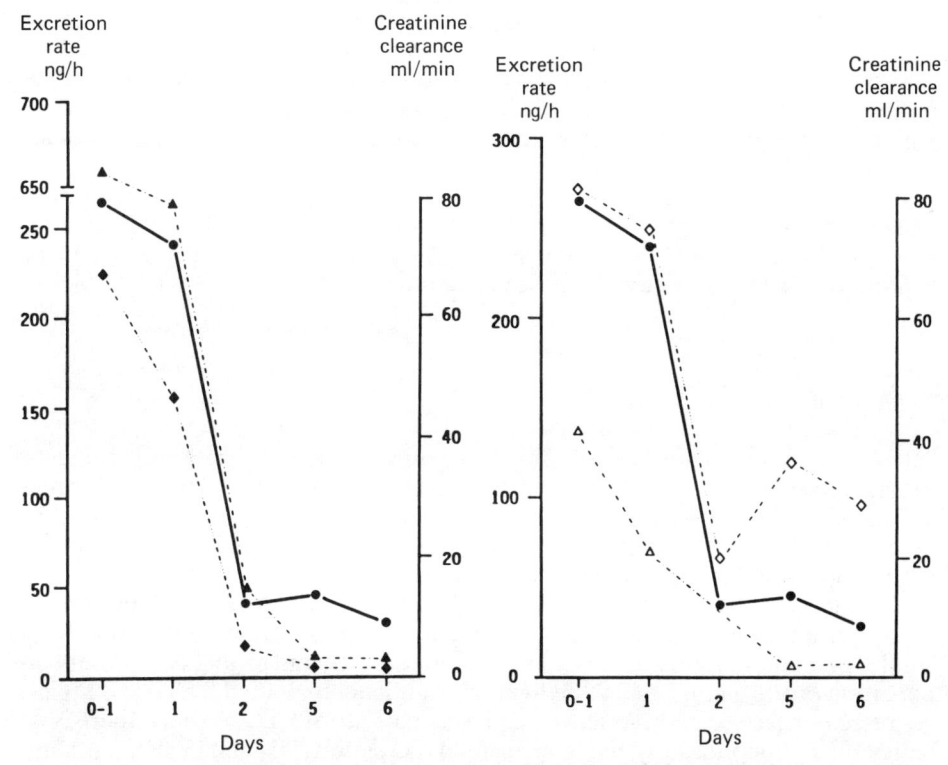

Fig. 13.3. Serial changes in excretion rate of TxB$_2$ (*filled diamond*: ◆), 6-keto-PGF$_{1\alpha}$ (*filled triangle*: ▲), 2,3-dinor TxB$_2$ (*open diamond*: ◇) and 2,3-dinor 6-keto-PGF$_{1\alpha}$ (*open triangle*: △) in a subject with acute alcoholic hepatitis developing hepatorenal syndrome. The creatinine clearance (*filled circle*) is represented by the *continuous line*. The excretion rate of all metabolites fell in parallel to creatinine clearance. Normal excretion rates for each metabolite <10–20 ng h^{-1}

recovered to leave hospital. Interestingly the excretion rate of these metabolites was as high as those with early HRS.

If the observation of changes in excretion rate in the one subject developing HRS can be carried over to similar subjects, there are three possible explanations for the decrease in excretion rate. First, renal excretion of TXB$_2$ and 6-keto-PGF$_{1\alpha}$ produced within the kidney is dependent on renal function, second, the majority of these metabolites are formed in the extrarenal circulation and their excretion rate is GFR dependent, third, the production of these eicosanoids falls during the onset of renal failure. One other study observed that in a large selection of cirrhotics with widely differing renal function, including those with renal failure, there was a linear relationship of 6-keto-PGF$_{1\alpha}$ and GFR (Guarner et al. 1986) and another group of workers has observed a similar but less linear relationship between PGE$_2$ excretion rate and GFR in cirrhotics (Arroyo et al. 1983). These and others have assumed that it is a decrease in the renal production of PGE$_2$ and 6-keto-PGF$_{1\alpha}$ that accounts for the fall in GFR. However, the temporal relationship could equally be explained by the possibility that excretion rate of these metabolites is GFR dependent. If there is a larger contribution of extrarenal TXB$_2$ and 6-keto-PGF$_{1\alpha}$ than has hitherto been recognized the question is why? One possible explanation is an increased systemic production of TXB_2 and 6-keto-$PGF_{1\alpha}$ secondary to low-grade intravascular coagulation. The observation that there was increased excretion of the dinor metabolites in these patients with HRS and those with severe hepatocellular dysfunction is compatible with this concept. If the β-oxidative capacity of the liver is exceeded then a higher proportion of urinary TXB_2 or 6-keto-$PGF_{1\alpha}$ would be systemically derived. The main argument against this latter possibility is the observation that administration of sulindac which is believed to have a sparing effect on renal prostaglandin synthesis, inhibits platelet/endothelial production, but does not affect urinary excretion of TXB_2 or 6-keto-$PGF_{1\alpha}$ in cirrhotics with ascites (Laffi et al. 1986b).

Leukotrienes

The cysteinyl leukotrienes are both potent renal vasoconstrictors and stimulate mesangial cell contraction (Badr et al. 1985; Dunn et al. 1986). They are formed via the 5-lipoxygenase pathway and glutathione detoxification pathway from arachidonic acid by a variety of cells or tissues including macrophages, Kupffer cells, lung, vascular tissue and possibly kidney. Following infusion of ^{3}H-labelled LTC_4 into man there is rapid excretion of metabolites into urine (Orning et al. 1985). The major identifiable urinary metabolite is LTE_4, which is relatively stable. Polar metabolites are also formed and excreted and probably represent ω-oxidation products formed by the liver. It is unlikely that any LTC_4 or LTD_4 are excreted unchanged in urine since the plasma half-life of LTC_4 is short, there is an active renal dipeptidase system converting LTD_4 into LTE_4 and in vitro both are converted into LTE_4 in human urine. Thus urinary LTE_4 excretion is believed to reflect systemic in vivo leukotriene production. The potential role of cysteinyl leukotrienes as mediators of hepatorenal syndrome was first suggested by Keppler et al. (1985). To date, however, there have only been preliminary reports of measurements of LTE_4 excretion in man (Huber et al. 1987; Moore et al. 1987).

We recently reported (at the EASL meeting, August 1988, Moore et al. 1988) our findings of urinary LTE_4 excretion in four groups of subjects: normal controls ($n=8$), compensated liver disease ($n=9$), decompensated liver disease, i.e. ascites or severe hepatocellular dysfunction ($n=19$), and hepatorenal syndrome ($n=11$). Urinary LTE_4 was assayed by high-pressure liquid chromatography (HPLC)–radioimmunoassay (RIA). All results were corrected for creatinine clearance (Cr.Cl) since we have previously shown that urinary excretion of LTE_4 is dependent on renal function. Patients with hepatorenal syndrome had the highest ratio of LTE_4/Cr.Cl (32.3 (11.5–141.4) pg LTE_4 ml^{-1} Cr.Cl) and this was significantly different from normal controls, compensated liver disease, and decompensated liver disease (0.6, 1.9 and 8.4 pg ml^{-1} Cr.Cl respectively).

The mechanism for increased urinary LTE_4 excretion in patients with decompensated liver disease is unknown. Impaired hepatobiliary excretion might enhance urinary leukotriene excretion in patients with severe liver disease. However, since only 8% of leukotrienes are faecally excreted in man, and several subjects with ascites and elevated urinary LTE_4 were anicteric at the time of study, this seems unlikely to account for some of the markedly elevated values observed in these subjects. Impaired cytochrome P450 activity by the liver will almost certainly increase the ratio of LTE_4 formed with respect to the ω-oxidation products.

However, it is likely that cysteinyl-leukotriene production is increased in decompensated liver disease. If local leukotriene production in the kidney or renal vasculature mirrors the overall increase observed then pathophysiological effects such as renal vasoconstriction, mesangial cell contraction and a fall in GFR would be expected. It is unlikely that systemically generated LTC_4 or LTD_4 is physiologically active on renal arterioles or glomerular function since their half-life is short and arterial levels are likely to be in the low picogram range similar to that of other eicosanoids.

It is hypothesized that in liver failure systemic endotoxaemia or other toxins stimulate synthesis of LTC_4 and LTD_4 by the renal arterioles resulting in vasoconstriction. If the glomeruli have the capacity to synthesize cysteinyl-leukotrienes, toxins may also stimulate the production of LTD_4 resulting in mesangial cell contraction and a further fall in GFR.

It is unlikely that any one mediator will prove to be the "cause" of hepatorenal syndrome and measures that have been tried against various single mediators and failed to influence the course of hepatorenal syndrome are shown in Table 13.3. It is more likely that there is a simultaneous activation of the powerful array of mediator pathways which act in concert and that renal failure develops when the time is "ripe". In addition to those pathways discussed there are many other areas which will no doubt prove of interest as potentially important factors involved in the pathogenesis of hepatorenal syndrome such as PAF, the epoxyeicosatrienoic acids, lipoxins, EDRF and perhaps even endothelin.

Table 13.3. Measures that have failed to reverse hepatorenal syndrome

Volume expansion:	Colloid (dextran, albumin)
	Mannitol
	Head out of water immersion
Treatment of ascites:	Paracentesis with reinfusion of ascites
	Le Veen shunt
	Portacaval shunt
Pressor agents:	Angiotensin II (AT II)
	Octapressin
Renal vasodilators:	Dopamine
	Saralasin (AT II antagonist)
	Acetylcholine
	Phentolamine (adrenergic blocker)
	Prostaglandin E_1
	Dazoxiben (thromboxane A_2 antagonist)
Detoxification:	Haemodialysis
	Cross circulation

References

Alverstrand A, Bergstrom J (1984) Glomerular hyperfiltration after protein ingestion, during glucagon infusion, and in insulin-dependent diabetes is induced by a liver failure hormone: deficient production of this hormone in hepatic failure causes hepatorenal syndrome. Lancet I: 195–197

Arroyo V, Planas R, Gaya J et al. (1983) Sympathetic nervous activity, renin–angiotensin system and renal excretion of prostaglandin E_2 in cirrhosis. Relationship to functional renal failure and sodium and water excretion. Eur J Clin Invest 13: 271–278

Badr KF, Baylis C, Pfeffer JM et al. (1985) Renal and systemic haemodynamic responses to intravenous infusion of leukotriene C_4 in the rat. Circ Res 54: 492–499

Bernadi M, Wilkinson SP, Wernze H et al. (1982) The renin–angiotensin–aldosterone system in fulminant hepatic failure. Clin Sci 62: 369–373

Dunn MJ, Simonson MS, Mene P (1986) The role of eicosanoids in the control of mesangial function. Trans Am Clin Climatol Assoc 98: 71–79

Epstein M, Berk DP, Hollenberg NK et al. (1970) Renal failure in the patient with cirrhosis: the role of active vasoconstriction. Am J Med 49: 175–185

Fitzgerald G, Healy C, Daugherty J (1987) Thromboxane A_2 biosynthesis in human disease. Fed Proc 46: 154–158

Gatta A, Milani L, Merkel C et al. (1981) Endotoxins and the hepatorenal syndrome. Lancet II: 101–102

Gentilini G, Laffi G (1988) Effects of OKY 046, a thromboxane synthase inhibitor, on renal function in non-azotemic cirrhotic subjects with ascites. Gastroenterology 94: 1470–1477

Gifford G, Flick D (1987) Natural production and release of TNF, TNF and related cytokines. Ciba Found Symp 131: 3–20

Govindarajan S, Nast C, Smith WL et al. (1987) Immunohistochemical distribution of renal prostaglandin endoperoxide synthase and prostacyclin synthase: diminished endoperoxide synthase in the hepatorenal syndrome. Hepatology 7: 654–659

Guarner C, Guarner F, Corzo J et al. (1986) Renal prostaglandins in cirrhosis of the liver. Clin Sci 70: 477–484

Hagmann WC, Denzlinger C, Keppler D (1985) Production of leukotrienes in endotoxin shock. FEBS Lett 180: 309–313

Huber M, Kastner S, Scholmerich J et al. (1987) Enhanced urinary excretion of cysteinyl leukotrienes in patients with hepatorenal syndrome. J Hepatol 5 (suppl 1): s34–s64

Iwatsuki S, Popovtzer MM, Corman JL et al. (1973) Recovery of hepatorenal syndrome after orthotopic transplantation. N Engl J Med 289: 1155–1159

Keppler D, Hagmann W, Rapp S et al. (1985) The relation of leukotrienes to liver injury. Hepatology 5: 883–891

Koppel MH, Coburn JW, Mims JW et al. (1969) Transplantation of cadaveric kidneys from patients with hepatorenal syndrome. Evidence for the functional nature of renal failure in advanced liver disease. N Engl J Med 280: 1367–1371

Laffi G, La Villa G, Pinzani M et al. (1986a) Altered renal and platelet arachidonic acid metabolism in cirrhosis. Gastroenterology 90: 274–282

Laffi G, Daskalopoulos G, Kronberg I et al. (1986b) Effects of sulindac and ibuprofen in patients with cirrhosis and ascites. Gastroenterology 90: 182–187

Michie HR, Manogue KR, Spriggs DR et al. (1988) Detection of circulating tumour necrosis factor after endotoxin administration. N Engl J Med 318: 1481–1486

Moore K, Taylor GW, Maltby N et al. (1987) Increased urinary excretion of leukotriene LTE_4 in decompensated liver disease. Clin Sci (suppl 18) 32: 117

Moore K, Taylor GW, Maltby N et al. (1988) EASL meeting. J Hepatol 7 (suppl 1): S61

Orning L, Kaijser L, Hammarstrom S (1985) In vivo metabolism of LTC_4 in man. Biochem Biophys Res Commun 130: 214–220

Pariente EA, Bataille C, Bercoff E, Lebrec D (1985) Acute effects of captopril on systemic and renal haemodynamics and on renal function in cirrhotic patients with ascites. Gastroenterology 88: 1255–1259

Rimola V, Arroyo V, Ginés P et al. (1986) Urinary excretion of 6-keto prostaglandin $F_{1\alpha}$, thromboxane B_2 and prostaglandin E_2 in cirrhosis with ascites. Relationship to functional renal failure (hepatorenal syndrome). J Hepatol 3: 111–117

Ring-Larsen H (1977) Renal blood flow in cirrhosis: relation to systemic and portal haemodynamics and liver function. Scand J Clin Lab Invest 37: 635–642

Schroeder ET, Anderson GH, Goldman SH et al. (1976) Effect of blockade of angiotensin II on blood pressure, renin and aldosterone in cirrhosis. Kidney Int 9: 511–519

Solis-Herruzo JA, Duran A, Favela V et al. (1987) Effects of lumbar sympathetic block on kidney function in cirrhotic patients with hepatorenal syndrome. J Hepatol 5: 167–173

Wilkinson SP, Arroyo V, Gazzard BG et al. (1974) Relation of renal impairment and haemorrhagic diathesis to endotoxaemia in fulminant hepatic failure. Lancet I: 521–524

Wilkinson SP, Moodie H, Stamatakis JD et al. (1976) Endotoxaemia in renal failure in cirrhosis and obstructive jaundice. Br Med J 2: 1415–1418
Zipser RD (1979) Prostaglandins: Modulators of renal function and pressor resistance in chronic liver disease. J Clin Endocrinol Metab 48: 895–900
Zipser RD, Martin K (1982) Urinary excretion of arterial blood prostaglandins and thromboxanes in man. Am J Physiol 242: E171–E177
Zipser RD, Radvan GH, Kronberg IJ et al. (1983) Urinary thromboxane B_2 and prostaglandin E_2 in the hepatorenal syndrome: Evidence for increased vasoconstrictor and decreased vasodilator factors. Gastroenterology 84: 697–703
Zipser RD, Kronberg I, Rector W et al. (1984) Therapeutic trial of thromboxane synthesis in the hepatorenal syndrome. Gastroenterology 87: 1228–1232

Discussion

Dr Parsons was asked whether the use of various filters might be useful as a means of improving the clearance of substances (such as leukotrienes) from the blood. Dr Parsons referred to a controlled clinical trial of charcoal haemoperfusion in acute liver failure which had been published recently in *Gastroenterology*. It appeared that this particular technique did not improve survival in patients with acute liver failure. Nevertheless, various groups of workers had reported a reduction in the level of mediators using absorption columns and filters and this was an avenue which required more exploration.

Dr Schrier emphasized how important it was to correct for the changes in renal function in the assessment of measurements of eicosanoids within the urine. Dr Arieff emphasized that a patient did not have to demonstrate overt liver failure before having a reduction in glomerular filtration rate reflecting the early onset of the hepatorenal syndrome. Dr Better and Dr Parsons both referred to the possibility of the existence of an unknown vasodilatory factor released by the liver with an effect on renal blood flow. Dr Better referred to work from Roberto Grossmann's laboratory which had demonstrated such a factor which caused an increase in renal blood flow. The pressure within the hepatic sinusoid seemed to be a key factor in this, and if this pressure is reduced by pre-hepatic portal ligation, then renal flow may suddenly increase.

Chapter 14

Drug-Induced Acute Renal Failure

A. L. Linton

There can be no doubt that adverse effects of drugs either cause or contribute to deterioration in renal function in a high proportion of cases of acute renal failure (ARF). Drugs produce renal damage by a variety of mechanisms, including dehydration, direct tubular toxicity, immunological disturbances and vasomotor actions; their effects may be extremely difficult to detect in patients in the intensive care setting, where so many other causes of renal dysfunction may be operating. Constant vigilance and careful evaluation of individual patients are required.

The list of drugs which may have nephrotoxic effects is very long, but the majority of clinically important drug-induced ARF follows the use of aminoglycosides or radiocontrast agents. Although the potential adverse effects of these agents has been known for many years, we still lack hard evidence on almost all aspects of their nephrotoxicity, from incidence, through pathophysiology to methods of avoidance or prevention. Some clinically important facets of the toxicity of these drugs will be reviewed, and renal impairment caused by some unexpected agents will be briefly described.

Aminoglycoside Nephrotoxicity

It is impossible to review the enormous literature on renal damage due to aminoglycosides (AG). In brief, all members of this group of antibiotics have at least some capacity to cause renal damage, but despite this, their clinical efficacy has ensured that they remain the mainstay of therapy for infections with Gram-negative organisms. The reported incidence of gentamicin nephrotoxicity varies from 0.5% to 30% of patients treated (Coggins and Fang, 1983a), with the nature, severity and duration of the ARF also widely variable. In contrast to this clinical uncertainty, pathological changes in renal tubular cells after gentamicin use are very common, and these may provide the basis for the claim that transmission electron microscopy of urinary sediment can contribute to the diagnosis of AG nephrotoxicity by revealing large numbers of myeloid bodies in necrotic tubular cells (Mandal et al. 1987). It has been suggested that the appearance of AG-induced renal damage may also be identified by the demonstration of enzymuria or microglobulinuria, but these may be seen in patients without reduction in renal function, and in patients with sepsis before antibiotics are administered (Richmond et al. 1982). Thus even diagnosis of AG-nephrotoxicity in the critically ill is a difficult task.

Pathophysiology

Basic pathophysiology of AG-nephrotoxicity remains obscure, although extensively studied in animals. The drugs accumulate in lysosomes in proximal tubular cells, inducing changes in volume and density, with deposition of so-called myeloid bodies. However, the relationship between AG accumulation and cell damage is not established, and in man these pathological changes occur early and frequently, often not associated with reduction in glomerular filtration rate (DeBroe et al. 1984). Some of the many animal studies have thrown up a number of possible ways of modifying the severity of the kidney damage. There is evidence to suggest that water and salt loading may be protective, but other animal studies suggest that if the sodium loading is done with sodium bicarbonate, the histological damage is more severe (Bennet et al. 1986). Moreover, rats with hereditary diabetes insipidus are not protected by their continuous diuresis, whereas rats with streptozotocin-induced diabetes mellitus are completely protected from AG-nephrotoxicity (Teixeira et al. 1982). Other animal studies have produced conflicting evidence on the effects of potassium, magnesium and calcium, of previous AG challenge, and even of castration of male rats (Whelton et al. 1981), but identification of feasible protective measures in man eludes us.

Clinical Aspects

AG-induced renal impairment commonly occurs after about a week of treatment, and recovery does not usually occur until about a week after stopping the drug. Many risk factors have been identified, of which the most important seem to be old age, renal or hepatic dysfunction, duration of treatment and peak or trough plasma levels (Smith et al. 1986). The type of AG used does not seem to alter the risk for renal damage (Meyer 1986). Since AGs are often absolutely indicated for treatment of severe infections, little can be done to avoid renal damage even if risk factors are present. Monitoring of blood levels is essential in high-risk patients, for it is clear that they predict incipient toxicity, particularly the trough level. Experimental toxicity is greater when total daily dose is given divided rather than as a single bolus, so dosage regimens should focus on more widely spaced bolus injections. But even simple monitoring of AG levels is beset with unexpected difficulties. In one major teaching hospital, recognition that reported AG blood levels (peak and trough) were often uninterpretable led to a study of accuracy of sampling and testing. The assay proved very accurate, but of 49 trough levels and 51 peak levels, only 10% were ordered for the correct time in relation to dose, and collected and recorded as such. Some 60% of all levels reported were uninterpretable (Bayliss, C, personal communication, 1988).

For the moment, the efficacy of AGs dictates that we continue to use them for serious infections. In every case, the possible risk factors should be evaluated, and if the cumulative risk is very high, alternative antibiotics should be sought. There is a need for greater awareness of AG nephrotoxicity, and closer monitoring, as well as an urgent need for more reliable data.

Contrast Nephropathy

Unlike AG nephrotoxicity, the risk of renal damage after injection of radiocontrast material may have been over-emphasized. After early case reports of ARF following radiological procedures in the 1960s, the 1970s produced large numbers of reports of renal impairment apparently related to the administration of contrast media as the use of these drugs increased. Despite this, hard evidence about incidence of contrast nephropathy remained scarce and reported figures ranged from 0 to over 70%. Much of this scatter is due to obvious factors such as the insensitivity of measures of renal function, different definitions of renal damage, different methodologies, lack of control groups and patient selection (Berkseth and Kjellstrand 1984).

Clinical Features

ARF following the administration of contrast agents ranges in severity from a non-oliguric slight rise in serum creatinine to fulminant renal failure. Most reported cases have followed intravenous urography (65%), with 30% following angiography and a few following computerized tomography. Preparation for intravenous urography followed by transient volume expansion then osmotic diuresis after contrast injection may produce acute changes in renal function, and ARF usually appears in 24–48 hours. Urinalysis is usually unhelpful, and neither urine osmolality nor fractional sodium excretion provide good diagnostic information, although the latter may be low, in contrast to vasomotor nephropathy (Fang et al. 1980). Rapid recovery with spontaneous diuresis usually occurs. Pathological changes occur in proximal tubular cells, with vacuolization and eventually necrosis. The pathogenesis of contrast nephropathy is also unclear. Hypotheses include direct cellular toxicity of contrast media, damage induced by increased uric acid or oxalate excretion, obstruction by proteinaceous casts or oxalate crystals, alterations in renal haemodynamics, changes in red cell morphology and even immunological injury due to circulating immune complexes (Coggins and Fang 1983b). There is little definitive evidence which might indicate methods of prevention or treatment.

Incidence and Risk Factors

The incidence of significant renal damage in healthy individuals receiving contrast media must be very low, for the numbers of such procedures performed are very large. Studies of selected populations have claimed to have identified patient groups at high risk, and the risk factors have included pre-existing renal disease, diabetes mellitus, dehydration and multiple myeloma (Berkseth and Kjellstrand 1984). Few of these studies were prospective, and fewer still controlled; much of this conventional wisdom has been challenged by more recent studies. Several prospective studies have revealed a very low incidence of renal damage after angiography, even in patients with both diabetes mellitus and chronic renal impairment (Kumar et al. 1981). Even in studies confined to intravenous urography, when a higher incidence of reduction in renal function was reported, the magnitude of change in serum creatinine levels was generally small, and seldom of clinical significance. Indeed, much of the change might be attributable to mild volume depletion after an osmotic diuresis (Teruel et al. 1981). Finally, in one of the few prospective and controlled studies, renal impairment occurred after CT scanning in 2.1% of cases, but was as frequent in those patients who did not receive contrast media for enhancement as in those who did (Cramer et al. 1985). This study also identified the risk of contrast nephropathy in hospital as 8:1000, and underlined the fact that because renal impairment is multifactorial, previous studies with no control group may have overestimated the risk.

The more recent studies have also failed to support many of the identified risk factors. Perhaps only pre-existing renal impairment still confers greater hazard, and warrants careful consideration of alternative investigative procedures, with careful monitoring if contrast must be used. Attempts to characterize contrast nephropathy by using more sensitive parameters of renal function than serum creatinine levels, such as urinary enzyme excretion, have produced more conflicting evidence. Use of these techniques has also failed to identify whether the new low-osmolality contrast media are any safer than the old (Jevnikar et al. 1988).

Other ARF Syndromes

A large number of drugs may produce other syndromes which may present as ARF, and their recognition is important for therapeutic purposes. The two most common such conditions are acute interstitial nephritis (AIN) and the syndrome of rhabdomyolysis; both occur and may be difficult to diagnose in the critically ill patient.

ARF from Interstitial Nephritis

Damage to the renal interstitium occurs as a result of many different conditions, but acute interstitial disease presenting as ARF is almost always due to an acute allergic response to drugs. The list of implicated drugs is long, but common causes are antibiotics (particularly penicillins, cephalosporins and suphonamides), diuretics (hydrochlorothiazide), non-steroidal anti-inflammatory agents and allopurinol. The syndrome may be suggested by the coincident appearance of ARF with a rash and arthralgias, but the latter symptoms are often transient or absent. Eosinophilia or eosinophiluria may be detected, but again are inconstant (Linton et al. 1980). Diagnosis of AIN is important, for renal function usually improves quickly following withdrawal of the offending agent, with or without steroid therapy – assistance may be obtained from ^{67}gallium scintigraphy, where intense, diffuse ^{67}Ga uptake by the kidneys strongly supports a diagnosis of AIN (Linton et al. 1985).

Non-Traumatic Rhabdomyolysis

Free myoglobin, released from muscle, is a potent cause of acute damage to renal function, although the precise mechanism is still uncertain. Rhabdomyolysis should be suspected if the following biochemical markers are found in unexplained ARF:

1. Disproportionate elevation of serum creatinine over BUN
2. Severe hyperuricaemia
3. Elevated CPK (MM isoenzyme)
4. Rapidly rising potassium and phosphate
5. Falling serum calcium and albumin

Rhabdomyolysis with renal damage often complicates trauma, but frequently also is caused by drugs, often in patients predisposed by chronic alcohol abuse and by muscle inertia in coma. Drugs involved have included all narcotics and sedatives, amphetamine, quinine, chlorpromazine and carbenoxolone. Treatment may be required for the specific biochemical disorders noted above, but although dialysis may be necessary, recovery is often swift after the acute muscle injury subsides (Koffler et al. 1976).

Other Nephrotoxic Drugs

Drugs with known adverse effects on renal function are numerous, but the following list will be restricted to those drugs likely to be used in an intensive care setting, and to those drugs more recently identified as potentially toxic. It is, however, worth noting that one class of drug seldom called for in acutely ill patients may profoundly affect renal function in patients who have recently become ill. These are the non-steroidal anti-inflammatory drugs (NSAIDs), now available widely without prescription, and consumed in amounts exceeding 2 billion tablets per year in the United States. Patients on NSAIDs exposed to surgery, trauma or acute illness are much more likely to develop acute renal impairment secondary to haemodynamic disturbances because of intrarenal prostaglandin suppression; they may also experience fluid retention, hyperkalaemia and renal papillary necrosis as a result of drugs taken just before the onset of acute illness (Zipser and Henrich 1986).

Anaesthetic Agents

Surgery and general anaesthesia are accompanied by reductions in renal blood flow and GFR, with reduced urine output and an increased filtration fraction. The extent to which trauma, anaesthetic agents and changes in fluid and electrolyte status contribute to this is uncertain, but anaesthesia alone, in well-hydrated patients, may produce very little change in renal function (Stanley et al. 1974).

Genuine nephrotoxicity does occur with methoxyflurane anaesthesia. Mild cases develop a renal concentrating defect, with polyuria unresponsive to vasopressin, but this may progress to oliguria and uraemia. Risk factors for toxicity include obesity (because of prolonged exposure to the lipid-soluble agent), volume depletion and pre-existing renal disease. The incidence of this ATN-like syndrome varies from series to series, but may be significant with prolonged administration at high concentration. It is believed that inorganic fluoride is the cause of the polyuric syndrome, the severity of which is related to peak serum fluoride levels achieved; the oliguric form of methoxyflurane nephrotoxicity may be due to deposition of another metabolite, oxalate, found extensively in the renal tubular cells (Cousins and Mazze 1973). Renal insufficiency may persist after methoxyflurane nephrotoxicity (Churchill et al. 1974). Episodes of renal insufficiency have also been reported after anaesthesia with halothane and enflurane, but these are extremely rare.

Amphotericin

Impairment of renal function occurs almost predictably after amphotericin administration, and the degree and duration of creatinine elevation are roughly proportional to the dose of the drug. After a cumulative dose of 2–3 g, casts appears in the urine, and hypokalaemia and loss of renal concentrating power may occur. Blood urea nitrogen and creatinine then rise, often without oliguria, and usually return to normal if the amphotericin is discontinued, although permanent renal damage can occur (Takacs et al. 1963). It is probable that sodium or volume depletion predispose to amphotericin toxicity, and both sodium loading and alkalinization may be protective, as may be the infusion of mannitol (Heidemann et al. 1983). These measures may allow treatment with amphotericin to be continued in the face of renal impairment, where it is considered vital.

Unexpected Causes of Reduced Renal Function

Nitroprusside

In patients who have cardiac failure, nitroprusside infusion decreases renal vascular resistance, but decreases systemic vascular resistance more. Regional flow studies have shown a marked increment in limb blood flow, and studies in dogs have suggested that the renal vascular dilatation is minor. This may then establish a "steal" syndrome causing reduction in renal blood flow, and progressive oliguria and azotaemia have been reported in man during nitroprusside administration (Reid and Muther 1987).

Amino Acids

Parenteral nutrition with amino acids is commonly employed in critically ill patients in an attempt to improve nutritional status. It has also been suggested that this may enhance the rate of recovery from ARF (Abel et al. 1973), although the proof is lacking. There is now increasing evidence to suggest that amino acids may have nephrotoxic potential, and the list of amino acids with detrimental tubular effects is lengthening. Both lysine and arginine produce tubular proteinuria and bicarbonaturia, and lysine infusion has been shown to induce ARF in rats and to reduce GFR in man (Zager 1987). It remains to be shown that ARF can be induced in man solely by amino acid infusion, but since ARF in the clinical setting is usually multifactorial, amino acids may certainly contribute. Animal studies suggest that amino acid infusion may sensitize rats to subsequent ischaemic injury, perhaps by synergistic toxicity. The net effect of amino acid feeding probably varies widely from patient to patient, and this greatly complicates therapeutic decisions.

Dextran and Albumin

Dextran is a polysaccharide used clinically as a volume expander. Its larger-molecular-weight fractions are poorly cleared from the blood, and may produce a hyperoncotic state. ARF related to dextran has been noted, and usually ascribed to ill-defined "toxic" effects of dextran on renal tubular cells. In a recently described case, however, renal impairment was thought to be related to a rise in plasma oncotic pressure, and it is theoretically possible that accumulation of any osmotically active substance in plasma could reduce GFR by opposing hydraulic effects in the glomerulus. Support for this mechanism came from the demonstration that acute reduction in plasma oncotic pressure by plasmapheresis produced a rapid recovery in renal function (Moran and Kapsner 1987). This interpretation has been challenged on the grounds that the colloid osmotic gradient across the glomerular walls would not be markedly increased. The renal effects of changes in colloid osmotic pressure produced by either albumin or dextran infusion are very complicated, and certainly warrant further study (Stein 1988).

Summary

This brief review highlights the problems faced by physicians managing critically ill patients. Few such patients will manage to avoid one or more of the known nephrotoxic agents described, and many other potential contributors to renal damage exist – other antibiotics, narcotics, prostaglandin inhibitors, vasoactive drugs and diuretics, to name only a few. Unceasing vigilance and careful study are required to reduce the toll of physician-induced disease.

References

Abel RM, Beck CH, Abbott WM, Ryan JA, Barnett GO, Fischer JE (1973) Improved survival from acute renal failure after treatment with intravenous essential L-amino acids and glucose. N Engl J Med 288: 695–699
Bennett WM, Wood CA, Houghton DC, Gilbert DN (1986) Modification of experimental aminoglycoside nephrotoxicity. Am J Kidney Dis 8: 292–296
Berkseth RO, Kjellstrand CM (1984) Radiologic contrast-induced nephropathy. Med Clin North Am 68: 351–370
Churchill D, Knaack J, Chirito E, Barre P, Cole G (1974) Persisting renal insufficiency after methoxyflurane anaesthesia. Am J Med 56: 575–581
Coggins CH, Fang LST (1983a) In: Brenner BM, Lazarus MG (eds) Acute renal failure. WB Saunders, Philadelphia, p 284
Coggins CH, Fang LST (1983b) In: Brenner BM, Lazarus MG (eds) Acute renal failure. WB Saunders, Philadelphia, pp 308–310
Cousins MJ, Mazze RI (1973) Methoxyflurane nephrotoxicity. Study of dose response in man. JAMA 225: 1611–1616
Cramer BC, Parfrey PS, Hutchinson TA et al. (1985) Renal function following infusion of radiologic contrast material. Arch Intern Med 145: 87–89
DeBroe ME, Paulus GJ, Verpooten GA et al. (1984) Early effects of gentamicin, tobramycin and amikacin on the human kidney. Kidney Int 25: 643–652
Fang LS, Sirota RA, Ebert TH, Lichtenstein NS (1980) Low fractional excretion of sodium with contrast media induced acute renal failure. Arch Intern Med 140: 531–535
Heidemann HT, Gerkens JF, Spickard WA, Jackson EK, Branch RA (1983) Amphotericin-B nephrotoxicity in humans decreased by salt repletion. Am J Med 75: 476–481
Jevnikar AM, Finnie KJC, Dennis B, Plummer DT, Avila A, Linton AL (1988) Nephrotoxicity of high- and low-osmolality contrast media. Nephron 48: 300–305
Koffler A, Friedler RM, Massry SG (1976) Acute renal failure due to non-traumatic rhabdomyolytis. Ann Intern Med 85: 23–28
Kumar S, Hull JD, Lathi S, Cohen AJ, Pletka PG (1981) Low incidence of renal failure after angiography. Arch Intern Med 141: 1268–1270
Linton AL, Clark WF, Driedger AA, Turnbull DI, Lindsay RM (1980) Acute interstitial nephritis due to drugs. Ann Intern Med 93: 735–741
Linton AL, Richmond JM, Clark WF, Lindsay RM, Driedger AA, Lamki LM (1985) Gallium[67] scintigraphy in the diagnosis of acute renal disease. Clin Nephrol 24: 84–87
Mandal A, Mize GN, Birnbaum DB (1987) Transmission electron microscopy of urinary sediment in aminoglycoside nephrotoxicity. Renal Failure 10: 63–81
Meyer RD (1986) Risk factors and comparisons of clinical nephrotoxicity of aminoglycosides. Am J Med 80 Suppl 6B: 119–125
Moran M, Kapsner C (1987) Acute renal failure associated with elevated plasma oncotic pressure. N Engl J Med 317: 150–153
Reid GM, Muther RS (1987) Nitroprusside-induced acute azotemia. Am J Nephrol 7: 313–315
Richmond JM, Sibbald WJ, Linton AM, Linton AL (1982) Patterns of urinary protein excretion in patients with sepsis. Nephron 31: 219–223
Smith CR, Moore RD, Lightman PS (1986) Studies of risk factors for aminoglycoside nephrotoxicity. Am J Kidney Dis VIII: 308–313
Stanley TH, Gray NG, Bidwai AV et al. (1974) The effects of high dose morphine and morphine plus nitrous oxide on urinary output in man. Can Anaesth Soc J 24: 379–384
Stein HD (1988) Letter to Editor. N Engl J Med 318: 253

Takacs FJ, Tomkeiwicz ZM, Merrill JP (1963) Amphotericin-B nephrotoxicity with irreversible renal failure. Ann Intern Med 59: 717–722
Teixeira RB, Kelley J, Alpert H, Pardo V, Vaamonde CA (1982) Complete protection from gentamicin-induced acute renal failure in the diabetes mellitus rat. Kidney Int 21: 600–612
Teruel JL, Marcen R, Onaindia JM, Serrano A, Quereda C, Ortuna J (1981) Renal function impairment caused by intravenous urography. Arch Intern Med 141: 1271–1274
Whelton A, Stout RL, Franklin W, Delgado F, Solez K (1981) Castration prevents gentamicin-induced acute renal failure and tubular necrosis in Fischer rats. Abstr Eighth Int Cong Nephrol (Athens) p 200
Zager RA (1987) Amino acid hyperalimentation in acute renal failure. A potential therapeutic paradox. Kidney Int 32 Suppl 22: S72–S75
Zipser RD, Henrich WL (1986) Implications of nonsteroidal anti-inflammatory drug therapy. Am J Med 80 Suppl 1A: 78–84

Discussion

Dr Kleinknecht opened the discussion by emphasizing that the data obtained from the French collaborative study demonstrated that nine out of the ten patients who developed acute renal failure in association with the administration of aminoglycosides, received these drugs on an incorrect basis – too great a dosage for too long, without close monitoring, and in the presence of several other risk factors for the development of renal dysfunction.

The discussion then turned to vasodilators in the intensive care unit; both Dr Bion and Dr Linton addressed the problem of dopamine. Dr Linton described it as somewhat akin to "holy water". There was a general concern that little evidence was available to support the notion that dopamine acts as a vasodilator in critically ill patients. Dr Myers described a study that his group had performed in patients following cardiac surgery. This study, published in *Kidney International* had demonstrated that following cardiac surgery patients who were vasodilated with nitroprusside had a decrease in their glomerular filtration rate and in the driving pressure from the glomerular capillary into Bowman's capsule in parallel with the decrease in arterial pressure. Dr Myers had also studied dopamine in this setting and claimed that there was no question that dopamine, when given in a so-called "renal protective dose", does not increase plasma flow. The Stanford group had measured plasma flow and it had remained unchanged. Nevertheless, there was, and often is, a rather striking diuresis and natriuresis which is almost certainly an action of dopamine and reflects the inhibition of water and sodium transport, mainly in the proximal tubule. Thus, an increase in urine flow rate associated with low-dose dopamine therapy is not necessarily a vasoactive effect; it is more likely that in shocked patients with a low cardiac output or a low blood pressure, the spontaneously activated vasoconstrictor influences associated with acute circulatory failure simply over-ride the dopaminergic action on the renal and splanchnic circulations.

Dr Myers then turned his attention to the dextran issue. He emphasized that the point of the paper published in the *New England Journal of Medicine* was to demonstrate that an increase in colloid osmotic pressure associated with dextran therapy, can prevent glomerular filtration just by reducing ΔP (the driving pressure from the glomerular capillary into the Bowman's capsule). From the measurements made in the patient reported, it appeared that when the blood colloid osmotic pressure rose to somewhere above 30–32 mmHg, anuria developed. Following plasmapheresis and the withdrawal of dextran therapy, glomerular filtration resumed at a colloid oncotic pressure of 28 mmHg. Thus, it seems that ΔP in man is somewhere between 28 and 32 mmHg.

The discussion turned to the nephrotoxicity traditionally associated with radiocontrast media. Dr Linton stated that he had undergone a conversion since he thought that contrast nephropathy was rare in clinical situations now. Whether it was different 5 years ago, was difficult to say, but Dr Solez reported that a debate at the Edmonton meeting had ended when most investigators including Carl Kjellstrand had agreed that contrast nephropathy had probably been over emphasized in the past.

Chapter 15

Nature of Postischaemic Renal Injury Following Aortic or Cardiac Surgery

B. D. Myers

Introduction

Three decades have elapsed since surgical correction of abdominal aortic aneurysms and cardiac valvular disease was first undertaken. Throughout the 1950s and early 1960s such surgery was associated with intense renal vasospasm. At least one-third of patients exhibited prolonged postoperative oligoanuria and 20% went on to die of acute renal failure (ARF). By 1963 this field of surgery was transformed by the discovery that intraoperative infusion of hypertonic mannitol largely prevented oliguria and ARF in patients undergoing abdominal aortic aneurysmectomy (Barry et al. 1961). Soon after, mannitol infusion was applied to open cardiac surgery. Once again, oligoanuria was overcome and the incidence of postcardiac surgical ARF sharply reduced (Dobernak et al. 1962). Today, the overall incidence of ARF following abdominal aortic or open cardiac surgery has been reduced to 5% or less in large, experienced centres (Abbott 1980; McCombs and Roberts 1979; Hilberman et al. 1979; Abel et al. 1976). However, because prophylactic mannitol together with other advances in anaesthesia and surgery have greatly increased the frequency of these surgical procedures, they remain among the commonest discrete causes of haemodynamically mediated ARF, nevertheless.

The past three decades have also witnessed an explosive growth in our knowledge and understanding of the pathophysiology of postischaemic renal injury. The development of analogues in experimental animals of the transient renal ischaemia that is encountered during aortic and cardiac surgery has revealed a complex postischaemic injury to both tubules and renal microvessels. This injury has been shown to dissipate glomerular transcapillary ultrafiltration pressure, resulting in a profound reduction in the rate of glomerular ultrafiltration (GFR) (Arendshorst et al. 1976; Tanner and Sophasan 1976; Hanley and

Davidson 1981; Burke et al. 1980). The capacity of the kidney to excrete nitrogenous and other waste solutes in final urine is compromised further by downstream backleak of filtered fluid through necrotic tubular walls (Arendshorst et al. 1976; Tanner and Sophasan 1976; Hanley and Davidson 1981; Burke et al. 1980). The reduction of ultrafiltration pressure and extent of backleak are most marked during the post-initiation or maintenance stage of ARF, and tend to improve during the subsequent stage of recovery (Eisenbach and Steinhausen 1973; Finn and Chevalier 1979). When protective measures, including mannitol and saline volume expansion, are taken prior to the ischaemic event, the severity of the injury is blunted and its course greatly abbreviated. Thus ARF in a setting of renoprotection differs substantially from unprotected ARF, despite an equivalent renal ischaemic insult. Differences include a high rather than low rate of urine flow, modest rather than extreme glomerular hypofiltration and a maintenance stage that persists for hours only rather than days or weeks (Hanley and Davidson 1981; Burke et al. 1980; Patak et al. 1979).

The purpose of this chapter is to review those mechanisms of filtration failure that operate in the postischaemic ARF that follows either abdominal aortic or open cardiac surgery. Access to the renal arteries and veins during abdominal aortic surgery greatly enhances the precision with which renal blood flow can be determined. I propose, therefore, to review first findings in our laboratory which elucidate the early initiation phase of ARF in patients undergoing such aortic surgery. I will then review findings in the postoperative period following open cardiac surgery. Although the approach used in this latter setting is more indirect, it helps clarify why some patients continue to develop a prolonged maintenance stage of ARF, notwithstanding the adoption of renoprotective measures during cardiopulmonary bypass.

Methods

Study Protocol

Abdominal Aortic Surgery

Thirty patients were studied during surgical repair of an aneurysmal or partially occluded atheromatous abdominal aorta. In 15, the repair procedure was associated with mechanical interruption of renal blood flow for 48 ± 8 min (mean$\pm$ISD) by suprarenal aortic clamping. The aorta was cross-clamped below the renal arteries in the remaining 15 patients. Neither age, 62 ± 9 vs 65 ± 9 years, nor total duration of surgery, 322 ± 63 vs 268 ± 58 min (mean$\pm$ISD) differed significantly between the two groups. Anaesthesia was maintained with ethrane or halothane; 12.5 g of 20% mannitol was administered hourly i.v. during preparation of the surgical field until the aorta was cross-clamped. Saline and/or Ringer's lactate was infused to lower haematocrit by between 12% and 16% below preoperative levels.

Open Cardiac Surgery

We have shown previously that only 5% of patients develop postoperative ARF following cardiopulmonary bypass, during which renal perfusion pressure is lowered to only approx. 50 mmHg, and renal perfusion rate falls by approx. 75% (Hilberman et al. 1979). Renoprotection during cardiopulmonary bypass is afforded by the same regimen of mannitol/crystalloid infusion as described above for abdominal aortic surgery. However, the postcardiac operative period differs from that following aortic surgery in that cardiac performance is frequently depressed in the former (Myers et al. 1980). This in turn, extends the period of renal underperfusion beyond that associated with the cardiac surgical procedure *per se*. Renoprotection in the early postoperative period includes cardiac preloading (volume expansion), afterload reduction (sodium nitroprusside infusion) and infusion of dopamine and frusemide in dosages designed to lower renovascular resistance and promote high rates of tubule fluid and urine flow. Fifty consecutive patients developing postoperative ARF under this regimen are the subjects of the present report. Renal physiological measurements were performed between postoperative days 4 and 7. A model of creatinine kinetics that has been described elsewhere (Moran and Myers 1985a) was used to classify the ARF in each patient into one of two types. Type A, or abbreviated ARF, refers to a course in which no maintenance stage is discernible; the initiation stage is followed directly by a stage of recovery. This was diagnosed in 27 instances. Type B, or overt ARF, refers to a course in which the initiation stage is followed by a maintenance stage that lasts for 7 days or more. It was encountered in the remaining 23 cases. Fifty additional patients making an uneventful recovery from cardiac surgery served as controls.

Physiological Determinations

Urinary clearances were performed during sustaining infusions of the clearance markers. Three or more urine collections were made at 30-min intervals through an indwelling bladder catheter. Blood was sampled from an intravascular radial arterial line at the midpoint of each urine collection. Inulin together with P-aminohippurate (PAH) were used to measure the glomerular filtration and renal plasma flow rates (RPF), respectively. RPF during aortic surgery was determined by dividing PAH clearance by its simultaneously measured renal arterio-venous extraction ratio. In control postoperative patients and those recovering from ARF (Type A) the PAH extraction ratio was assumed to be 0.8 and 0.7, respectively (Myers et al. 1984). All patients were also infused with a polydispersed solution of neutral dextran 40 (130 mg kg^{-1}). The fractional clearance of dextrans of graded size (relative to inulin) was determined after subjecting blood and urine to gel permeation chromatography, and assaying the dextran concentration in each eluate with anthrone (Myers et al. 1984). Arterial hydraulic pressure was determined by connecting the radial arterial line to a transducer. Cardiac pressures and flows were measured by standard techniques as described elsewhere (Myers et al. 1980). Oncotic pressure of arterial plasma was taken to be the same as that in afferent glomerular arterioles (π_a) and determined directly by membrane osmometry using a Weil oncometer (IL no. 196, Lexington, MA). Finally, plasma renin activity and a renal renin secretion ratio (RSR) were determined before and after application of the aortic cross-clamp; RSR = [Vr−Ar/Ar] × 100, where Vr and Ar are respectively renin activity in renal venous and radial arterial plasma.

Data Analysis

Normal values for glomerular filtration rate and its determinants were obtained by studying 21 healthy, adult volunteers while at bed rest. Differences from normal in fractional dextran clearances of patients undergoing aortic surgery were interpreted in terms of a theoretical model of transcapillary solute flux that has been described previously (Myers et al. 1988). It is based on a hydrodynamic theory of transport of neutral macromolecules through an isoporous glomerular capillary wall (Chang et al. 1975). The model assumes that pore radius (computed to be 56 Å in normal subjects) is not altered during aortic or following cardiac surgery. It also includes mass balance relations that predict variations in concentrations and fluxes of the probe dextran molecules along the length of the glomerular capillary. Since GFR, RPF and π_a are known, it becomes possible to use a curve-fitting technique to predict the reciprocal changes in transcapillary hydraulic pressure difference (ΔP) and the ultrafiltration coefficient (K_f) that are required to explain observed alterations in the transglomerular flux of water (inulin clearance) and solutes (fractional dextran clearance) (Myers et al. 1988). The significance of differences in measured pressures and flows were evaluated with an analysis of variance (ANOVA) using the CLINFO system. All results are expressed as the means±SEM.

Findings and Comments

Infrarenal Aortic Clamping

Intra- and postoperative findings are compared to those of healthy controls in Table 15.1. All tabulated intraoperative findings were determined between 20 and 120 min following release of the aortic clamp. Mannitol/saline infusion had resulted in an elevated serum osmolality (291±3 vs a preoperative level of

Table 15.1. Filtration dynamics during aortic infrarenal clamping

	Hct	Δ Weight	V̇	GFR	RPF	MAP	π_a
	(%)		(ml min^{-1} 1.73 m^{-2})			(mmHg)	
Healthy controls	45 ± 1	–	6.2±1.0	105±5	574±33	88±2	24.2±0.9
Aortic Surgical Patients							
Intraoperative	35±2[a]	ND	3.2±0.8[a]	59±7[a]	407±66[a]	82±2	14.3±0.7[a]
24 h postoperative	39±1[b]	+6.7±0.1	1.8±0.5[b]	84±8[b]	467±67	95±4[b]	17.7±0.7[b]

Hct, haematocrit; V̇, urine flow rate; GFR, glomerular filtration rate; RPF, renal plasma flow rate; MAP, mean arterial pressure; π_a, afferent oncotic pressure.
  [a] $p<0.01$, intraoperative vs controls.
  [b] $p<0.01$, post- vs intraoperative.

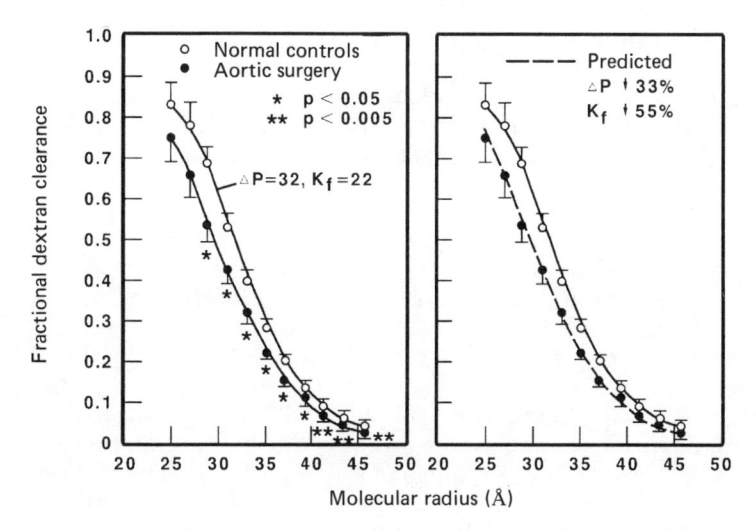

Fig. 15.1. *Left panel*: fractional dextran clearances during aortic surgery are compared with those of normal controls. *Right panel*: a theoretical model predicts (*heavy dashed line*) that a decline in ΔP by 33% and of K_f by 55% below control values will replicate the depression of fractional clearances observed during aortic surgery.

281±1 mosm (kg H_2O)$^{-1}$, $p<0.01$) and haemodilution (Hct 35±2 vs 42±1% preoperatively, $p<0.01$). A high rate of urine flow and access to the renal vein permitted accurate determination of GFR and RPF. The former was depressed respectively below control and unanaesthetized postoperative levels by 44% and 30%. Corresponding depression of RPF was more modest, 29% and 13%, respectively. Haemodilution lowered intraoperative π_a to only 14.3 mmHg, a finding that should have increased intraoperative GFR and filtration fraction, and not depressed them as was observed. It follows that depression of ΔP and/or K_f must have been implicated in the intraoperative hypofiltration.

Intraoperative fractional dextran clearances are compared to those of healthy, conscious controls in Fig. 15.1. As shown, transglomerular dextran transport was depressed over virtually the entire range of molecular radii examined. When measured GFR, RPF and π_a are taken into account, the value of ΔP that minimizes the sum of chi squares between the fractional dextran clearances measured in healthy controls and those depicted by the isoporous model is 32 mmHg. Although this value may not be accurate to within a few mmHg, it provides a basis for estimating the magnitude of change in ΔP following infrarenal aortic clamping. As indicated by the heavy dashed line in the right panel of Fig. 15.1, the fractional dextran clearance profile during aortic surgery is replicated by the model when ΔP is allowed to fall below the putative control value by 33% (to 22 mmHg); the predicted, corresponding decline in K_f is by 55% (from a control value of 22.2 to 9.9 ml (min mmHg)$^{-1}$). Thus ultrafiltration pressure in these mannitol/saline loaded patients was maintained high by an effect of lowered π_a to offset the reduction in ΔP during aortic surgery. Maintenance of a high ultrafiltration pressure permitted a relatively rapid GFR despite the lowered K_f. The efficacy of renoprotection is evidenced by a nearly normal GFR 24 hours postoperatively (Table 15.1), and by the absence of azotaemia in all patients throughout the first postoperative week.

Suprarenal Aortic Clamping

Aortic surgery associated with suprarenal clamping lowered GFR more profoundly than with infrarenal clamping. As shown in Fig. 15.2, GFR declined by more than 50% in 13/15 patients *before* application of the suprarenal cross-clamp (left lower panel). The corresponding number in whom GFR declined by >50% before application of the infrarenal cross-clamp was only 5/15 (left upper panel). Following release of the cross-clamp GFR returned to >50% of the preoperative value in all but 3 of the infrarenal group (right upper panel). In contrast, postclamp GFR remained profoundly depressed in all 15 members of the suprarenal group (right lower panel).

Potential determinants of postischaemic GFR reduction following suprarenal clamping are summarized in Table 15.2. Whereas GFR was only 39% of the corresponding value following infrarenal clamping, RPF was reduced only slightly. Thus, suprarenal clamping leads to a profound fall in filtration fraction (0.07 ± 0.01 vs 0.17 ± 0.02, $p<0.001$). As shown in Table 15.2, π_a is low and not different between the two groups, and so cannot be invoked to explain the depressed GFR and filtration fraction following suprarenal clamping. By exclusion, either reduction of ΔP or K_f, or some combination of the two could be implicated in the hypofiltration. A significant impairment of PAH extraction and urinary concentration points to an attendant injury to proximal and distal tubules

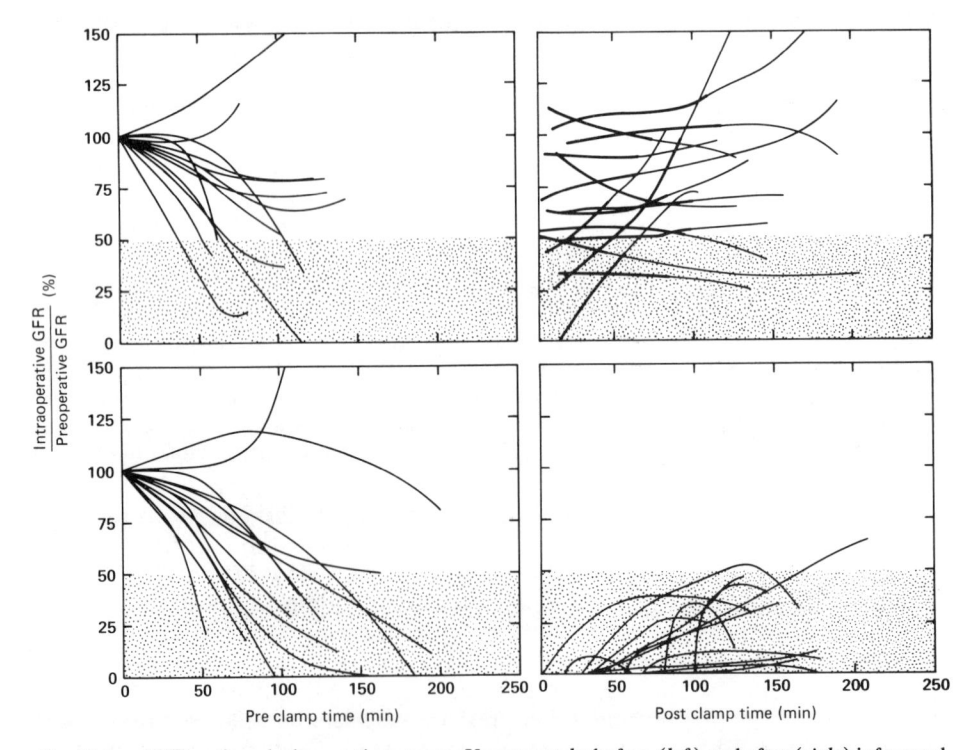

Fig. 15.2. GFR vs time during aortic surgery. *Upper panels*: before (*left*) and after (*right*) infrarenal clamping. *Lower panels*: before (*left*) and after (*right*) suprarenal clamping. A curve-smoothing technique has been used to reflect change in serial inulin clearances.

(Table 15.2). The combination of filtration failure and tubular injury is typical of postischaemic ARF. Because transtubular backleak is likely to be associated with such injury, we have not attempted to compute the extent of $\Delta P/K_f$ reduction from the dextran sieving profile.

Table 15.2. Vascular and tubular effects of suprarenal aortic clamping (30–120 min postclamp)

	Infrarenal	Suprarenal	p value
RPF (ml min^{-1} 1.73 m^{-2})	406 ± 66	331 ± 71	NS
GFR (ml min^{-1} 1.73 m^{-2})	59 ± 7	23 ± 5	<0.001
Filtration fraction	0.17 ± 0.02	0.07 ± 0.01	<0.001
π_a (mmHg)	14.3 ± 0.7	14.6 ± 0.8	NS
PAH extraction	0.70 ± 0.04	0.43 ± 0.07	<0.005
U/P osmolality	1.42 ± 0.09	1.15 ± 0.05	<0.02

The trend towards transient hypofiltration in the infrarenal group and the more marked GFR reduction in the suprarenal group were associated with extreme elevation in plasma renin activity and renal RSR (Fig. 15.3). Given the normal renal perfusion pressure and state of volume expansion (Table 15.1) it seems likely that enhanced activity of the renin–angiotensin system even before application of a cross-clamp, reflects an increase in renal sympathetic efferent nerve traffic consequent upon anaesthesia, laparotomy and manipulation of the aorta. Although no clear difference in renin activity and RSR is evident between members of the infrarenal and suprarenal groups, it is conceivable that sympathetic nervous influences upon GFR are more intense when the upper abdominal aorta and origin of the renal arteries are manipulated, as was the case in the suprarenal group.

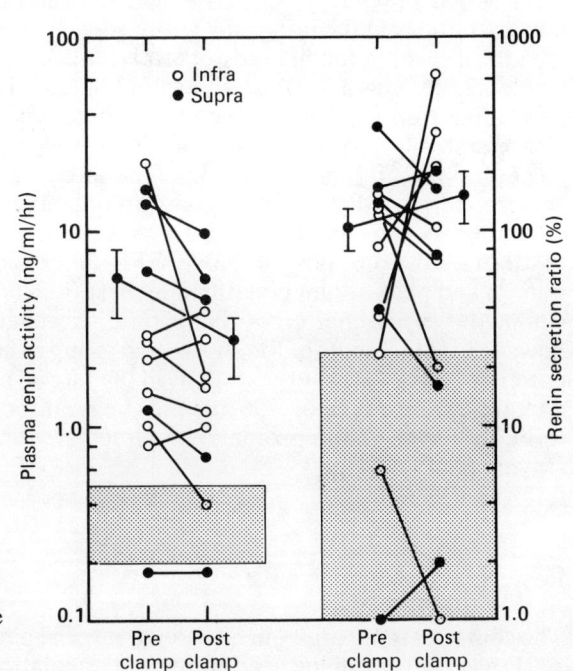

Fig. 15.3. Plasma renin activity (*left*) and renin secretion ratio (*right*) before and after aortic clamping. The *shaded zones* represent the normal range on a high Na$^+$ intake.

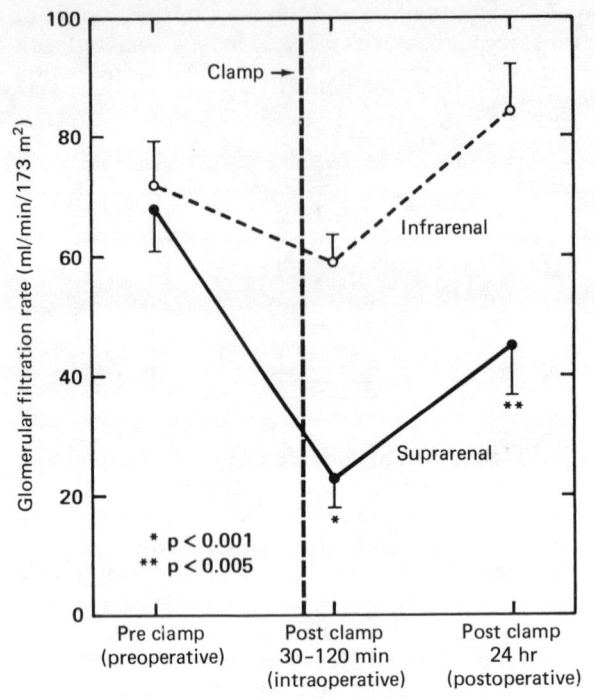

Fig. 15.4. GFR vs time following infrarenal (○) or suprarenal (●) aortic clamping.

As stated previously, the GFR had returned to a nearly normal range 24 h postoperatively in the infrarenal group (Fig. 15.4). The peak postoperative serum creatinine level in the first postoperative week was the same as the preoperative level, 1.2 ± 0.1 mg dl^{-1}. Also shown in Fig. 15.4 is the course of injury following suprarenal clamping. The onset of the recovery stage was clearly evident 24 h postoperatively. Mean GFR had increased from 23 ± 5 intraoperatively to 45 ± 8 ml min^{-1} 1.73m^{-2} ($p<0.01$). The latter value was significantly below the corresponding GFR following infrarenal clamping, however. Mean serum creatinine level peaked at 2.3 ± 0.4 vs a preoperative level of 1.2 ± 0.1 mg dl^{-1} ($p<0.01$). Of note, postoperative GFR depression was most marked (8–20 ml min^{-1}) and peak serum creatinine highest (4.2–5.8 mg dl^{-1}) in 4 of 5 patients in whom the suprarenal cross-clamp time exceeded 50 min. Without exception, however, all members of the suprarenal group exhibited an abbreviated (Type A) pattern of ARF. This suggests that, in the face of mannitol/saline renoprotection, a total ischaemic time of >90 min may be required for the initiation stage of ARF to be followed by the prolonged maintenance stage that typifies Type B ARF (Myers et al. 1984).

Postcardiac Surgical ARF

The course of renal injury in 50 cardiac surgical patients developing postoperative ARF has been computerized using a mathematical model of creatinine kinetics

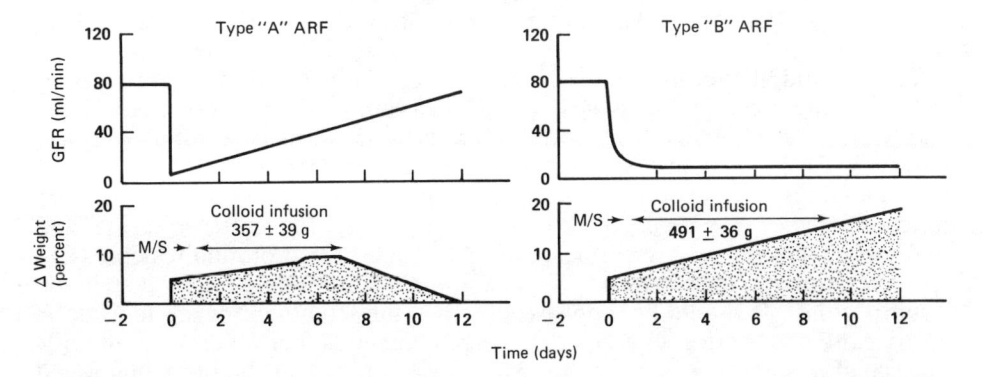

Fig. 15.5. Course of ARF following cardiac surgery in 50 patients. Twenty-seven patients exhibited Type A injury (*left*) and 23 Type B injury (*right*). Changes in computed GFR are in upper panel. Weight change and fluid infusion regimens are in lower panel. M/S, mannitol/saline expansion.

(Moran and Myers 1985a). As shown in Fig. 15.5, 27 cases exhibited an abbreviated Type A injury, which is characterized by a step decrement in GFR associated with cardiopulmonary bypass, followed promptly by a ramp-like recovery. As may be seen below the GFR panel in Fig. 15.5, mannitol/saline volume expansion to 5% body weight on the day of surgery was replaced on subsequent days by colloid volume expansion. On average 353 g of protein was infused by postoperative day 7, with an attendant increase in body weight by 9%. A more protracted Type B injury was observed in the remaining 23 patients. An exponential decline in GFR was followed after postoperative day 2 by a low GFR plateau, representing the maintenance stage of ARF. A greater infusion of colloid (491 g protein) was required to maintain an adequate circulation, and resulted in a 15% increase in body weight above preoperative values. Despite the greater preloading and a comparable afterload, cardiac performance was clearly inferior to that associated with Type A renal injury (Fig. 15.6). Profound reduction of stroke volume and stroke work indices point to prolonged and severe

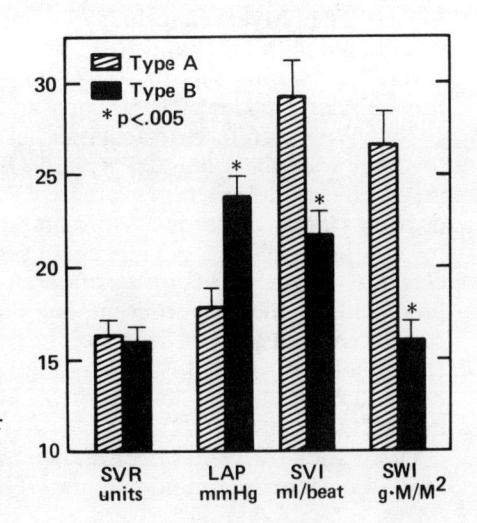

Fig. 15.6. Cardiac performance on postoperative day 4–7 in patients with Type A (*hatched bars*) vs Type B (*black bars*) ARF. SVR, systemic vascular resistance; LAP, left atrial filling pressure (from occlusion pulmonary artery pressure); SVI, stroke volume index; SWI, stroke work index.

postoperative left ventricular dysfunction in those who exhibited Type B renal injury.

Tubular and glomerular function are summarized in Table 15.3. Both groups were non-oliguric, a finding typical of ARF in a setting of renoprotection (Myers and Moran 1986; Myers et al. 1982). Reflecting more marked tubular injury, however, Type B patients exhibited isosthenuria, and excreted a high fraction of the filtered sodium load. By contrast, and in keeping with recovering tubular function, Type A patients elaborated a relatively concentrated urine and reabsorbed filtered sodium efficiently. Although still profoundly depressed, inulin clearance in the recovering Type A group was three-fold higher than in the Type B group. It should be emphasized that serum creatinine levels in Type A injury continued to rise for 4 or 5 days despite the linear daily increment in GFR illustrated in Fig. 15.5. It is not surprising, therefore, that the aforementioned urinary indices frequently lead to a misdiagnosis of prerenal failure in Type A ARF (Moran and Myers 1985a).

Table 15.3. Tubular and glomerular function in postoperative acute renal failure

	Controls	Type A ARF	Type B ARF
Urine flow (ml min^{-1})	1.9 ± 0.2	1.7 ± 0.3	1.6 ± 0.2
Urine-to-plasma osmolality	1.94 ± 0.07	1.35 ± 0.05[a]	1.06 ± 0.03[ab]
Urine-to-plasma inulin	80.8 ± 10.6	30.2 ± 6.2[a]	12.0 ± 3.0[ab]
Fractional excretion of sodium (%)	1.2 ± 0.2	1.9 ± 0.6	7.7 ± 1.5[ab]
Glomerular filtration rate (ml min^{-1} 1.73 m^{-2})	97 ± 3	36 ± 3[a]	11 ± 1[ab]
PAH clearance (ml min^{-1} 1.73 m^{-2})	473 ± 23	297 ± 46[a]	74 ± 10[ab]
Afferent oncotic pressure (mmHg)	20.3 ± 0.3	21.5 ± 0.5	25.3 ± 0.8[a]
Mean arterial pressure (mmHg)	87 ± 2	79 ± 1[a]	78 ± 2[a]

[a] $p<0.01$ vs normal.
[b] $p<0.01$ vs Type B vs Type A.

We have shown previously that the maintenance stage of Type B injury is probably associated with transtubular backleak of clearance markers (Moran and Myers 1985b; Myers et al. 1979). Accordingly, inulin and PAH clearances cannot be equated with GFR and RPF, respectively. In contrast, Type A injury that is several days into the recovery stage should no longer be associated with transtubular backleak (Eisenbach and Steinhausen 1973; Finn and Chevalier 1979). We, therefore, calculated RPF from PAH clearance and applied it together with the values of π_a and GFR listed in Table 15.3 to the isoporous membrane model, so as to evaluate ΔP and K_f in recovering Type A injury by the dextran sieving technique. Our computations are illustrated in Fig. 15.7, which reveals that dextran sieving coefficients in Type A patients were uniformly elevated above those of postoperative controls. The best fit sieving curve predicted by the isoporous model suggests that an increase in diffusive and convective transport of dextran is best accounted for by a decline in ΔP by 13% combined with the 48% of reduction in estimated RPF. A simultaneous depression of K_f contributes to the low GFR observed in recovering Type A injury (Deen et al. 1972).

Depression of ΔP has been shown by micropuncture determinations to be the most important determinant of low GFR in animals with experimental postischae-

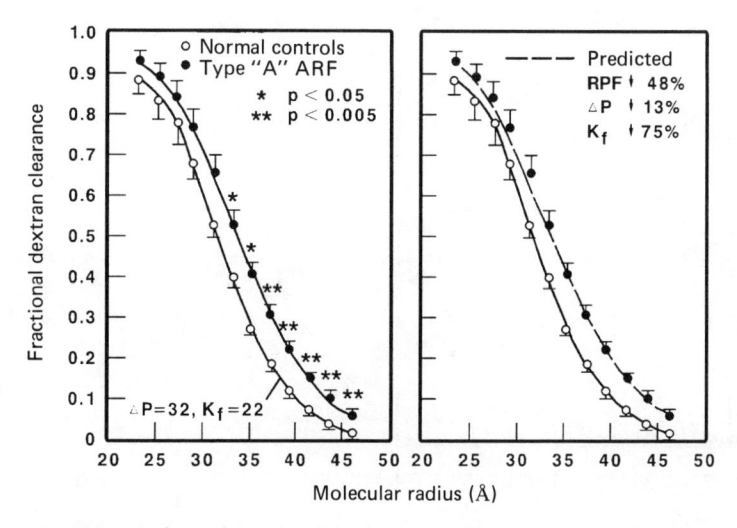

Fig. 15.7. *Left panel*: fractional dextran clearances in Type A ARF are compared with postoperative controls. *Right panel*: a theoretical model predicts (heavy dashed line) that a decline in ΔP by 13% combined with a fall in K_f by 75% and the measured depression of RPF by 48% replicates the elevation of fractional clearances observed in Type A ARF.

mic ARF (Arendshorst et al. 1976; Burke et al. 1980). It seems reasonable to infer that ΔP in Type B patients was if anything, lower than the 28 mmHg computed for Type A injury. It is especially noteworthy, therefore, that our practice of colloid volume expansion in the postoperative period led to elevation of π_a in the Type B group to 25.3 mmHg on average (Table 15.3). It follows that the net pressure for ultrafiltration at the afferent end of the glomerular capillary network ($\Delta P - \pi_a$) must have been depressed to below 3 mmHg, thereby contributing substantially to the profoundly low inulin clearance of only 11 ml min^{-1} 1.73m^{-2}. Inspection of Fig. 15.8 reveals that π_a exceeds 28 mmHg in a substantial fraction of Type B patients, a phenomenon not observed in postoperative controls, and potentially capable of abolishing net ultrafiltration pressure entirely. From the sieving data in milder Type A injury, we infer that profound depression of ultrafiltration pressure combined with low K_f accounts for the sustained hypofiltration that characterizes the maintenance stage of postoperative Type B ARF.

Conclusions

The adoption of renoprotective measures appears to have increased the threshold above which the kidney will exhibit postischaemic injury that is clinically detectable following aortic or cardiac surgery. Should the surgical procedure itself constitute the only ischaemic insult, the ensuing ARF is observed to be abbreviated (Type A) and to lack a discernible maintenance stage. More sustained perioperative renal ischaemia (for example, the preoperative rupture

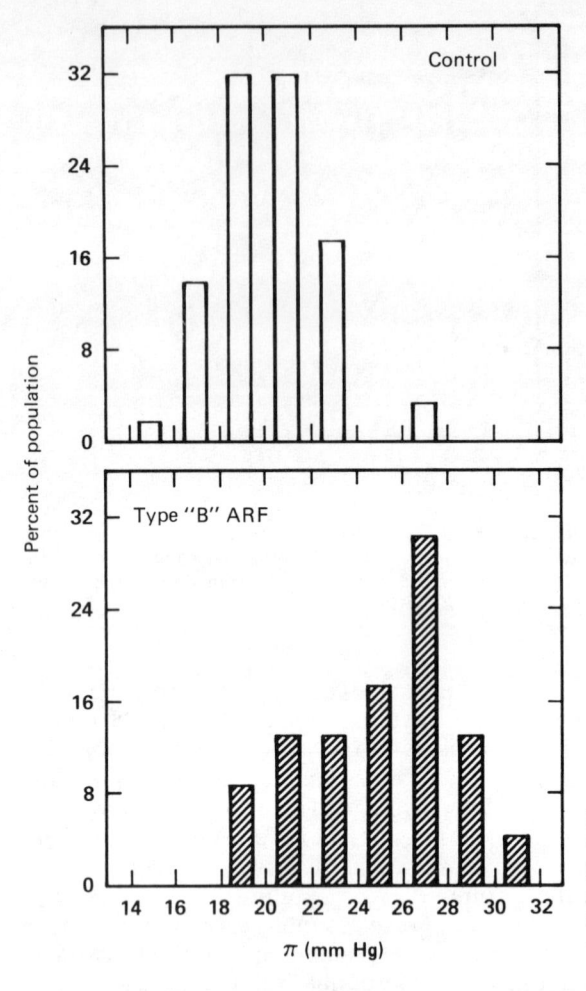

Fig. 15.8. Distribution of plasma oncotic pressure in non-azotaemic, postcardiac surgical controls (*upper panel*) compared with massively colloid-infused patients with Type B ARF (*lower panel*).

of an aortic aneurysm or a prolonged low cardiac output state in the postoperative period) seems to be a necessary condition for the development of ARF that is accompanied by a protracted maintenance stage (Type B). Even under these conditions renoprotection offers therapeutic benefit. A non-oliguric course and preservation of a useful, albeit low level of GFR, greatly facilitates patient management.

Renoprotection is widely held to operate by lowering renovascular resistance and preserving tubular cell integrity. Whereas these effects are without doubt important, the potential role of π_a in the filtration failure that typifies ARF has been largely neglected. This is because micropuncture studies of ARF in experimental animals have been performed under standardized conditions during which π_a has varied little. Our findings clearly indicate that the GFR-sparing effect of intraoperative renoprotection with mannitol/saline volume expansion is partly a consequence of haemodilution, with an ensuing reduction of intraglomerular capillary oncotic pressure (Tables 15.1 and 15.2). This particular protective effect is likely to be short-lived if massive colloid infusion is employed in the postoperative period, however. When recovery from a postischaemic renal injury is not rapid, ΔP is likely to remain at a fixed low level, partly because of preglomerular vasoconstriction, and partly because of tubular obstruction (Arendshorst et al. 1976; Tanner and Sophasan 1976; Burke et al. 1980; Tanner and Knopp 1986). An effect of colloid infusion rapidly to increase π_a could then dissipate the net pressure for ultrafiltration, thereby lowering GFR and perhaps prolonging the ARF (Deen et al. 1972). The use of colloid volume expansion to minimize positive fluid balance is widespread in the setting of haemodynamically mediated ARF. Because it can contribute to prolonged filtration failure, we propose that the place of colloid infusion in the management of patients with postischaemic ARF be carefully reappraised.

Acknowledgement. This study was supported by National Institutes of Health grant AM29985.

References

Abel RM, Buckley MJ, Austen WG et al. (1976) Etiology, incidence, and prognosis of renal failure following cardiac operations. J Thorac Cardiovasc Surg 71: 333–343
Abbott WM (1980) Renal failure complicating vascular surgery. In: Bernhard VM, Towne JB (eds) Complications in vascular surgery. Grune & Stratton, New York, pp 363–377
Arendshorst WJ, Finn WF, Gottschalk CW (1976) Micropuncture study of acute renal failure following temporary renal ischemia in the rat. Kidney Int 10, Suppl 6: S100–S105
Barry KG, Cohen A, Knochel JP et al. (1961) Mannitol infusion. II. The prevention of acute functional renal failure during resection of an aneurysm of the abdominal aorta. N Engl J Med 264: 967–971
Burke TJ, Cronin RE, Duchin KL et al. (1980) Ischemia and tubule obstruction during acute renal failure in dogs: mannitol in protection. Am J Physiol 238: F305–F314
Chang RLS, Robertson CR, Deen WM et al. (1975) Permselectivity of the glomerular capillary wall to macromolecules. I. Theoretical considerations. Biophys J 15: 861–886
Deen WM, Robertson CR, Brenner BM (1972) A model of glomerular ultrafiltration in the rat. Am J Physiol 223: 1178–1183
Dobernak RD, Reiser MP, Lillehie CW (1962) Acute renal failure after open-heart surgery utilizing extracorporeal circulation and total body perfusion. Analysis of 1000 patients. J Thorac Cardiovasc Surg 43: 441–452
Eisenbach GM, Steinhausen M (1973) Micropuncture studies after temporary ischemia of rat kidneys. Pflugers Arch 343: 11–25
Finn WF, Chevalier RL (1979) Recovery from postischemic acute renal failure in the rat. Kidney Int 16: 113–123
Hanley MJ, Davidson K (1981) Prior mannitol and furosemide infusion in a model of ischemic acute renal failure. Am J Physiol 241: F556–F564
Hilberman M, Myers BD, Carrie BJ et al. (1979) Acute renal failure following cardiac surgery. J Thorac Cardiovasc Surg 77: 880–888
McCombs PR, Roberts B (1979) Acute renal failure following resection of abdominal aortic aneurysm. Surg Gynecol Obstet 148: 175–178
Moran SM, Myers BD (1985a) Course of acute renal failure studied by a model of creatinine kinetics. Kidney Int 27: 928–937
Moran SM, Myers BD (1985b) Pathophysiology of protracted acute renal failure in man. J Clin Invest 76: 1440–1448
Myers BD, Moran SM (1986) Hemodynamically mediated acute renal failure. N Engl J Med 314: 97–105
Myers BD, Chui F, Hilberman M et al. (1979) Transtubular leakage of glomerular filtrate in human acute renal failure. Am J Physiol F319–325
Myers BD, Carrie BJ, Yee RR et al. (1980) Pathophysiology of hemodynamically mediated acute renal failure in man. Kidney Int 18: 495–504

Myers BD, Hilberman M, Spencer RJ et al. (1982) Glomerular and tubular function in non-oliguric acute renal failure. Am J Med 72: 642–649

Myers BD, Miller DC, Mehigan JT et al. (1984) Nature of the renal injury following total renal ischemia in man. J Clin Invest 73: 329–341

Myers BD, Peterson C, Molina CR et al. (1988) Role of cardiac atria in the human renal response to changing plasma volume. Am J Physiol F562–573

Patak RV, Fadem SZ, Lifschitz MD et al. (1979) Study of factors which modify the development of norepinephrine-induced acute renal failure in the dog. Kidney Int 15: 227–237

Tanner GA, Knopp LC (1986) Glomerular blood flow after single nephron obstruction in the rat kidney. Am J Physiol 250: F77–F85

Tanner GA, Sophasan S (1976) Kidney pressures after temporary renal artery occlusion in the rat. Am J Physiol 230: 1173–1181

Discussion

Dr Myers was asked how much of the decrease in ΔP was related to an increase in intratubular pressure. He replied that an analysis by mass balances of the back leak suggested that this could account for about half the reduction in inulin clearance. However, it was impossible to sort out in man whether a change in ΔP was related to an obstructive element within the tubule or the effect of tubular glomerular feedback with spasm of the afferent arteriole and a decrease in intraglomerular pressure.

Professor Cameron referred to a study performed at Guy's Hospital in which renal venous blood was sampled in some patients and renal plasma flow (measured by para-amino hippurate clearance) correlated with the cardiac output. There was a very close correlation and he thought that the problem following cardiac surgery was essentially one of pump failure. Providing the cardiac output can be restored, then the kidney will recover over a variable period of time. Dr Myers was then asked about the concept of colloid osmotic pressure and the correlation of the pressure exerted by a protein in vivo, where the reflection coefficient (sigma, Σ) will reflect the presence and quantity of a negative charge on the capillary membrane, compared with measurements made in vitro using an uncharged Amicon filter. Dr Bihari suggested that the effective oncotic pressure might be quite different in vivo compared with measurements made in vitro. Dr Myers did not agree with this suggestion. Since the technique measured the transmembrane hydraulic pressure exerted by the movement of saline into the colloid-containing sample. This measurement had nothing to do with charge on the surface of capillary endothelium and was a physical force. Nevertheless, he agreed that the duration of cardiopulmonary bypass and aortic cross clamping was of considerable importance. There was no doubt that a prolonged bypass time was associated with changes in capillary permeability and if bypass was more than 320 minutes, then the incidence of other organ failure greatly increased. Dr Bihari then suggested that complement activation and the other changes associated with bypass might alter charge distribution within the microcirculation of various tissues and this could reduce the effectiveness of negatively charged proteins to exert a colloid oncotic effect, which would not be detected in vitro using an uncharged membrane.

Chapter 16

Acute Renal Failure in Sepsis

A. L. Linton

Acute deterioration in renal function is an extremely common clinical event and one which presents problems both of diagnosis and of treatment. As long ago as 1883 Andrew Clark in London, England described patients in whom "the kidney without any sensible alteration of structure cannot produce healthy urine" (Clark 1883). He also noted that the urine which was produced was of low density and low volume; this condition or one similar to it was extensively described by Bywaters and Beal (1941) in patients with crush injuries suffered during the London Blitz. This type of acute renal failure came to be known as acute tubular necrosis because of the pathological appearances found in the kidneys examined at that time.

Over the past two decades the literature on acute renal failure has been somewhat confused, partly because of semantic difficulties and partly because various experimental models behave differently in terms of pathogenesis, pathology, intervention and outcome. It has become generally accepted, however, that if one defines acute renal failure to include any cause of rapid deterioration in renal function whether or not oliguria is present, the process of differential diagnosis is primarily to decide whether the reduction in renal function is due to prerenal causes, renal causes or postrenal causes. Acute reduction in renal function can obviously follow a reduction in blood volume, reduction in cardiac output or hypotension with failure of renal autoregulation – these constitute the prerenal causes. Postrenal causes of acute deterioration in renal function consist of any of the multiple causes of obstruction to the urinary tract, while renal causes include acute tubular necrosis (or vasomotor nephropathy), primary parenchymal renal disease, and obstruction to the renal vasculature.

It is not within the scope of this chapter to discuss primary glomerular causes of acute renal failure since these can usually be readily distinguished by the different onset, the association with hypertension, and the presence of red cell casts in the urine. It is worth emphasizing that in any unexplained renal failure it is vital to consider the possibility that obstruction might be present and there are now a number of imaging methods which can be used – again this aspect of differential diagnosis will not be discussed here. When a patient exhibits an unexplained reduction in renal function the usual problem is to distinguish between prerenal causes and acute tubular necrosis (ATN – this term will be used in preference to vasomotor nephropathy throughout this chapter).

Current dogma has it that patients with prerenal failure can be identified by the presence of continuing ability to concentrate the urine and the ability to retain sodium; in contrast, those patients with ATN exhibit isosmolar serum and urine and excrete inappropriately large amounts of sodium in the urine. Various numbers are used in arriving at this distinction and these are outlined in Table 16.1. It is obvious that some patients will fall in a grey zone and clinical experience suggests that this may in fact be a majority of patients developing acute renal insufficiency. This in turn may be in part due to the administration of drugs which confuse the issue such as diuretics, or to the concurrent presence of other disease notably cardiac failure, hepatic failure or sepsis. Patients who fall clearly into one or other diagnostic group may confidently be treated by standard methods but the time has come to examine the realities of this issue more closely.

Table 16.1. Urinary diagnostic indices in acute renal failure

	Prerenal	ATN
Urine osmolality (mOsm kg^{-1})	>500	300
Urine/plasma osmolality	>1.5/1	<1.1/1
Urine Na (mEq l^{-1})	<10	>40
FE_{Na} (%)	<1	>3

A Revised Approach to Diagnosis

There is increasing evidence to suggest that the simple diagnostic algorithm outlined above is now inadequate for the type of patient commonly referred with acute deterioration in renal function. In a recent review of 100 cases of acute renal failure seen in our intensive care unit, 43% of the patients had urinary indices which did not give a clear diagnostic answer by the criteria outlined above. Recently also a spate of papers has appeared identifying patients with acute renal insufficiency often of sufficient severity and duration to require dialysis in whom some concentrating power had been preserved and urinary sodium was low. Clinical situations in which this has been reported include sepsis, haemoglobinuria, hepatic cirrhosis, burns, allograft rejection, drug-induced renal failure and renal failure following surgery (Zarich et al. 1985). It is suggested, therefore, that diagnostic possibilities considered when renal function acutely deteriorates should continue to include prerenal causes, defined as by the urinary indices noted above, classical ATN with loss of concentrating power and marked urinary sodium leak, and finally a group of patients usually with complex underlying conditions, with urinary indices which are indeterminate but in which acute renal failure is established and is accompanied by urinary sodium retention. Clinical experience suggests that this type of acute renal failure may be very resistant to therapy and obviously the pathophysiology is probably very different from classical ATN.

Correlation between Structure and Function in ARF

Further support for the view that the pathophysiology of acute renal insufficiency may be diverse comes from recent re-examination of the pathology in acute renal failure. For many years it has been accepted that the clinical syndrome of ATN was not necessarily accompanied by pathological necrosis of tubular cells. This view was largely based on pathological studies in the 1950s, one of which was that published by Finkh and which has recently been re-examined by Solez (1983). That re-examination has suggested that when modern pathological techniques are used and suitable statistical methods introduced, those patients who clinically had ATN also had significant pathological changes in the tubules. In contrast, the clinical syndrome of ARF with sodium retention does not seem to be accompanied by important evidence of direct tubular damage (Walker et al. 1986).

ARF and Sepsis

One of the commonest clinical settings in which renal impairment accompanied by sodium retention occurs is that of generalized sepsis. The fact that sepsis and ARF commonly co-exist is well established in the literature (Kleinknecht et al. 1972). It is clear that sepsis often causes death in ARF but it is also certain that generalized sepsis produces impairment of renal function very frequently. That this should be so is not surprising bearing in mind the multiple adverse effects of endotoxin (Wardle 1982). These are listed in Table 16.2. Since the pathogenesis of renal impairment in sepsis is still a mystery, the relative contribution of individual factors cannot be assessed. Animal studies attempting to delineate the pathogenesis of ARF in sepsis have in general suffered from the fact that when sepsis is induced in animals by intravenous infusion of either live *Escherichia coli* or endotoxin the clinical syndrome produced is characterized by vasoconstriction and reduced cardiac output; there is no doubt that renal failure does occur but the haemodynamic disturbance is quite unlike that seen in the early phases of human sepsis. The latter condition is characterized by a vasodilated high cardiac output condition in which renal failure also occurs (MacLean et al. 1967).

Table 16.2. Adverse effects of endotoxin

1. Sympathetic vasoconstriction 2. Local angiotensin generation 3. Plasma volume reduction 4. Disseminated intravascular coagulation	? contribute to onset phase of ARF
5. Endothelial cell damage 6. Loss of endothelial prostacyclin 7. Platelet/WBC aggregation 8. Fibrin thrombi 9. Interstitial oedema	? contribute to maintenance phase of ARF

We have recently described an animal model of generalized sepsis which appears to mimic closely the haemodynamic and renal disturbances seen in man. The model has been described in detail elsewhere (Richmond et al. 1985; Walker et al. 1986). In this model, generalized sepsis is induced in sheep by caecal perforation and serial monitoring of cardiac output, systemic resistance, blood pressure and pulmonary capillary wedge pressure is maintained for a period of 48 hours. Fluid is given at a rate adequate to maintain the baseline pulmonary capillary wedge pressure and these animals all show a sharp reduction in systemic vascular resistance and a marked rise in cardiac output. Results of the haemodynamic monitoring and evaluation of renal function are shown in Table 16.3. It can be seen that despite volume loading adequate to maintain pulmonary capillary wedge pressure and CVP, the animals demonstrated a significant decrease in glomerular filtration rate. This was accompanied by oliguria, a low urinary sodium excretion, well-maintained urine osmolarity and increased plasma renin activity. These animals therefore exhibit a paradox; the reduced sodium excretion and maintained urine osmolarity suggest that the reduction of GFR was due to hypoperfusion but this was directly contradicted by the evidence of well-maintained blood pressure and pulmonary capillary wedge pressure associated with increased cardiac output and reduced peripheral resistance. Other observations included an increase in clearance of lysozyme and low-molecular-weight protein suggesting some degree of tubular damage, but histological examination of the kidneys revealed no visual evidence to support this. Immunofluorescence of the kidneys was entirely negative and there was no evidence of glomerular damage.

Table 16.3. Haemodynamic data and renal function in sheep with generalized sepsis

	Baseline	24 h	48 h
BP (mmHg)	111 ± 13	105 ± 11	113 ± 8
Cardiac index (l min^{-1} m^{-2})	4.9 ± 1.0	5.3 ± 1.8	6.9 ± 3.5[a]
SVRI (d s cm^{-5} m^2)	1909 ± 386	1636 ± 441	1435 ± 460[a]
Serum creatinine (mg dl^{-1})	0.85 ± 0.12	1.2 ± 0.24	2.04 ± 0.85[a]
Glomerular filtration rate (ml min^{-1})	130 ± 55	98 ± 31	34 ± 21[a]
FE$_{Na}$ (%)	2.07 ± 0.72	0.50 ± 0.44[a]	0.40 ± 0.36[a]

[a] Significantly different from baseline ($p<0.05$).

We believe that this model of acute renal failure in generalized sepsis closely mimics that seen in man. We believe also that it constitutes a model of ARF in which reduced GFR is accompanied by sodium retention and absence of histological evidence of acute tubular necrosis; we suggest that this condition differs in pathogenesis from classical ATN. It is possible that this type of ARF seen in sepsis has a similar pathogenesis to that seen in other conditions where the GFR falls and sodium retention occurs. These conditions would include the hepatorenal syndrome, ARF after burns, after some nephrotoxic agents, after episodes of haemoglobinuria and in some episodes of allograft rejection. The model further mimics sepsis in man in that the sheep develop low-molecular-weight proteinuria indicative of some tubular cell damage whether or not the GFR decreases. The explanation of the paradoxical observations is still elusive. There is conflicting evidence on the effect of sepsis on renal blood flow in the

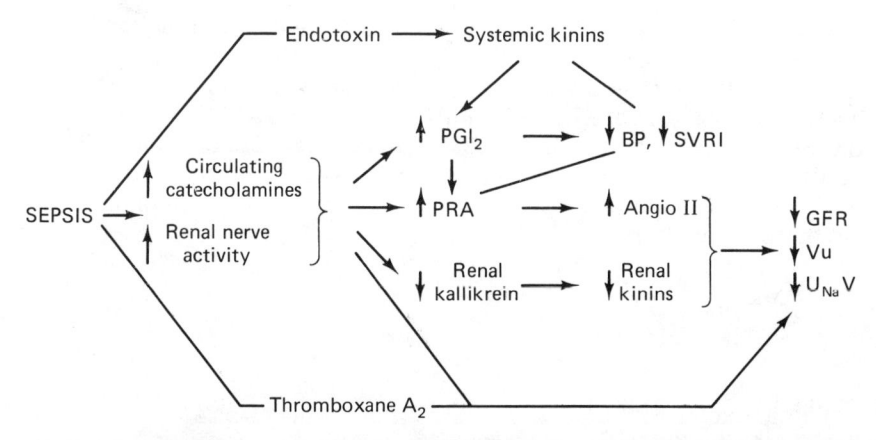

Fig. 16.1. Hypothetical interaction of factors which may contribute to renal dysfunction in sepsis.

literature and its effect on the intrarenal distribution of blood. It appears that in this form of animal sepsis the kidney somehow 'perceives' volume contraction from an unidentified signal despite well-maintained blood pressure and perfusion. While the afferent signal is not clear, there is convincing evidence that the sodium retention observed is induced by any one of a number of sodium-retaining mechanisms including elevated plasma renin and angiotensin levels and probably elevated plasma catecholamine levels. There is some evidence that there is also increased efferent renal sympathetic nerve activity and all in all the model bears a close resemblance to the haemodynamic disturbance seen in the hepatorenal syndrome.

Further studies in our sheep model of renal failure associated with sepsis have revealed that renal functional changes correlated well with other manifestations of severe sepsis – GFR reduction and sodium retention correlated significantly with increased cardiac index, decreased system vascular resistance, pulmonary arterial hypertension, leukopenia, hypoproteinaemia and hypoglycaemia. In sheep with the most severe sepsis and consequently the most severe renal impairment, plasma renin activity was increased and urinary kallikrein excretion was decreased. PRA correlated inversely with GFR, urine volume and sodium excretion; urinary kallikrein excretion correlated positively with urine volume and sodium excretion. Urinary excretion of 6-keto-$PGF_{1\alpha}$ was increased and correlated inversely with mean arterial pressure. During sepsis urinary thromboxane B_2 excretion was increased and thromboxane synthetase inhibition conferred protection for renal function (Cumming et al. 1988, 1989).

Analysis of this evidence and other data from the literature has allowed us to develop the hypothetical interaction of factors shown in Fig. 16.1 which may contribute to renal dysfunction in sepsis.

Conclusions

ARF continues to present an extremely difficult therapeutic problem. This may in part be due to our failure in the past to recognize that a significant percentage of patients presenting with a sudden decrease in GFR are suffering neither from volume depletion nor from classical ATN, but from a haemodynamic disturbance which reduces GFR and causes the retention of sodium simultaneously. It is very likely that the pathogenesis and by extension the prevention and treatment of this condition will differ considerably from those required for either prerenal ARF or acute tubular necrosis. It is possible that the emergence of complicated patients with this type of renal impairment is in part responsible for our continuing lack of success in the treatment of ARF.

References

Bywaters EGL, Beall D (1941) Crush injuries with impairment of renal function. Br Med J i: 427–435
Clark A (1883) An address on renal inadequacy. Br Med J February 24
Cumming AD, Driedger AA, McDonald JWD, Lindsay RM, Solez K, Linton AL (1988) Vasoactive hormones in the renal response to systemic sepsis. Am J Kidney Dis 11: 23–32
Cumming AD, McDonald JW, Lindsay RM, Solez K, Linton AL (1989) The protective effect of thromboxane synthetase inhibition on renal function in systemic sepsis. Am J Kidney Dis 13: 114–119
Kleinknecht D, Jungers P, Chanard J (1972) Uraemic and non-uraemic complications in acute renal failure. Kidney Int 1: 190–196
MacLean JD, Mulligan WG, MacLean APH (1967) Patterns of septic shock in man – a detailed study of 56 patients. Ann Sug 166: 543–558
Richmond JM, Walker JF, Avila A, Sibbald WJ, Linton AL (1985) Renal and cardiovascular response to non-hypotensive sepsis in a large animal model with peritonitis. Surgery 97: 205–214
Solez K (1983) Pathogenesis of acute renal failure. Int Rev Exp Pathol 24: 277–333
Walker JF, Cumming AD, Lindsay RM, Solez K, Linton AL (1986) The renal response produced by nonhypotensive sepsis in a large animal model. Am J Kidney Dis 8: 88–97
Wardle N (1982) Acute renal failure in the 1980s: the importance of septic shock and of endotoxaemia. Nephron 30: 193–200
Zarich S, Fang LST, Diamond JR (1985) Fractional excretion of sodium. Exceptions to its diagnostic value. Arch Intern Med 145: 108–111

Discussion

Dr Bihari asked Dr Linton about the liver function of the sheep. He emphasized that one of the first defects observed in severe sepsis was one of abnormal liver function and Dr Linton confirmed that the sheep model demonstrated a rise in bilirubin and a fall in serum albumin. Dr Bihari drew attention to the similarity between the haemodynamic effects of sepsis and those abnormalities observed in cirrhosis. He wondered whether the hepatic dysfunction of sepsis might actually contribute to the renal abnormalities observed in this condition and he proposed that this form of renal dysfunction might be a milder presentation of the hepatorenal syndrome. Dr Schrier emphasized that the major regulator for renal sodium and water excretion was fullness of the arteriovascular tree. In all sodium-

and water-retaining states that are unrelated to a decrease in cardiac output, there is evidence of peripheral arterial vasodilatation. This includes cirrhosis, an arteriovenous fistula, sepsis, high output cardiac failure, pregnancy and the use of vasodilators. Dr Schrier emphasized that the regulation of renal sodium and water excretion was not related to filling of the venous side of the circulation, nor the total blood volume, but rather reflected an interaction between peripheral arterial resistance and cardiac output as the two determinants of the fullness of the arteriovascular tree. The lack of response to fluid replacement usually reflects a capillary leak so that it is very difficult to fill the arteriovascular tree by giving normal saline alone. Dr Schrier warned against generalizing from one situation to the next. Whilst the fullness of the arteriovascular tree might form a common hypothesis in the explanation of salt and water excretion, it was quite clear that the contribution of the various mediators was different in different conditions. For instance, in sepsis the kallikrein–kinin system may be activated, whereas in cirrhosis there is portal hypertension with a low colloid oncotic pressure. Thus, whilst one might have a common hypothesis, each condition has to be analysed separately since they all have unique characteristics.

Dr Lopez-Novoa mentioned the possibility that platelet-activating factor might be an important mediator in both sepsis and cirrhosis in the decrease of GFR. Dr Linton was then asked about the administration of non-steroidal anti-inflammatory drugs in his animal model. He reported that the non-steroidal anti-inflammatory drugs were given 1 hour before the induction of sepsis and the sheep died within a very short time after sepsis was established. Several participants thought this was very interesting because there had been reports in the literature of non-steroidal anti-inflammatory drugs, in particular ibuprofen, protecting against the effects of endotoxin in sepsis. This appeared to be mediated through an inhibition of synthesis of various arachidonic acid metabolites. On the other hand Dr Bihari pointed out, that since the effects of endotoxin in sepsis appeared to be mediated through various cytokines, particularly tumour necrosis factor, it might be that non-steroidal anti-inflammatory drugs could increase the release of these compounds. Dr Bihari referred to some evidence that PGE_2 and PGI_2 were important prostaglandin compounds which had a negative feedback role in the activated macrophage such that they reduced the synthesis and release of tumour necrosis factor and interleukin-1 from these cells.

Dr Macias referred to evidence that oxygen free radicals were important in the renal damage associated with endotoxic shock. He reported experiments in animals, in which allopurinol protected against the effects of septic shock, and also referred to data in the literature suggesting that glutathione might protect in this situation. Professor Cameron emphasized that the kidney in septic shock was the "victim", not the "villain" of the piece. Clearly this victimization reflected a battering from mediators, platelet activating factor, various cytokines, free radicals of oxygen and other unrecognized mediators. Professor Cameron then turned to the problem of prolonged acute tubular necrosis (ATN) in patients in the intensive care unit. He suggested that sepsis might prolong the illness and of course the administration of many nephrotoxic drugs may produce further injury. There was no doubt that if acute tubular necrosis and the period of oliguria were prolonged to 30 days or more, the patient was very likely to die. Dr Bihari mentioned that as a practising specialist in intensive care, the biggest insult the patient might receive in this period of oligoanuria, was a visit from the haemodialysis machine. He emphasized that patients being treated during this period with intermittent haemodialysis had episodes of hypotension on a daily basis which required treatment with colloid infusions and inotropic support with catecholamines. This episodic hypotension during the course of the illness could be one factor which contributed to the prolongation of the course of ATN. Professor Cameron agreed that episodes of hypotension were certain to affect renal function and Dr Schrier referred to work from his laboratory, which had demonstrated that the failed ATN kidney of the rat was unable to autoregulate its blood flow, such that there were large falls in blood flow with small reductions in mean arterial pressure. Both Dr Bihari and Professor Cameron emphasized that uraemia itself was a very toxic state and caused profound immunosuppression. Whilst there was little evidence that treating the blood urea and serum creatinine on its own improved survival, the uraemic state had to be removed if a patient was to be given the best chances of survival. Most participants agreed that this concept of treating uraemia was in fact an act of faith rather than something based on a mass of scientific data.

Steroids were dismissed for the treatment of endotoxic shock on the basis of recently reported controlled clinical trials which were thought to show no benefit in terms of outcome. Dr Myers reminded participants that a high dose of methylprednisolone was a very potent inhibitor of cytokine release from macrophages stimulated with endotoxin. However, this was only possible if the monocyte or macrophage was pre-treated with steroids before it was stimulated with endotoxin. Everyone agreed that this reflected a major problem in the prevention of organ failure since many of the studies of the protective effect of various agents had been done in animals and in vitro models in which the protective agent was administered before the insult. One of the participants mentioned the use of steroids in the treatment of smoke inhalation injury and referred to data obtained in the Falklands war. Dr Noone replied that whilst few patients had suffered from severe smoke inhalation to the respiratory tract, it was found that the infection rate from burn wounds was significantly higher in the group of patients who had been treated with large doses of corticosteroids. Sex differences, and reasons why the paediatric age group were relatively resistant to Gram-negative septicaemia were discussed, but no conclusions drawn.

Finally, some reference was made to the crystalloid/colloid debate and the use of various fluids in resuscitation from shock. Dr Bihari referred to a commonly held belief that very often the kidneys have to be sacrificed so that the lungs do not become oedematous. He emphasized that the administration of too little fluid during resuscitation from septic shock was a much more common mistake than too much fluid and whilst arguments have centred on the relative risks of pulmonary oedema in patients resuscitated with colloid, compared with those resuscitated with normal saline or Hartmann's solution, there was no good evidence to suggest that one fluid was better than the other. It did appear, however, that in the management of burns in North America, where crystalloid is routinely used to resuscitate the patient, acute renal failure is rare, with acute respiratory failure being more frequent. By contrast in burns units located in the United Kingdom where colloid is the primary agent used during resuscitation, acute respiratory failure is less frequently found, but renal dysfunction occurs more commonly. Dr Linton referred to the data of Lucas from the 1970s which had demonstrated a detrimental effect of plasma compared with crystalloid used during resuscitation. Both lung function and renal function appeared to be worse in patients and animals treated with colloids. Dr Myers emphasized again the problems of raising colloid osmotic pressure to a level which might reduce glomerular filtration, but the conclusion of the discussion reaffirmed the most obvious factor in the process of resuscitation – that is, it is not so much the form of fluid used to resuscitate the septic patient, but rather the quality of the "monkey" with his finger on the drip controller.

Section IV
Clinical Features of Acute Renal Failure in the Intensive Therapy Unit

Chapter 17

Strategies in Management of Acute Renal Failure in the Intensive Therapy Unit

R. W. Schrier, W. T. Abraham and J. Hensen

Introduction

Acute renal failure (ARF) may be defined as an abrupt decrease in previously stable renal function sufficient to result in retention of nitrogenous waste, e.g. blood urea nitrogen (BUN) and creatinine, in the body. Acute renal failure is commonly encountered in the hospital setting. The incidence of ARF is largely dependent on the patient population. A prospective study of general medical and surgical inpatients showed an incidence of almost 5% (Hou et al. 1983). A higher frequency of occurrence is encountered in selected clinical settings, particularly, an incidence of 15%–25% is seen in the Intensive Therapy Unit (ITU) (Wilkins and Faragher 1983). The mortality of patients presenting with ARF alone is 8%. However, the overall mortality of patients with ARF in the setting of the Intensive Therapy Unit still averages 60% or more, despite improvements in monitoring, diagnostics, and therapy (Brunner et al. 1986; Frankel et al. 1983; Stott et al. 1972). Thus, ARF remains a special challenge for the ITU physician.

In this chapter, we will discuss the causes, diagnostic approach, and pathogenesis of ARF, and emphasize current strategies in its management with respect to the Intensive Therapy Unit.

Differential Diagnosis

In a few clinical situations, an elevation in the serum creatinine level does not represent a true decrease in the glomerular filtration rate (GFR). These situations arise when a substance either competes with creatinine for secretion by the renal tubule cells (trimethoprim-sulphamethoxazole, cimetidine) (Berglund et al. 1975; Freston 1982a, b) or interferes with the creatinine assay using spectrophotometric methods (acetoacetate due to ketoacidosis, cefoxitin) (Gerard and Khayam-Bashi 1985; Saah et al. 1982). On the other hand, there are examples where a normal creatinine level does not indicate normal filtration, e.g. aging with loss of muscle mass. This limits the diagnostic utility of the plasma creatinine level and argues for monitoring of creatinine clearances as an estimate of GFR (Tonnesen 1988).

Once the diagnosis of true ARF is established, the anatomic site of the problem must be localized. The classic approach is to categorize the cause as either postrenal, prerenal, or intrarenal.

Postrenal Azotaemia

Postrenal or obstructive causes of ARF are secondary to urethral obstruction, bilateral ureteral obstruction, unilateral ureteral obstruction in a solitary kidney, or diffuse occlusion of the intrarenal collecting system, as in uric acid nephropathy, and are seen in 2%–5% of all cases of ARF (Ellis and Arnold 1982; Hou et al. 1983; Gross and Anderson 1986; Sos et al. 1983). Patients with obstruction of the urinary tract may have fluctuating urine output and urinary indices that mimic prerenal azotaemia during the first few hours. Although patients with obstructive uropathy may be anuric, an "adequate" urine output does not preclude this diagnosis. Renal ultrasonography, reported to be 93% sensitive and specific for urinary tract obstruction, is an excellent screening test (Talner et al. 1981). However, ultrasonography is user dependent and even in the best circumstances never 100% sensitive. Therefore, when obstruction is strongly suspected on clinical grounds, retrograde pyelography should be performed even when the ultrasound shows minimal or no hydronephrosis. A random urine uric acid to creatinine ratio of greater than one (when expressed in mg dl^{-1}) may be helpful in making the diagnosis of acute uric acid nephropathy (Kelton et al. 1978).

Prerenal Azotaemia

Prerenal azotaemia represents the reversible renal response to fluid or haemodynamic derangements. It is most frequently caused by relative or absolute volume depletion resulting in a decrease in renal blood flow with a resultant fall in glomerular capillary filtration pressure. Early correction of hypovolaemia by administration of colloid or crystalloid fluids immediately reverses this form of ARF and prevents progression to the slowly reversible parenchymal form of ARF, acute "intrinsic" renal failure, i.e. "acute tubular necrosis". A recent prospective study found prerenal azotaemia to be the single most common cause of ARF in a general medical–surgical hospital (Hou et al. 1983). In our experience prerenal forms account for 40%–80% of ARF (Anderson et al. 1977; Dixon and Anderson 1985; Gross and Anderson 1986; Miller et al. 1978). Moreover, prolonged renal hypoperfusion, e.g. associated with trauma or surgery, is the most common cause of tubular injury and will be discussed separately. Various clinical situations are associated with renal hypoperfusion (Table 17.1). Patients with an elevated serum creatinine and a history and physical examination suggestive of volume depletion (orthostatic hypotension, poor skin turgor, dry mucous membranes) are easily recognized. However, a number of causes of prerenal azotaemia are much more difficult to diagnose clinically, and have mechanisms of decreased renal blood flow that are less obvious.

Table 17.1. Causes of prerenal azotaemia

I. Volume depletion
   A. Extracellular fluid loss
      1. Gastrointestinal losses (e.g. diarrhoea, vomiting)
      2. Urinary losses (e.g. due to administration of diuretics, salt-wasting nephropathy)
      3. Skin and sweat losses (e.g. burns)
      4. Haemorrhage
   B. Extracellular fluid sequestration ("third-space" losses)
      1. Pancreatitis
      2. Hypoalbuminaemia (e.g nephrotic syndrome, malnutrition, advanced liver disease)
      3. Trauma (e.g. crush injuries)
      4. Peritonitis

II. Low cardiac output
   A. Congestive heart failure or cardiogenic shock
      1. Ischaemic heart disease (e.g. acute myocardial infarction)
      2. Valvular heart disease
      3. Arrhythmias
      4. Other cardiomyopathies (e.g. hypertensive, idiopathic)
   B. Impaired cardiac filling
      1. Pericardial tamponade
      2. Constrictive pericarditis
      3. Massive pulmonary embolism
      4. Positive pressure ventilation

III. Decreased peripheral or increased renal vascular resistance
   A. Peripheral vasodilation
      1. Medications (e.g. vasodilators, antihypertensives)
      2. Sepsis
      3. Anaphylactic shock
      4. Miscellaneous (e.g. adrenal cortical insufficiency, hypermagnesaemia, hypercapnia, hypoxaemia, CNS-mediated hypotension)
   B. Renal vasoconstriction
      1. Medications (e.g. alpha-adrenergic agonists, non-steroidal anti-inflammatory agents)
      2. Sepsis
      3. Hepatorenal syndrome

Patients with severe congestive heart failure can have prerenal azotaemia, a manifestation of decreased "effective arterial blood volume", despite evidence of gross total body fluid overload (peripheral and/or pulmonary oedema). Patients with severe liver disease complicated by the hepatorenal syndrome have an extreme form of prerenal azotaemia characterized by increased renal vascular resistance. Patients with severe bilateral renal artery stenosis may develop prerenal ARF when treated with the group of drugs known as angiotensin-converting enzyme inhibitors (Hricik et al. 1983). The decrease in GFR is felt to be caused by a decrease in efferent arteriolar resistance which results in a fall in glomerular ultrafiltration pressure. Withdrawal of the offending drug usually results in a prompt return of renal function. Non-steroidal anti-inflammatory drugs produce a number of renal syndromes, presumably by their ability to block prostaglandin synthesis (Clive and Stroff 1984). Prerenal ARF may result when these drugs are administered to patients with a decreased effective blood volume. Under these conditions, intrarenal prostaglandins appear to be important in maintaining renal blood flow and GFR (Clive and Stroff 1984). In most instances, the ARF is reversible when the drug is discontinued.

Most patients with prerenal azotaemia have an increased BUN to creatinine ratio, (>20:1, when expressed in mg dl^{-1}), a low urine sodium (<20 mEq l^{-1}), and a low fractional excretion of sodium (<1%) (Espinel 1976). However, many other factors influence these parameters, and there are various causes for both a low and a high fractional excretion of sodium (FE$_{Na}$) in patients with ARF (Table 17.2) (Zarich et al. 1985).

Table 17.2. FE$_{Na}$ in acute renal failure

FE$_{Na}$ <1%	FE$_{Na}$ >1%
Prerenal azotaemia	Diuretic use
Acute glomerulonephritis	Late obstructive uropathy
Early obstructive uropathy	Non-reabsorbable solute
Early sepsis	– glucose
10%–15% of non-oliguric AIRF	– bicarbonate
especially:	– mannitol
– contrast-induced	Chronic renal failure
– myoglobinuria-induced	AIRF

Intrarenal Azotaemia

A variety of renal and extrarenal disturbances can result in intrarenal forms of ARF (Table 17.3). Intrarenal forms of ARF can be categorized as acute intrinsic renal failure (AIRF), acute interstitial nephritis, acute glomerulonephritis or small vessel vasculitis, and acute renovascular disease (Brezis et al. 1986). In hospitalized adults in whom reversible prerenal and postrenal azotaemia have been excluded, ARF is usually due to acute intrinsic renal failure (Frankel 1983; Tonnesen 1988).

Acute Intrinsic Renal Failure

AIRF can be induced by renal hypoperfusion (ischaemia) or nephrotoxins (endogenous or exogenous), and frequently by a combination of both (Brezis et al. 1986). It is not immediately reversed upon discontinuation of the insult and is associated with some tubular dysfunction and cell damage (Brezis et al. 1986). Although the term "acute tubular necrosis" has been extensively used in the literature to describe this form of ARF, tubular necrosis may not be seen histologically (Brezis et al. 1986), and it should, therefore, be used as a pathological description only. The tubular dysfunction presents as the inability to dilute or concentrate the urine appropriately resulting from abnormalities in tubular function, as well as altered response to vasopressin.

Table 17.3. Common causes of the various forms of intrarenal ARF

I. Acute intrinsic renal failure
   A. Renal ischaemia ("prolonged prerenal", see Table 17.1)
   B. Nephrotoxins (e.g. aminoglycosides, radiocontrast agents, heavy metals, organic solvents)
   C. Pigmenturia (e.g. myoglobinuria, haemoglobinuria)

II. Acute glomerulonephritis (GN) and small vessel vasculitis
   A. Postinfectious GN
   B. Membranoproliferative GN
   C. Rapidly progressive GN
   D. Vasculitis

III. Acute interstitial nephritis
   A. Medications (e.g. penicillins, sulphonamides, rifampin, cimetidine, captopril, thiazides, frusemide, allopurinol)
   B. Hypercalcaemia
   C. Infections
   D. Infiltration (e.g. sarcoid, lymphoma)
   E. Connective tissue disease

IV. Acute renovascular disorders
   A. Malignant hypertension
   B. Renal artery occlusion
   C. Renal vein thrombosis

Underlying disorders that predispose to AIRF are listed in Table 17.3. Most patients with AIRF have multiple acute insults resulting in the development of ARF (Rasmussen and Ibels 1982; Rigden et al. 1982). In recent series, 40%–60% of cases of AIRF occurred in a postoperative or trauma setting whereas the remainder were observed in medical settings (Gross and Anderson 1986; McMurray et al. 1978; Minuth et al. 1976). A recent analysis of risk factors in the development of AIRF retrospectively studied 143 patients who developed an acute increase in serum creatinine of more than 2.2 mg dl^{-1} and who did not have prerenal or postrenal azotaemia, glomerulonephritis or interstitial nephritis (Rasmussen and Ibels 1982). The following were considered possible acute insults: hypotension (74%), sepsis (31%), contrast media and aminoglycosides (25%), pigmenturia (22%) and dehydration (35%). Of the 143 patients 64% had more than one acute insult prior to AIRF.

Patients with AIRF may be oliguric (urine output <400 ml day^{-1}) or non-oliguric (urine output >400 ml day^{-1}) (Anderson et al. 1977). The urine sodium concentration is typically >40 mEq l^{-1}, but occasionally may be <20 mEq l^{-1} in non-oliguric patients. The FE$_{Na}$ is usually >1% in both oliguric and non-oliguric patients, resulting from the impairment in sodium reabsorption. Whereas reabsorption of sodium and water is high in prerenal failure and results in high urinary creatinine concentrations, in AIRF decreased tubular sodium and water reabsorption leads to a decrease in urinary creatinine concentration (Espinel 1976; Zarich et al. 1985).

Mortality is high in this patient population with AIRF. When ARF develops in patients in intensive therapy units, the reported survival rate is less than 25% (Brunner et al. 1986; Frankel et al. 1983; Stott et al. 1972). Overall, patients with non-oliguric ARF do better than patients with oliguric disease, the death rates being 26% and 50%, respectively (Anderson et al. 1977).

Despite greater awareness of their toxicity and more intensive monitoring of antibiotic blood levels, aminoglycoside antibiotics remain a common cause of hospital-acquired AIRF (Humes et al. 1982). Although aminoglycoside blood levels are useful in ensuring adequate antibacterial activity, their value in predicting renal toxicity remains controversial. However, sustained high serum levels are associated with increased toxicity (Humes et al. 1982; Smith et al. 1978). Factors that appear to predispose patients to aminoglycoside nephrotoxicity include dose and duration of drug administration, pre-existing renal impairment, intravascular volume depletion, concurrent nephrotoxins, potassium depletion, and advanced age (possibly because true GFR is often overestimated in these patients when calculating drug dosages) (Humes et al. 1982; Smith et al. 1978). Most cases of aminoglycoside induced AIRF are non-oliguric and occur 7–10 days after initiation of treatment. Dialysis is usually not required (Humes et al. 1982; Smith et al. 1978), but may become necessary if oliguria develops. The impaired renal function is usually reversible, although it may take weeks to months for the serum creatinine to return to baseline (Smith et al. 1978).

Exposure to contrast material is a common cause of AIRF (Berkseth and Kjellstrand 1984). Although most physicians avoid excretory urography in patients with significant renal disease, many other procedures subject patients to radiocontrast material including angiography (peripheral and coronary), computer tomographic (CT) scanning with contrast, and digital subtraction angiography. Apparently at highest risk are patients with pre-existing renal impairment, especially if secondary to diabetic nephropathy (Berkseth and Kjellstrand 1984). While most cases of contrast-induced AIRF are reversible and do not require dialysis, insulin-dependent diabetic patients with serum creatinine levels of >5 mg dl^{-1} may develop irreversible ARF (Berkseth and Kjellstrand 1984). Other reported risk factors are more controversial. These include intravascular volume depletion, multiple myeloma, large contrast load and type of contrast agent used, proteinuria, hypertension, and hyperuricaemia.

Diseases of Glomeruli and Small Blood Vessels

Acute glomerular injury is often associated with hypertension and an active urinary sediment characterized by proteinuria and haematuria, pyuria, and often red blood cell casts. Acute glomerulonephritis (GN) is an uncommon cause of hospital-acquired ARF but may account for a greater percentage of outpatients presenting with ARF. Together with avid salt and water retention, these patients often have a low urinary sodium concentration and FE_{Na} which is similar to patients with prerenal azotaemia (Espinel 1976). Percutaneous renal biopsy may be indicated if the aetiology of ARF is unknown and the existence of a systemic disease (e.g. vasculitis) is suspected but not proven.

Interstitial Nephritis

An increasingly recognized cause of intrarenal ARF is allergic interstitial nephritis (AIN). Drugs most commonly implicated are listed in Table 17.3. Patients may manifest a syndrome of fever, skin rash, arthralgias, and peripheral and urinary eosinophilia or they may have none of these features (Wilson et al. 1976). In the latter case, the diagnosis may be made by a renal biopsy showing interstitial infiltration by lymphocytes, plasma cells and eosinophils. Patients suspected of having AIN should have their urine carefully examined for the presence of eosinophils. With the Wright stain, eosinophils appear basophilic with bilobed nuclei and large granules that may or may not take up eosin (Galpin et al. 1978). More recently, use of the Hansel's stain has been advocated to search for urinary eosinophils. With this technique, the granules stain eosinophilic (Nolan et al. 1986). Hansel's stain is less pH dependent than Wright's stain.

Renal Vascular Disorders

Vascular causes of ARF are uncommon. Malignant hypertension which results in fibrinoid necrosis of intrarenal arterioles can be a cause of ARF. Characteristically, these patients have a markedly elevated blood pressure (diastolic usually >120 mmHg) and evidence of end-organ damage. Grade IV hypertensive retinal changes with haemorrhages and papilloedema are usually present together with haematuria and proteinuria. Renal artery occlusion due to emboli or atherosclerotic plaques and renal artery or vein thrombosis may result in ARF (Dash et al. 1983; Delans et al. 1982; Madias et al. 1982; Scully et al. 1984; Shaw and Golpalka 1982; Sos et al. 1983). These lesions generally must be bilateral or occur in a solitary kidney. ARF secondary to renal artery thrombosis usually occurs after blunt abdominal trauma whereas embolization to the renal arteries may come from a dissecting aortic aneurysm, a cardiac mural thrombus, or a valvular source. Cholesterol emboli, a rare cause of ARF, should be considered in elderly patients with diffuse vascular disease, especially if there is evidence of peripheral embolization or recent manipulation of the aorta. This variety of ARF may be associated with eosinophilia and is often irreversible. Bilateral renal vein thrombosis is also an unusual cause of ARF. It should be considered in patients with the nephrotic syndrome, especially if secondary to membranous GN or membranoproliferative GN, with an acute deterioration in renal function or in the presence of pulmonary emboli.

Pathogenesis

A better understanding of the pathogenesis of ARF in the setting of ischaemic and nephrotoxic insults (acute intrinsic renal failure) may help in understanding its management. Several hypotheses have been suggested. Factors other than a reduction in total renal blood flow seem to be important in the severe reduction in GFR in this setting as total renal blood flow has been shown to be reduced comparably in advanced chronic renal failure and acute renal failure (Reubi et al. 1964), and yet only the latter situation requires dialysis to sustain life.

Vascular Theories

The cessation or profound diminution of glomerular filtration is one of the most important defects in ARF. At least three vascular events may be important in the initiation phase of ARF. These events are (a) constriction of the afferent arteriole, (b) dilatation of the efferent arteriole, and (c) decreased permeability of the glomerular membrane.

Afferent Arteriolar Constriction

Severe vasoconstriction of the afferent arteriole could diminish glomerular filtration pressure to the degree that very little filtrate would be formed. This especially may play a role during the initiation phase of ARF. The glomeruli are primarily located in the renal cortex and thus any persistent blood flow might pass through the medullary regions of the kidney. This then would explain the finding of near cessation of measurable glomerular filtration in spite of some persistence of renal blood flow in ARF (Chedru et al. 1972; Jaenike 1967, 1969; Oken et al. 1966; Thiel 1967, 1970). Various clinical and experimental observations have been made which support this mechanism in ARF. Poor filling of the terminal cortical vasculature has been demonstrated angiographically (Hollenberg et al. 1968). Collapse of proximal tubular lumina of many nephrons and pallor of the cortical region are common histological findings (Finckh et al. 1962; Oken et al. 1966). Silicone-rubber vascular injections into animals with uranyl nitrate-induced ARF as well as inert gas washout studies in rats with glycerol-induced ARF and in rats and dogs with uranyl nitrate-induced ARF have demonstrated progressive cortical ischaemia (Chedru et al. 1972; Flamenbaum 1973; Flamenbaum et al. 1972). This vascular pattern of cortical ischaemia in experimental renal failure is similar to that observed in patients with ischaemic or nephrotoxic ARF when the ^{133}xenon washout technique is used to estimate renal blood flow (Hollenberg et al. 1968, 1970). It should be emphasized that the demonstration of cortical ischaemia in experimental and clinical ARF provides only inferential evidence in support of a vascular pathogenesis of ARF.

Efferent Arteriolar Dilatation

Dilatation of the efferent arteriole while afferent arteriolar tone remains unchanged, thus reducing glomerular hydrostatic pressure, may diminish glomerular filtration. However, the diminution of blood flow to the superficial renal cortex observed in ARF cannot be explained by this mechanism alone.

Decreased Glomerular Membrane Permeability

Although glomeruli in the kidneys of patients with ARF appear normal by light microscopy (Finckh et al. 1962), an experimental model of ARF in the dog using a 2-hour noradrenaline infusion consistently showed abnormality of the glomerular epithelial structures by transmission and scanning electron microscopy (Cox et al. 1974). However, a more recent study using the 2-hour noradrenaline infusion model did not reproduce these electron microscopic morphological abnormalities (Bulger et al. 1980). Direct measurement of glomerular dynamics in different models of ARF in rats demonstrated small but significant decreases in glomerular ultrafiltration coefficients (Blackshear et al. 1983). Whether the decrement in ultrafiltration coefficient observed in these studies was due to an actual decrease in glomerular permeability or surface area or both could not be determined.

Mediators of Vasoconstriction

Several investigators have demonstrated that plasma renin activity is elevated in patients with ARF (Kokot and Kuska 1969; Oken et al. 1966; Vertel and Knochel 1967). The theory suggesting a role for the renin–angiotensin system in the pathogenesis of ARF, proposed by Schnermann et al. (1966), suggests that the tubular dysfunction that results from ischaemic or nephrotoxic injury would increase intraluminal or intracellular sodium chloride concentration or both at the macula densa. This would in turn stimulate the release of renin and thus the generation of angiotensin. The increased angiotensin activity would then be the mediator of the afferent arteriolar constriction, which has been proposed as the initiating event in the pathogenesis of ARF. Evidence in support of this hypothesis comes from micropuncture studies that have demonstrated that increased sodium concentration in the tubular fluid near the macula densa is associated with activation of renin in the juxtaglomerular apparatus of the same nephron (Granger et al. 1972). Recent evidence, however, suggests that chloride may be the more important solute activating the tubuloglomerular feedback mechanism (Briggs et al. 1980). It remains to be shown that a similar mechanism is involved in the pathogenesis of ARF. Indeed, acute renal failure in several experimental models is not prevented by the infusion of either angiotensin antagonists (Baranowski et al. 1974; Powell-Jackson et al. 1972) or an inhibitor of angiotensin converting enzyme (Baranowski et al. 1974).

Other vasoconstrictor substances that are proposed to play a role in the initiation phase of ARF are vasopressin, thromboxane, and catecholamines. Also, a role for a decrease in renal vasodilators such as atrial natriuretic factor (ANF) or renal prostaglandins has been suggested. The beneficial effects of calcium channel blockers in noradrenaline-induced ARF is thought to be partly due to their vasodilator properties (Tonnesen 1988). However, other vasodilatory agents such as secretin or acetylcholine, are not protective (Schrier and Hensen 1988), suggesting a specifically protective effect of "calcium channel arrest" (Hochachka 1986; Schrier and Hensen 1988).

Potential Role of Cell Swelling

Regulation of intracellular volume is known to be dependent on a supply of metabolic energy, and this energy is used primarily to pump sodium from the cell interior to the extracellular fluid (ECF) space (Leaf 1956; Wilson 1954). As cellular membranes are permeable to sodium, the high ECF sodium concentration (140–145 mEq l^{-1}) creates a steep concentration gradient for the passive diffusion of sodium into the cell which has a sodium concentration of approximately 10 mEq l^{-1}. In the absence of active pumping of sodium from the cell, the osmolality within the cell would exceed that of the ECF and induce water movement into cells. Swelling of the glomerular epithelial cells in the rat has been demonstrated to be a consistent consequence of obstruction of the renal artery for

60–90 min (Flores et al. 1973). Further investigation into the role of cell swelling in the pathogenesis of ARF is needed.

Backleak Theory

This hypothesis proposes that in ARF normal glomerular filtration actually persists but that, because of disruption of the integrity of tubular epithelium, the glomerular filtrate, including any normally unreabsorbable markers such as inulin, is totally reabsorbed (Bank et al. 1967; Flamenbaum et al. 1971). The minimal urinary excretion of creatinine or inulin by patients with ARF would thus indicate that despite normal glomerular filtration, tubular disruption (i.e. tubular necrosis) allowed the creatinine and inulin to "backleak" from the tubular lumen into the peritubular circulation. An anatomic basis for this hypothesis has been provided by the observation of tubular necrosis in clinical cases and experimental models of ARF (Bank et al. 1967; Flamenbaum et al. 1971; Oliver et al. 1951). Micropuncture studies, performed as early as 1929, in frogs poisoned by mercuric chloride showed that phenolsulphonphthalein "leaked" out of damaged tubules (Richards 1929). More recent micropuncture studies have provided further support for this theory (Bank et al. 1967; Steinhausen et al. 1969); however, other similar studies have failed to confirm a role for backleak in the pathogenesis of ARF (Conger et al. 1981; Flamenbaum et al. 1971). Since severe tubular necrosis is not a common finding in the clinical syndrome of ARF in man, it is not clear that this mechanism plays an important role in human ARF (Finckh et al. 1962; Olsen and Skjoldborg 1967).

Tubular Obstruction Theory

Tubular obstruction by intraluminal debris, cast formation, cytoplasmic blebs, and/or interstitial oedema has been proposed as a cause of the decreased glomerular filtration in ARF (Baker and Dodds 1925; Mason et al. 1963; Meroney and Rubini 1959; Peters 1945). Oedematous enlargement of the kidneys and intraluminal cast formation are not infrequent findings in clinical and experimental ARF. Moreover, abnormal dilatation of the proximal tubular lumina of nephrons may also be a prominent histological feature of ARF (Schrier and Cronin 1978). Intraluminal pressures have been measured in several experimental models of ARF, including failure induced by noradrenaline (Conger et al. 1981), by renal artery cross-clamping (Arendshorst et al. 1975; Tanner and Sophasan 1976), and by the administration of methaemoglobin (Hollenberg et al. 1970; Jaenike 1967; Ruiz-Guinazu et al. 1967), and glycerol (Oken et al. 1966, 1970; Suzuki and Mostofi 1970). Taken together, the results of these studies demonstrate that intraluminal pressure may be increased but not uniformly in all nephrons of experimental models. Increased intraluminal pressure has been most consistently found in ischaemic and methaemoglobin-induced forms of ARF, thus it appears to be an important pathogenic factor in these models but to have a less prominent role in nephrotoxin-induced forms of the disease.

In summary, tubular obstruction, which occurs both as the consequence of tubular cell necrosis and diminished transglomerular pressure, may play an important role in the maintenance phase of ARF. An increase in intraluminal pressure in experimental ARF is most readily demonstrated when renal blood flow has been returned to normal with saline loading or a renal vasodilator.

Mechanism of Cellular Ischaemia

Decreased blood flow to the proximal tubule or the thick ascending limb results in decreased oxygen delivery to these hypoxia-sensitive cells with a subsequent fall in ATP levels. Despite activation of anaerobic glycolysis (Pasteur effect), energy insufficiency and loss of membrane transport functions, e.g. impaired pumping of the Na,K-ATPase membrane pump, occurs. When inhibitors of Na,K-ATPase (ouabain) were infused prior to hypoxia or when ion-pumping work was reduced prior to hypoxia, the sensitivity to hypoxia was minimized. In other words, when cells were partially "metabolically arrested", their tolerance to hypoxia increased (Hochachka 1986).

Another physiological concept which is important in the understanding of new possible treatments of ARF is the "channel arrest concept" (Hochachka 1986). Recent investigations into the mechanism of tubular dysfunction have suggested a potential role for cellular calcium homeostasis in ischaemia-related injury. These investigations have been summarized in a recent review (Schrier and Hensen 1988). The remarkably low free intracellular calcium concentration is normally maintained directly or indirectly by ATP-dependent pumps. Intracellular organelles, namely mitochondria and endoplasmic reticulum, actively increase their calcium uptake during extraordinary intracellular conditions, such as those probably induced by ischaemia. Limitation in energy supply (ATP) results in a large uncontrolled influx in calcium, which at high cytosolic concentrations acts as a cellular toxin (Hochachka 1986; Rubin et al. 1985; Schrier and Hensen 1988). The term "calcium channel arrest" describes manoeuvres to inhibit uncontrolled calcium fluxes in order to increase protection against the hypoxia-induced deleterious increase in intracellular calcium (Hochachka 1986). Data from studies using calcium channel blockers in experimentally induced ARF strongly support this hypothesis (Schrier et al. 1987; Schrier and Hensen 1988).

Management of Acute Renal Failure

Because of the high mortality of ARF in the ITU extraordinary efforts should be made to prevent ARF (Cameron 1986). In this respect, volume loading is still one of the most consistently protective manoeuvres, e.g. in the perioperative setting in man (Bush et al. 1981).

The first principle of therapy is to exclude any cause of acute azotaemia remediable to specific therapy. Obstructive uropathy should be treated by placement of a Foley catheter, ureteral stints, or nephrostomy tubes, resulting in rapid improvement of renal function. Acute uric acid nephropathy with intratubular crystal deposition may occur after treatment of lymphoreticular malignancy as part of a tumour lysis syndrome. Treatment consists of forced diuresis with alkalinization of the urine. In severe cases, haemodialysis may be indicated to reduce the large uric acid load (Kjellstrand et al. 1974). Hypercalcaemia may cause ARF, again usually in the setting of a malignancy or massive calcium and vitamin D ingestion. Saline and frusemide diuresis is usually adequate therapy although dialysis may be indicated when renal function is significantly impaired. Finally, a few of the causes of rapidly progressive glomerular nephritis (RPGN) and systemic vasculitis associated with ARF are treatable but a discussion of these rare entities is beyond the scope of this chapter.

Fluids and Electrolytes

Once ARF has developed, compensation for renal function has to be accomplished by the ITU physician. In the setting of the ITU, invasive haemodynamic monitoring is usually performed in critically ill patients, and allows a more accurate assessment of fluid balance than non-invasive methods such as assessment of skin turgor and jugular venous filling. Prerenal azotaemia when secondary to volume depletion is easily diagnosed and rapidly reversible with restoration of the euvolaemic state. However, in the case of prolonged hypoperfusion with resulting tubular damage, ARF is not immediately reversible when the initiating disturbance is eliminated, suggesting renal parenchymal damage awaiting cell regeneration for functional recovery (Brezis et al. 1986).

The management of fluid and electrolyte balance is complex, especially in the case of non-oliguric ARF. In general, fluid intake should be balanced against total output plus insensible losses. Venous filling should be maintained in the normal to upper normal range. Failure to provide adequate fluid and electrolyte replacement may, in fact, convert a non-oliguric into an oliguric ARF. If venous overfilling with pulmonary congestion occurs, haemodialysis or haemofiltration might be needed. Serum electrolytes, including calcium, phosphorus, and magnesium levels should be followed, and patients should be placed on a potassium restricted diet. Many patients require oral phosphate binders, while magnesium-containing antacids should be restricted to prevent severe hypermagnesaemia. However, severe hypophosphataemia has been reported in the course of ARF, which might be due to a hyperalimentation (carbohydrate)-stimulated, insulin-induced intracellular shift of phosphorus (Kurtin and Kouba 1987). To overcome this effect, consideration should be given to the use of parenteral fat (Kurtin and Kouba 1987).

Nutrition

Moderate protein restriction is sometimes advocated to forestall the need for dialysis. This decision must be made with an understanding of the patient's nutritional status and the expected course of his illness. Forestalling dialysis at the expense of malnutrition is clearly unwarranted and will increase endogenous catabolism. To avoid negative nitrogen and calorie balance replacement of amino acids and calories by enteral or intravenous hyperalimentation was introduced in the treatment of the acutely ill patient with ARF. Whether this aggressive hyperalimentation with carbohydrates and fat solutions is better than moderate protein and calorie support is a matter of dispute (Knochel 1985). However, in the age of "early" and "intensive" dialysis, it is felt that vigorous protein and caloric replacement is "possibly the most important factor in improved survival in critically ill patients" (Lazarus 1986). In addition, removal of amino acids (10–20 g day^{-1}) by intensive haemodialysis must also be taken into consideration in calculation of protein supplementation.

Dialysis

Absolute indications for dialysis are overt uraemia (as manifested by pericarditis, central nervous system disturbances, and/or gastrointestinal haemorrhage), refractory hyperkalaemia, and fluid overload. However, the objective is to avoid, rather than treat, uraemic complications. Even though, to our knowledge, no sizable prospective controlled study has proven the value of prophylactic dialysis, many reports as well as clinical experience strongly support this approach (Kleinknecht et al. 1972). A recent controlled study failed, however, to show any significant benefit from intensive dialysis, when one group was dialysed to maintain BUN ≤100 mg dl^{-1}, and the BUN of the other group was kept at <60 mg dl^{-1} (Gillum et al. 1986). Clearly, volume overload, progressive acidosis, and electrolyte abnormalities need to be controlled, and the uraemic symptoms of confusion, lethargy, and anorexia avoided. There is, however, experimental evidence that the haemodynamic alterations that often occur during dialysis may delay the recovery of renal function (Myers and Moran 1986). Especially in diabetic patients with autonomic neuropathy, the rapid fluid shifts with haemodialysis are not well tolerated, and severe hypotension may occur (Grenfell 1986). In this regard, continuous or pump-assisted arteriovenous haemofiltration might offer some advantages (Grenfell 1986). It is for the above-mentioned reasons that there are no specific serum concentrations of nitrogenous wastes at which dialysis should be started. Most nephrologists, however, institute dialysis when the blood urea nitrogen approaches 80–100 mg dl^{-1} (28–35 mmol^{-1}) and the serum creatinine approaches 8–10 mg dl^{-1} (600–800 µmol e^{-1}), unless spontaneous recovery is occurring. The mode of dialysis used (haemodialysis, peritoneal dialysis, haemofiltration) should be based on local experience, the patient's haemodynamic status, and specific contra-indications such as recent abdominal surgery or high risk for systemic anticoagulation. In some catabolic states (e.g. rhabdomyolysis, burns, sepsis) even the continuous use of peritoneal dialysis is inadequate to prevent uraemic symptoms (Nolph et al. 1969; Schrier and Cronin 1978). Haemodialysis may be needed in salicylate, ethylene glycol, and methanol poisoning. Diabetic patients may rarely need haemodialysis rather than peritoneal dialysis because of impaired metabolic clearance of the peritoneum.

Diuretics

Several reports suggest that early aggressive treatment with mannitol, high doses of frusemide (up to 3 gu day^{-1}) or frusemide and dopamine may convert oliguric ARF into non-oliguric ARF (Burke et al. 1983; Cantarovich et al. 1971; Graziani et al. 1984; Levinsky et al. 1980). Mannitol, if used before or soon after the renal insult, may be more effective in improving renal function than frusemide (Levinsky et al. 1980). However, the morbidity seems not to be convincingly altered when mannitol was prophylactically utilized (Ridgen et al. 1984).

Moreover, there is little evidence that prophylactic diuretics (e.g. mannitol) have any major advantage over routine intravascular volume expansion in high-risk situations (Brezis et al. 1986; Levinsky et al. 1980). Other studies have failed to show any benefit of frusemide (Kleinknecht et al. 1976) and support the view that patients who appear to respond to this form of treatment had less severe renal injury initially. Furthermore, diuretic-induced conversion into non-oliguric ARF may not mimic the better prognosis of spontaneously non-oliguric ARF. In summary, frusemide and mannitol seem to be of limited value in prevention and treatment of ARF. Non-oliguric ARF, however, may be easier to manage than oliguric ARF. When the non-oliguric state is maintained with diuretic therapy, care should be taken to avoid inducing volume depletion.

Dopamine

Infusion of low-dose dopamine (about 1 µg kg^{-1} min^{-1}) (Kjellstrand et al. 1988) results in increased renal plasma flow, GFR, and sodium excretion (Elgholzi et al. 1984). Administration of dopamine in patients with ARF improves urine flow and sodium excretion. However, the effect on prognosis remains to be proven (Henderson et al. 1980). A trial of low-dose dopamine may be especially useful in oliguric ARF patients with volume overload or heart failure.

Specific Recommendations

A reasonable clinical approach for patients with a serum creatinine of 5 mg dl^{-1} or less was recently delineated by Kjellstrand et al. (1988). They recommend that patients with ARF should be treated with a combination of dopamine infused at a rate of 1 µg kg^{-1} min^{-1} and rapidly escalating doses of frusemide, approximately 2–5–10 mg kg^{-1} infused at hourly intervals over a 15–20 min period to decrease the ototoxicity of a high peak level. If diuresis is established, these authors recommend maintenance of diuresis by continued mannitol and frusemide infusions. In a normal-sized adult, infusion at a rate of 20 ml h^{-1} of 500 ml of 20% mannitol containing the frusemide dose to which the patient responded, was suggested. If diuresis is accomplished, it usually eases considerably the conservative management of ARF. However, the patient must be carefully monitored for side effects of mannitol (hyperosmolality) and frusemide (pancreatitis, deafness). Mannitol should be given in 0.45% saline solution to replace urinary electrolyte losses. In the presence of a normal volume status, the osmotic diuresis with mannitol is substantially greater, and thus probably more protective, then with isotonic saline infusion alone.

Experimental "Aetiological" Treatments (Kjellstrand et al. 1988)

A number of other procedures, deduced from the pathophysiological concepts outlined above, have been shown to be beneficial in prevention or management in ARF in experimental animals. Vasodilatation by PGE$_2$ (Neumayer et al. 1985), inhibition of thromboxane synthesis (Lelcuk et al. 1985), induction of a hypothyroid state (Paller and Sikora 1986), reduced protein intake (Andrews

1986), infusion of amino acids (Abel et al. 1973), treatment with free oxygen radical scavengers (Paller 1985), indirect antagonism of vasopressin by lithium or demedocycline (Solez 1983), antithrombin III infusion (prevention of intravascular coagulation) (Ono et al. 1984), blockade of AMP conversion into adenosine (Gerkens et al. 1982), and infusion of ATP-Mg^{2+} (energy replacement) (Siegel et al. 1980), have all been demonstrated to exert beneficial effects on the initial or maintenance phase of ARF. Their usefulness under clinical conditions has yet to be proven. It is noteworthy, however, that some of these proposed treatments are potentially dangerous. Because of their potential usefulness in clinical situations two novel aetiologically based treatments are briefly considered below.

Calcium Channel Blockers and ANF

As outlined above, calcium channel blockers have been shown to possess a protective effect in experimental models of ARF (Schrier et al. 1987; Schrier and Hensen 1988). In addition to their effects on cellular calcium homeostasis, these drugs tend to increase renal blood flow with a concurrent increase in GFR, similar to infusion of dopamine (Loutzenhizer and Epstein 1987). For these reasons, calcium channel blockade may play an important role in the future treatment of ARF.

ANF has recently been shown to ameliorate ischaemic ARF in vivo and in vitro (Nakamoto et al. 1988). This effect could not be solely attributed to its vasodilating properties on the glomerular capillaries. We recently demonstrated that ANF prevents hormone-induced intracellular calcium mobilization in cultured glomerular mesangial cells (Meyer-Lehnert et al. 1988). A clinical study, evaluating the effect of intrarenal ANF infusion on the course of ARF is currently being performed by our group.

References

Abel RM, Beck CH, Abbott WM et al. (1973) Improved survival from acute renal failure after treatment with intravenous essential L-amino acids and glucose. N Engl J Med 288: 695
Anderson RJ, Linas SL, Berns AS et al. (1977) Nonoliguric acute renal failure. N Engl J Med 296: 1134
Andrews PM (1986) Dietary protein prior to renal ischemia dramatically effects postischemic recovery. Kidney Int 30: 299
Arendshorst WJ, Finn WF, Gottschalk CW (1975) Pathogenesis of acute renal failure following temporary renal ischemia in the rat. Circ Res 37: 558
Baker SL, Dodds EC (1925) Obstruction of the renal tubules during excretion of hemoglobin. Br J Exp Pathol 6: 247
Bank N, Mutz BF, Aynedjian HS (1967) The role of "leakage" of tubular fluid in anuria due to mercury poisoning. J Clin Invest 46: 695
Baranowski RL, O'Conner GJ, Kurtzman NA (1974) The effect of 1-sarcosine, 8-leucyl angiotensin II on the pressor effect of infused angiotensin II. Arch Int Pharmacodyn Ther 209: 75
Berglund F, Killander J, Pompeius R (1975) Effect of trimethoprim-sulfamethoxazole on the renal excretion of creatinine in man. J Urol 114: 802
Berkseth RO, Kjellstrand CM (1984) Radiologic contrast-induced nephropathy. Med Clin North Amer 68: 351
Blackshear JL, Davidman M, Stillman T (1983) Identification of risk for renal insufficiency from non-steroidal anti-inflammatory drugs. Arch Intern Med 143: 1130

Brezis M, Rosen S, Epstein FH (1986) Acute renal failure. In: Brenner BM, Rector FC (eds) The kidney, 3rd edn. W. B. Saunders, Philadelphia, p 735

Briggs JP, Schnermann J, Wright FS (1980) Failure of tubule fluid osmolality to affect feedback regulation of glomerular filtration. Am J Physiol 8: F427

Brunner F, Broyer M, Brynger H et al. (1986) Combined report on regular dialysis and transplantation in Europe XV, 1984. Proc Eur Transplant Assoc, vol 22

Bulger RE, Cronin RE, Dobyan DC (1980) Glomerular architecture changes after a two-hour infusion of norepinephrine. Am J Anat 159: 379

Burke TJ, Arnold PE, Schrier RW (1983) Prevention of ischemic acute renal failure with impermeant solutes. Am J Physiol 244: F646

Bush HL Jr, Huse JB, Johnson WC et al. (1981) Prevention of renal insufficiency after abdominal aortic aneurysm resection by optimal volume loading. Arch Surg 116: 1517

Cameron JM (1986) Acute renal failure in the intensive care unit today. Intensive Care Med 12: 64

Cantarovich F, Fernandez JC, Locatelli A, Loredo JP, Cristhot J (1971) Frusemide in high doses in the treatment of acute renal failure. Postgrad Med J 47 (Suppl): 13

Chedru MF, Baethke R, Oken DE (1972) Renal cortical blood flow and glomerular filtration in myohemoglobinuric acute renal failure. Kidney Int 1: 232

Clive DM, Stroff JS (1984) Renal syndromes associated with nonsteroidal antiinflammatory drugs. N Engl J Med 310: 563

Conger JD et al. (1981) The effect of acetylcholine on the early phase of reversible norepinephrine-induced acute renal failure. Kidney Int 19: 399

Cox JW et al. (1974) Studies on the mechanism of oliguria in a model of unilateral acute renal failure. J Clin Invest 53: 1546

Dash H, Little JR, Zaino R et al. (1983) Metastatic periosteal osteosarcoma causing cardiac and renal failure. Am J Med 75: 145

Delans RJ, Ramirez G, Farber MS et al. (1982) Renal artery thrombosis: a cause of reversible acute renal failure. J Urol 128: 1287

Dixon BS, Anderson RJ (1985) Nonoliguric acute renal failure. Am J Kidney Dis 6: 71

Elgholzi JL, Earnhardt JT, Meyer P (1984) Dopamine: vascular and renal effects and alterations in hypertension. In: Grunfeld JP, Maxwell MH (eds) Advances in nephrology, vol 13. Year Book Medical Publishers, Chicago, p 135

Ellis EN, Arnold WC (1982) Renal failure secondary to bilateral ureteric obstruction: review of 50 cases. Can Med Assoc J 127: 601

Espinel CH (1976) FE_{Na} test: Use in the differential diagnosis of acute renal failure. JAMA 236: 579

Finckh ES, Jeremy D, Whyte HM (1962) Structural renal damage and its relation to clinical features in acute oliguric renal failure. Q J Med 31: 429

Flamenbaum W (1973) Pathophysiology of acute renal failure. Arch Intern Med 131: 911

Flamenbaum W, McDonald FD, DiBona GF et al. (1971) Micropuncture studies of renal tubular factors in low-dose mercury poisoning. Nephron 8: 221

Flamenbaum W, McNeil JS, Kotchen TA et al. (1972) Experimental acute renal failure induced by uranyl nitrate in the dog. Circ Res 31: 682

Flores JE et al. (1973) The role of cell swelling in ischemic renal injury. In: Friedman EA, Eliahou HE (eds) Proceedings of the Conference on Acute Renal Failure. Department of Health, Education, and Welfare, New York, p 19

Frankel MC, Weinstein AM, Stenzel KH (1983) Prognostic patterns in acute renal failure: The New York Hospital, 1981–1982. Clin Exp Dial and Apheresis 7: 145

Freston JW (1982a) Cimetidine: I. Developments, pharmacology, and efficacy. Ann Intern Med 97: 573

Freston JW (1982b) Cimetidine II. Adverse reactions and patterns of use. Ann Intern Med 97: 728

Galpin JE, Shinaberger JH, Stanley TM et al. (1978) Acute interstitial nephritis due to methicillin. Am J Med 65: 756

Gerard SK, Khayam-Bashi H (1985) Characterization of creatinine error in ketotic patients. Am J Clin Pathol 84: 659

Gerkens JF, Heidemann HT, Jackson EK (1982) Effects of aminophylline on amphotericin B nephrotoxicity in the dog. J Pharmacol Exp Ther 224: 609

Gillum DM, Dixon BS, Yanover MJ et al. (1986) The role of intensive dialysis in acute renal failure. Clin Nephrol 25: 249

Granger P, Dahlheim H, Thurau K (1972) Enzyme activities of the single juxtaglomerular apparatus of the rat kidney. Kidney Int 1: 78

Graziani G, Cantalupp A, Casati S et al. (1984) Dopamine and furosemide in oliguric acute renal failure. Nephron 37: 39

Grenfell A (1986) Acute renal failure in diabetics. Intensive Care Med 12: 6
Gross PA, Anderson RJ (1986) Acute renal failure and toxic nephropathy. In: Klahr S, Massry SG (eds) Contemporary nephrology, vol 3. Plenum, New York
Henderson IS, Beattie TJ, Kennedy AC (1980) Dopamine hydrochloride in oliguric states. Lancet I: 827
Hochachka PW (1986) Metabolic arrest. Intensive Care Med 12: 127
Hollenberg NK, Epstein J, Rosen SM et al. (1968) Acute oliguric renal failure in man: evidence for preferential renal cortical ischemia. Medicine 47: 455
Hollenberg NK, Adams DF, Oken DE et al. (1970) Acute renal failure due to nephrotoxins: renal hemodynamic and angiographic studies in man. N Engl J Med 282: 1329
Hou SH, Bushinsky DA, Wish JB, Cohen JJ, Harrington JT (1983) Hospital-acquired renal insufficiency: A prospective study. Am J Med 74: 243
Hricik DE, Browning PJ, Kopelman R, Goorno WE, Madias NE, Dzau VJ (1983) Captopril-induced functional renal insufficiency in patients with bilateral renal-artery stenoses or renal-artery stenosis in a solitary kidney. N Engl J Med 308: 373
Humes HD, Weinberg JM, Knauss TC (1982) Clinical and pathophysiologic aspects of aminoglycoside nephrotoxicity. Am J Kidney Dis 2: 5
Jaenike JR (1967) The renal lesion associated with hemoglobinemia: a study of the excretory defect in the rat. J Clin Invest 46: 378
Jaenike JR (1969) Micropuncture study of methemoglobin-induced acute renal failure in the rat. J Lab Clin Med 73: 459
Kelton J, Kelley WN, Holmes EW (1978) A rapid method for the diagnosis of acute uric acid nephropathy. Arch Intern Med 138: 612
Kjellstrand CM, Campbell DC 2d, von Hartitzsch B, Buselmeier TJ (1974) Hyperuricemic acute renal failure. Arch Intern Med 133: 349
Kjellstrand CM, Berkseth RO, Klinkmann H (1988) Treatment of acute renal failure. In: Schrier RW, Gottschalk KW (eds) Diseases of the kidney. Little, Brown, Boston/Toronto, pp 1501–1542
Kleinknecht D, Jungers P, Chanard J, Barbanel C, Ganeval D (1972) Uremic and non-uremic complications on acute renal failure: Evaluation of early and frequent dialysis on prognosis. Kidney Int 1: 190
Kleinknecht D, Ganeval D, Gonzalez-Duque LA, Fermanian J (1976) Furosemide in acute oliguric renal failure. A controlled trial. Nephron 17: 51
Knochel JP (1985) Complications of total parenteral nutrition. Kidney Int 27: 489
Kokot F, Kuska J (1969) Plasma renin activity in acute renal insufficiency. Nephron 6: 115
Kurtin P, Kouba J (1987) Profound hypophosphatemia in the course of acute renal failure. Am J Kidney Dis 10: 346
Lazarus JM (1986) Acute renal failure. Intensive Care Med 12: 61
Leaf A (1956) On the mechanism of fluid exchange of tissue *in vitro*. Biochem J 62: 241
Lelcuk S, Alexander F, Kobzik L et al. (1985) Prostacyclin and thromboxane A_2 moderate postischemic acute renal failure. Surgery 98: 207
Levinsky NG, Bernard DB, Johnston PA (1980) Enhancement of recovery of acute renal failure: effects of mannitol and diuretics. In: Brenner BM, Stein JM (eds) Contemporary issues in nephrology, vol 6. Churchill Livingstone, New York, p 163
Loutzenhizer R, Epstein M (1987) Calcium antagonists and the kidney. Hosp Pract 22: 63
Madias NE, Kwon OJ, Millan VG (1982) Percutaneous transluminal renal angioplasty. Ann Intern Med 142: 693
Mason AD Jr, Teschan PE, Muirhead EE (1963) Studies in acute renal failure: III. Renal histologic alterations in acute renal failure in the rat. J Surg Res 3: 450
McMurray SD, Luft FC, Maxwell DR et al. (1978) Prevailing patterns and predictor variables in patients with acute tubular necrosis. Arch Intern Med 138: 950
Meroney WH, Rubini ME (1959) Kidney function during acute tubular necrosis: clinical studies and a theory. Metabolism 8: 1
Meyer-Lehnert H, Caramelo C, Tsai P, Schrier RW (1988) Interaction of atriopeptin III and vasopressin on calcium kinetics and contraction of aortic smooth cells. J Clin Invest 82: 1407–1414
Miller TR, Anderson RJ, Berns AS et al. (1978) Urinary diagnostic indices in acute renal failure: a prospective study. Ann Intern Med 88: 47
Minuth AN, Terrell JB, Suki WN (1976) Acute renal failure: a study of the course and prognosis of 104 patients and of the role of furosemide. Am J Med Sci 271: 317
Myers BD, Moran SM (1986) Hemodynamically mediated acute renal failure. N Engl J Med 314: 97
Nakamoto M, Shapiro JI, Shanley PF, Chan L, Schrier RW (1988) *In vitro* and *in vivo* protective effect of atriopeptin III on ischemic acute renal failure. J Clin Invest 80: 698

Neumayer H-H, Wagner K, Groll J et al. (1985) Beneficial effects of long term prostaglandin E_2 infusion on the course of postischemic acute renal failure. Long-term studies in chronically instrumented conscious dogs. Renal Physiol 8: 159

Nolan C 3d, Anger M, Kelleher S (1986) Eosinophiluria: a new method for detection and definition of the clinical spectrum. N Engl J Med 315: 1516

Nolph KD, Whitcomb ME, Schrier RW (1969) Mechanisms for inefficient peritoneal dialysis in acute renal failure associated with heat stress and exercise. Ann Intern Med 71: 317

Oken DE, Acre ML, Wilson DR (1966) Glycerol-induced hemoglobinuric acute renal failure in the rat: I. Micropuncture study of the development of oliguria. J Clin Invest 45: 724

Oken DE, DiBona GF, McDonald FD (1970) Micropuncture studies of the recovery phase of myohemoglobinuric acute renal failure in the rat. J Clin Invest 49: 730

Oliver J, MacDowell M, Tracy A (1951) The pathogenesis of acute renal failure associated with traumatic and toxic injury: Renal ischemia, nephrotoxic damage and the ischemic episode. J Clin Invest 30: 1307

Olsen TS, Skjoldborg H (1967) The fine structure of the renal glomerulus in acute anuria. Acta Pathol Microbiol Scand 70: 205

Ono I, Ohura T, Azami K et al. (1984) Anticoagulation therapy for renal insufficiency after burns. Burns 11: 104

Paller MS (1985) Free radical scavengers in mercuric chloride induced acute renal failure in the rat. J Lab Clin Med 105: 459

Paller MS, Sikora JJ (1986) Hypothyroidism protects against free radical damage in ischemic renal failure. Kidney Int 29: 1162

Peters JT (1945) Oliguria and anuria due to increased intrarenal pressure. Ann Intern Med 23: 221

Powell-Jackson JD, Brown JJ, Leaver AF et al. (1972) Protection against acute renal failure in rats by passive immunization against angiotensin II. Lancet I: 774

Rasmussen HH, Ibels LS (1982) Acute renal failure: multivariate analysis of causes and risk factors. Am J Med 73: 211

Reubi RC, Gossweiler N, Gurtler R (1964) The renal blood flow in acute renal failure. In: Shaldon S, Cooke GC (eds) Acute renal failure. Davis, Philadelphia, p 25

Richards AN (1929) Direct observations of change in function of the renal tubule caused by certain poisons. Trans Assoc Am Physicians 44: 64

Ridgen SP, Dillon MJ, Kind PRN et al. (1984) The beneficial effect of mannitol on postoperative renal function in children undergoing cardiopulmonary bypass surgery. Clin Nephrol 21: 148

Rigden SPA, Barratt TM, Dillon MJ et al. (1982) Acute renal failure complicating cardiopulmonary bypass surgery. Arch Dis Child 57: 425

Rubin RP, Weiss GP, Putney JP Jr (eds) (1985) Calcium in biological fluids. Plenum Press, New York, pp 391–490

Ruiz-Guinazu A, Coelho JB, Paz RA (1967) Methemoglobin-induced acute renal failure in the rat: *in vivo* observation, histology and micropuncture measurements of intratubular and postglomerular vascular pressures. Nephron 4: 257

Saah AJ, Kock TR, Drusano GL (1982) Cefoxitin falsely elevates creatinine levels. JAMA 247: 205

Schnermann J, Nagel W, Thurau K (1966) Die frühdistale Natriumkonzentration in Rattennieren nach renaler Ischämie und haemorrhagischer Hypotension. Pflugers Arch 287: 296

Schrier RW, Cronin RE (1978) Acute renal failure. In: Coggins CH, Cummings NB (eds) Fogarty International Center Monograph on Prevention of Kidney and Urinary Tract Disease. US Government Printing Office, Washington DC

Schrier RW, Hensen J (1988) Cellular mechanism of ischemic acute renal failure: role of Ca^{2+} and calcium entry blockers. Klin Wochenschr 66: 800–807

Schrier RW, Arnold PE, Van Putten VJ, Burke TJ (1987), Cellular calcium in ischemic acute renal failure: role of calcium entry blockers. Kidney Int 32: 312–321

Scully RE, Marks EJ, McNeely BU (1984) Case records of the Massachusetts General Hospital. N Engl J Med 310: 244

Shaw AB, Golpalka SG (1982) Renal artery thrombosis caused by antihypertensive treatment. Br Med J 285: 1617

Siegel NJ, Glazier WB, Chaudry IH (1980) Enhanced recovery from acute renal failure by the postischemic infusion of adenine nucleotides and magnesium chloride in rats. Kidney Int 17: 338

Smith CR, Maxwell RR, Edwards CQ, Rogers JF, Lietman PS (1978) Nephrotoxicity induced by gentamicin and amikacin. Johns Hopkins Med J 142: 85

Solez K (1983) Pathogenesis of acute renal failure. Int Rev Exp Pathol 24: 277

Sos TA, Pickering TG, Phil D et al. (1983) Percutaneous transluminal renal angioplasty in renovascular hypertension due to atheroma or fibromuscular dysplasia. N Engl J Med 309: 274

Steinhausen M, Eisenbach GM, Helmstadter V (1969) Concentration of lissamine green in proximal tubules of antidiuretic- and mercury-poisoned rats and the permeability of these tubules. Pflugers Arch 311: 1

Stott RB, Cameron JS, Ogg CS, Bewick M (1972) Why the persistant high mortality in acute renal failure? Lancet I: 75

Suzuki T, Mostofi FK (1970) Electron microscopic studies of acute tubular necrosis: early changes in lower tubules of rat kidney after subcutaneous injection of glycerin. Lab Invest 23: 15

Talner LB, Scheible W, Ellenbogen PH, Beck CH Jr, Gosink BB (1981) How accurate is ultrasonography in detecting hydronephrosis in azotemic patients? Urol Radiol 3: 1

Tanner GA, Sophasan S (1976) Kidney pressure after temporary renal artery occlusion. Am J Physiol 230: 1173

Thiel G, Wilson DR, Acre ML et al. (1967) Glycerol-induced, hemoglobinuric acute renal failure in the rat: II. The experimental model, predisposing factors, and pathophysiologic features. Nephron 4: 276

Thiel G, McDonald FD, Oken DE (1970) Micropuncture studies of the basis for protection of renin depleted rats from glycerol-induced acute renal failure. Nephron 7: 67

Tonnesen AS (1988) Acute renal failure. In: Gallagher TJ, Shoemaker WC (eds) Critical care – state of the art. Society of Critical Care Medicine, Fullerton, California, pp 177–222

Vertel RM, Knochel JP (1967) Non-oliguric acute renal failure. JAMA 200: 598

Wilkins RG, Faragher EB (1983) Acute renal failure in an intensive care unit: incidence, prediction and outcome. Anesthesia 38: 628

Wilson TH (1954) Ionic permeability and osmotic swelling of cells. Science 120: 104

Wilson DM, Turner DR, Camerson JS, Ogg CS, Brown CB, Chantler C (1976) Value of renal biopsy in acute intrinsic renal failure. Br Med J 2: 459

Zarich S, Fang LST, Diamond JR (1985) Fractional excretion of sodium. Exceptions to its diagnostic value. Arch Intern Med 145: 108

Discussion

Dr Schrier was asked to discuss in more detail some of the new strategies that are not yet available in clinical practice, but which might perhaps change the history of acute renal failure in the ICU. From the very first Dr Schrier emphasized that since there was an 80% mortality from acute renal failure in patients with other organ dysfunction, it is highly ethical to look for other strategies which might improve outcome. Thus there was no ethical concern about early intervention, even when it was highly invasive, such as catheterization of the renal artery. He likened this technique to the techniques of the cardiologists when thrombolytic therapy was first introduced with its infusion directly into the coronary arteries. Similarly he felt that nephrologists would in the future be very aggressive about the prevention of acute renal failure and might well introduce renal artery catheterization as a specific intervention in the care of such cases. He emphasized that intervention would have to be early, and would have to be based on an understanding of the pathogenesis of acute renal failure. He mentioned that a prospective, randomized, multi-centre study, already in progress in Denver, was looking at some interventions which required intrarenal infusions. This technique had not been a problem so far but of course was contra-indicated if some sort of bleeding disorder was present.

Dr Schrier reiterated a general conclusion of the workshop; since two factors are involved in the pathogenesis of ischaemic acute renal failure – a vasomotor element together with tubular necrosis leading to tubular obstruction – successful intervention would require the use of agents that have a vascular effect as well as an effect on the tubule. He then went on to emphasize the role of changes in intracellular calcium levels as a factor that might be common to both abnormalities in tubular epithelial cell function and vascular smooth muscle function. Studies in the dog of ischaemic acute renal failure associated with a noradrenaline infusion suggested that the administration of a calcium blocker, verapamil or nifedipine, might provide protection against the development of acute renal failure. Timing of the administration of the calcium blocker was crucial in so far as protection was much less obvious if the calcium antagonist was administered 30 minutes after the insult. Dr Schrier emphasized that diagnosis of acute renal failure in the ICU can be made relatively early using the urinary indices; in the presence of a creatinine level of 180 µmol l^{-1}, a urinary sodium of more than 30 mmol l^{-1}, together with a urine:plasma ratio for creatinine of 20 or less, in the absence of diuretics or mannitol, then that patient is going to go on and progress to a full-blown acute renal failure syndrome. He thought it might be quite possible to infuse verapamil into the renal artery in a patient with incipient acute renal failure on the basis of the clinical picture and the urinary indices and this might not only prevent the fall in GFR, but also at the subcellular level, reduce mitochondrial calcium uptake and improve cellular function. Indeed a group in Berlin has used diltiazem in a prospective randomized study of kidneys used for cadaver transplantation. They had shown improved function in the calcium blocked kidney compared with grafts which did not receive the calcium blocker. The studies were done by giving the calcium blocker to the recipient of the graft but the same group has gone on to show that perfusing the donor organ before removal and during transport with a calcium antagonist improves its function. Dr Schrier emphasized that calcium blockers might work not only on tubular cells, but also on vascular smooth muscle cells and on mesangial cells. He emphasized that the various vasoconstrictors released in acute circulatory failure – angiotensin-II, noradrenaline and vasopressin – all act through the same post-receptor signal transduction mechanism. This is a calcium-dependent process involving the hydrolysis of phosphatidylinositol which can be prevented by the administration of these calcium blockers.

Again the work of John Conger from Colorado was mentioned. Dr Conger has demonstrated in a rat model of acute renal failure associated with intrarenal noradrenaline that renal blood flow is very poorly autoregulated. In the normal rat kidney there is preservation of renal blood flow despite falls in renal perfusion pressure. This is mediated through changes in renal vascular resistance. On the other hand in rats with ischaemic acute renal failure after 1 week, there is a virtual absence of renal autoregulation. Apparently this had also been shown in the dog and whilst no studies have been done in the human, all discussants agreed that haemodialysis might prolong the duration of acute renal failure by providing a source of episodes of hypotension. Since mortality is directly related to the duration of acute renal failure and oliguria, prolongation of the oliguric phase might well be a contributing factor to the high mortality. Dr Solez mentioned that he had shown by biopsy at 4 weeks, that an acutely failed kidney may demonstrate fresh necrotic lesions late on in the course of renal failure. Very modest alterations in blood pressure may well cause a degree of ischaemia which could prolong the course of ischaemic acute renal failure. Dr Schrier emphasized that studies in Conger's animal model suggest that defective autoregulation can be prevented by treatment with a calcium antagonist. Similarly hypersensitivity to renal nerve stimulation, which occurs in animals with ischaemic acute renal failure, can be abolished by the administration of calcium antagonists.

Dr Schrier then turned his attention to atrial natriuretic factor. He observed that the fall in blood pressure detected with atrial natriuretic factor in normal conscious animals reflected a fall in cardiac output related to a reduction in preload. On the other hand, in patients with heart failure and other forms of acute circulatory failure with increased circulating levels of noradrenaline, angiotensin-II and vasopressin, atrial natriuretic factor appears to reduce arterial vascular resistance. He thought that in patients with acute renal failure, the major effect of atrial natriuretic factor would probably be the blocking of the effects of circulating vasoconstrictors.

Atrial natriuretic factor had been shown to protect animals from acute renal failure and it acted on both blood vessels and tubules. Perhaps the combination of a calcium antagonist with atrial natriuretic factor might be the optimal form of prevention in patients with incipient acute renal failure and indeed this combination could be infused directly into the renal artery. Dr Schrier went on to discuss more studies with calcium antagonists which demonstrated a cytoprotective effect within the renal tubule itself. He emphasized the importance of the re-perfusion injury and the increase in extracellular calcium concentration as blood flow is increased during the phase of resuscitation. It was emphasized that the kidney was no different from the brain or the heart in which re-perfusion injury is so often the sequel to a period of ischaemic hypoxia.

Following on from this, many participants doubted that the moment of intervention at which intrarenal infusion of the protective agent would be initiated, could be identified as readily as Dr Schrier had suggested. Dr Neild drew attention to the fact that calcium antagonists had been studied primarily in models of ischaemic acute renal failure, and he wondered whether one could generalize from that to all other forms seen in human beings. Together with Dr Linton he doubted that it was possible to identify the group of patients who required treatment with the intrarenal infusion of any renal protective regimen, whatever that might be, just upon the basis of urinary indices. Dr Myers emphasized that Dr Schrier had not been talking about protection. In fact, if the GFR is 2 ml min^{-1} in each kidney and this is to be increased by intervention to 5 ml min^{-1} on each side, then one is intervening following an injury which has caused firmly established acute renal failure. Again, he felt that the urinary indices depended almost entirely on what day they were measured following the injury. Dr Myers thought that a selective intervention within the renal circulation was unpromising unless some systemic intervention was also introduced at the same time to reverse respiratory failure, to improve myocardial function and to reduce oedema in the gastrointestinal tract. Dr Neild asked Dr Schrier what his strategy was at present for renal protection, specifically for a patient with diabetic renal failure who has angina and requires a coronary angiogram followed by surgery. Dr Schrier replied that mannitol was their main protective agent. This was given at 1 g kg^{-1} at the time of injection of the contrast medium. It was also given during surgery to patients at risk of developing acute renal failure. Dr Bihari and Professor Cameron both agreed that it was difficult to use urinary indices to define groups of patients in most intensive care units since the majority of patients had received dopamine, frusemide and mannitol. Dr Linton re-emphasized his observation that many patients with sepsis had a low urinary sodium, whilst their serum creatinine was rising. Dr Schrier replied that they were in prerenal failure and if the tubules were able to concentrate the urine such that the urinary sodium was 4 or 5 mmol l^{-1}, then the tubules' integrity was intact. Dr

Linton emphasized that all such patients were volume expanded with oedema and high wedge pressures. Dr Schrier replied that this may well have been the case, but since they were peripherally vasodilated, this might account for underfilling of the arteriovascular tree leading to the sodium retention. Dr Bihari was concerned about another controlled study of intervention in an attempt to prevent organ failure with the administration of one single substance. He felt that since a number of mediators were involved in the tissue damage, it might be more appropriate to intervene with a cocktail of substances designed to prevent cellular injury. Presently, mannitol, low-dose dopamine and frusemide are used in the prevention and treatment of acute renal failure and it might be more appropriate to assess the effects of combining a calcium blocker with these plus atrial natriuretic factor all at the same time.

Chapter 18

Acute Renal Failure and Crush Injury

O. S. Better

Introduction

The Rambam Hospital is the main civilian and military hospital in Northern Israel. The great majority of the casualties in the Lebanese and Syrian campaigns in the last 25 years have been evacuated to this centre. Our geographic proximity to the front and the extensive use of rescue helicopters have allowed us to examine and treat victims of trauma often within 30 minutes of their injury. In some instances we have been able to start treatment in subjects with crush injury even before the completion of the extrication of the subject trapped under fallen masonry.

The purpose of this short review is to summarize our experience with the prevention of acute renal failure following crush injury with emphasis on some of the more interesting aetiological and clinical aspects of crush injury that have received only scant attention in the literature. Detailed accounts of the prevention of acute renal failure in traumatic rhabdomyolysis (Ron et al. 1984) as well as the orthopaedic management of crushed limbs (Reis and Michaelson 1986) have been published previously from this institution.

In-depth reviews summarizing vast clinical experience in rhabdomyolysis and acute renal failure have been published in the last several years (Gabow et al. 1982; Honda 1988; Knochel 1981a). From these studies it appears that rhabdomyolysis is not rare and that mechanical compression of muscle is aetiologically important in almost 40% of patients with rhabdomyolysis (Gabow et al. 1982). In a recent series, acute renal failure developed in 16.5% of patients with rhabdomyolysis, whereas the mortality in this subgroup exceeded 40% (Ward 1988).

The History, Description and Management of Myoglobinuric Renal Failure

Although the nephrotoxic potential of crush injury was mentioned in the early German literature of this century (Gabow et al. 1982) it was the classic studies by

Bywaters and Beall (1941) during the Blitz of London that brought to international attention the devastating effects on the kidney of extensive crush injury. The search and efforts of Bywaters and colleagues to find a link between trauma to muscle and kidney failure culminated in the demonstration that the nephrotoxic agent that leaked from damaged muscle was myoglobin (Bywaters and Popjak 1942). Moreover, they went on to demonstrate the therapeutically important phenomenon that myoglobin is nephrotoxic only in acid but not in alkaline urine (Bywaters and Stead 1944). Had this insight, gained in 1944, been available to Bywaters in 1941 he could have prevented acute renal failure in some of his patients by utilizing solute alkaline diuresis and thus perhaps have saved their lives in that predialysis era.

Eneas et al. (1979) demonstrated the usefulness of mannitol–bicarbonate diuresis in protecting the kidney against myoglobinuric damage. We have shown that if instituted immediately after extrication (or even during extrication) massive volume replacement followed by mannitol–bicarbonate diuresis may completely prevent acute renal failure in victims suffering from extensive crush injury. This was true even in subjects trapped under debris for more than 24 hours! (Ron et al. 1984).

Aetiology of Myoglobinuric ARF

Theoretically, the following may be involved in the pathogenesis of myoglobinuric renal failure (Honda 1988): ischaemia of the kidney; injury to the glomerular filtering apparatus; tubular obstruction by myoglobin and urate casts; tubular epithelial injury by reabsorbed myoglobin and backleak of filtrate. In some cases, glomerular injury may be aggravated by disseminated intravascular coagulation.

Based on the post-mortem demonstration of massive pigment plugs in the renal tubuli of victims of crush injury, the prevailing feeling in the 1940s was that tubular obstruction was the main cause of this type of renal failure. Today, this concept has been modified to include involvement of the entire nephron and its circulation in this process.

The muscles are the bulkiest organ system in the body, comprising almost 40% of body weight. During extensive injury to muscles, their uptake of extracellular fluid volume and ions and the release of intracellular enzymes, metabolites and ions may reach the most extreme levels seen in clinical medicine in salvageable patients. In no other condition may the level of creatine kinase in the plasma reach the level of from 10^4 to 10^6 IU l^{-1} (Gabow et al. 1982; Schulze 1962).

It is rarely appreciated how massive the "prerenal" component may become in rhabdomyolysis. In our experience it is quite common in extensive traumatic rhabdomyolysis for the muscles to sequester approximately 12 litres or more in a 75 kg adult over a period of 48 h (i.e. the order of magnitude of the entire extracellular fluid volume). If inadequately corrected, this potentially fatal hypovolaemia may cause renal ischaemia by activation of the battery of constrictor hormones such as angiotensin II, catecholamines, arginine vasopressin and intrarenal thromboxane. We, in unpublished reports, and others have seen indirect evidence of renal ischaemia even when volume depletion has been corrected. Thus, perfusion as measured by a ^{99}Tc mDPTA radionuclide scan may be absent in myogobinuric renal failure, suggesting renal ischaemia (in this setting absence of ^{99}Tc mDPTA uptake by the kidney may not be a grave prognostic sign) (Pham et al. 1987). Others have shown markedly diminished urinary sodium excretion in myoglobinuric renal failure, suggesting a component of renal ischaemia in this condition (Crowin et al. 1984).

In parallel with the amply described central role of myoglobin (and perhaps additional unidentified proteins derived from muscles and erythrocytes) other metabolites may have nephrotoxic potential (Fig. 18.1). Amongst them are purines, which are released in large quantities from disintegrating muscle and converted by the liver into uric acid. The release of organic acids from the same source may lead to profound metabolic acidosis (Gabow et al. 1982; McCarron et al. 1979), thus potentiating the nephrotoxic and obstructive potential of both myoglobin and urate particularly on the background of the oliguria and urinary concentration seen in the "prerenal" phase of rhabdomyolysis.

Finally, the acute hyperphosphataemia seen in rhabdomyolysis may increase the Ca × P product, thus creating a systemic tendency to metastatic calcification. The kidney may be adversely involved in this process. This may be aggravated by induced metabolic alkalosis in overzealous and injudicious efforts to alkalinize the urine as protection against myoglobinuric and hyperuricosuric tubular injury.

The time elapsed from the extrication to the initiation of i.v. fluid load is critical to the kidney following crush injury. Delays of 12 hours (and probably somewhat less than that) are associated with renal failure (Reis and Michaelson 1986).

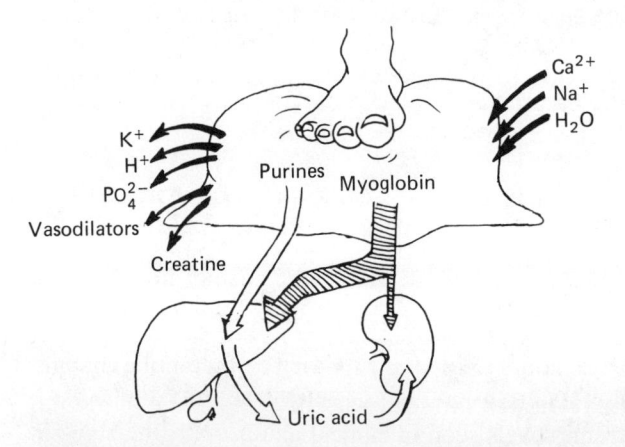

Fig. 18.1. The injured muscles may act as a huge sink for extracellular fluid and ions. This may cause a profound hypovolaemia and contribute to the hypocalcaemia. The crushed muscles also leak massive quantities of intracellular metabolites, enzymes, organic acids and probably also unidentified vasodilatory substances (Blachar et al. 1981). In the prerenal phase of rhabdomyolysis the urine is concentrated and acid. This renders the kidney susceptible to the toxic and obstructive effects of the load of myoglobin and urate originating from the muscles. Myoglobin is cleared from the bloodstream within less than 22 min of its appearance there by degradation in the kidney and by uptake by the reticuloendothelial system. There it is converted into bilirubin (Koskelo et al. 1963) and excreted by the liver.

Compounds released during muscle damage and not shown here are: (a) muscle enzymes particularly creatine kinase (some containing the MB "myocardial" fraction) (Siegel et al. 1983); and (b) thromboplastin which may contribute to the tendency for disseminated intravascular coagulation sometimes seen in rhabdomyolysis.

Abnormalities in Mineral and Electrolyte Metabolism

Rhabdomyolysis may lead to profound hypocalcaemia (reaching less than 1.2 mmol e^{-1}). This is due to a variety of causes acting synergistically. Amongst these are: massive deposition of calcium in injured muscles (Meroney et al. 1957), hyperphosphataemia and decreased production of renal 1,25-dihydroxycholecalciferol (Llach et al. 1981). This hypocalcaemia presents a therapeutic dilemma. On the one hand, it aggravates the cardiotoxic effect of hyperkalaemia. On the other hand, attempts at correction of the hypocalcaemia with an exogenous calcium load may worsen the tendency for metastatic calcification and for the development of hypercalcaemia during recovery (Knochel 1981b).

Severe hyperkalaemia may complicate rhabdomyolysis. It is surprising that hyperkalaemia is not seen more often in this condition, in view of the massive amounts of potassium stored in the muscles (75% of body potassium) (De Fronzo and Bia 1985), and the predilection to acute renal failure seen in this condition. Of interest is the fact that we encountered hyperkalaemia (mean 6.2 mEq l^{-1}; range 4.5–8.3 mEq l^{-1}) in seven victims of crush syndrome with normal kidney function. This transient "non-azotaemic hyperkalaemia" was, therefore, almost entirely due to disruption of the internal potassium balance. This illustrates the well-known inability of the intact kidney to handle acute potassium loads (De Fronzo and Bia 1985). Parallel limitations are seen in the excretion of acute endogenous loads of phosphate and of urate, resulting, respectively, in hyperphosphataemia and hyperuricaemia, despite normal renal function.

The hypokalaemic effect of glucose and insulin may be impaired in rhabdomyolysis (Honda 1988; Schulze 1962). Thus the traditional first and second line of defence against hyperkalaemia (i.e. i.v. Ca^{2+} followed by glucose and insulin) may not be appropriate on the background of rhabdomyolysis.

Therapeutic Considerations in the Crush Syndrome

When people are trapped under heavy rubble those who sustain injury to the trunk and head probably die instantaneously. Those who are rescued may have suffered crush injury of the limbs. Victims of crush injury may be saved even after having been trapped for up to 28 hours (Ron et al. 1984). The metabolic changes and the internal volume losses apparently do not commence before the extrication and decompression of limbs. Therefore, intensive search for live trapped subjects should continue for at least 48 hours and perhaps even longer. The extrication process must be carried out with extreme caution in order to prevent further trauma from the impact of moving debris. When a limb with access for a venous line has been exposed and becomes available, an i.v. infusion of saline should be started immediately. It may then take another 45 minutes to complete the removal of the trapped subject from under the rubble.

Patients with extensive traumatic rhabdomyolysis may present with flaccid paralysis of the affected muscle and with widespread sensory loss in the overlying skin. This condition may mimic paraplegia secondary to a spinal cord lesion. Useful diagnostic signs suggesting an intact spinal cord are normal urinary bladder function and normal anal sphincter tone.

In the hospital, the infusion started on site is followed by massive volume replacement averaging 12 litres a day in order to achieve a diuresis of approximately 8 litres per day (internal losses into muscle may reach over 18 litres in 60 hours) (Ron et al. 1984). Administration of mannitol (approximately 160 g day^{-1}) and sodium bicarbonate (approximately 240 mEq day^{-1}) help to secure solute alkaline (UpH > 6.5) diuresis. Metabolic alkalosis (BpH more than 7.45) is prevented with acetazolamide (average 150 mg day^{-1}). This regimen is utilized until the disappearance of myoglobin from the urine and the tapering off of the negative potassium balance.

In our experience, myoglobinuric renal failure may be prevented with correction of volume losses and institution of the described vigorous mannitol-alkaline diuresis. This measure by itself may also correct the hyperkalaemia. However, there is no need to give frusemide to prevent the renal failure associated with the crush syndrome.

Although the proposed regimen in our experience has proved successful in preventing renal failure, it is quite possible that less-aggressive solute alkaline diuresis might have achieved the same results. Thus, following the correction of the hypovolaemia, urinary outputs of 4 litres per day may be adequate to protect the kidney in the crush syndrome. This will obviate the need to use bladder catheterization, required when higher urine outputs are achieved. Whether or not the use of mannitol and bicarbonate may be omitted from the therapeutic protocol is not certain at present. However, *we* do not recommend the abandonment of these important tools in the management of the crush syndrome.

A recent preliminary report has suggested that in neurosurgical patients mannitol may cause acute renal failure (Dorman et al. 1988). We have not encountered such a complication and feel that when proper precautions are used (monitoring urine flow, plasma osmolality and central venous pressure), mannitol is a relatively safe agent in the doses recommended.

As far as the treatment of the local injury is concerned, a conservative approach seems warranted. Since the skin has an extraordinary capacity to withstand pressure and is a good barrier against infection, every effort should be made to avoid the conversion of a closed injury into an open one. In particular, the excision of non-infected dead muscle is not essential. When the orthopaedic surgeon is compelled to perform a fasciotomy to relieve intracompartmental pressure and restore the distal circulation, he should bear in mind that intense bleeding is not evidence of viability of the underlying muscle. Dead muscle may also bleed profusely. Therefore, demarcation between live and necrotic muscle can only be achieved by the application of mechanical or electrical stimulation.

Summary

In rescue operations for people trapped under fallen debris, intravenous replenishment of the massive internal volume losses should be started as soon as physical contact has been established with the injured subject. This should be followed by induced forced alkaline–mannitol diuresis. This regimen will stabilize the impaired haemodynamics and will prevent myoglobinuric and hyperuricosuric renal failure and correct the hyperkalaemia and metabolic acidosis often seen in rhabdomyolysis. This treatment is effective even in subjects rescued after having been trapped for 28 hours.

Local treatment of the crushed limbs should be conservative. Closed injury should not be converted into an open one unless distal arterial perfusion has been compromised.

References

Blachar Y, Fong JSC, De Chadarevian JP, Drummond KN (1981) Muscle extract infusion in rabbits: a new experimental model in the crush syndrome. Circ Res 49: 114–124
Bywaters EGL, Beall D (1941) Crush injuries with impairment of renal function. Br Med J i: 427–432
Bywaters EGL, Popjak G (1942) Experimental crushing injury. Surg Gynecol Obstet 75: 612
Bywaters EGL, Stead JK (1944) The production of renal failure following injection of solutions containing myohaemoglobin. Q J Exp Physiol 33: 53
Crowin HL, Schreiber MJ, Fang LST (1984) Low fractional excretion of sodium occurring with hemoglobinuric and myohemoglobinuric induced acute renal failure. Arch Intern Med 144: 981–982
De Fronzo RA, Bia MB (1985) Extrarenal potassium homeostasis. In: Seldin DW, Giebisch G (eds) The kidney: physiology and pathophysiology. Raven Press, New York, pp 1179–1206
Dorman H, Sondheimer J, Cadnapaphornchai P (1988) Characteristics of mannitol-induced (MI) acute renal failure. Kidney Int 33: 188 (abstract)
Eneas JF, Schonfeld PY, Humphreys MH (1979) The effect of infusion of mannitol-sodium bicarbonate on the clinical course of myoglobinuria. Arch Intern Med 139: 801–805
Gabow PA, Kaehny WD, Kelleher SP (1982) The spectrum of rhabdomyolysis. Medicine 61: 141–152
Honda N (1988) Acute renal failure and rhabdomyolysis. Nephrology Forum. Kidney Int 23: 888–898
Knochel JP (1981a) Rhabdomyolysis and myoglobinuria. In: Suki WN, Eknoyan G (eds) The kidney in systemic disease, 2nd edn. John Wiley, New York, pp 263–284
Knochel JP (1981b) Serum calcium derangement in rhabdomyolysis. Editorial. N Engl J Med 305: 161–162
Koskelo P, Kekki M, Wager O (1963) Kinetic behavior of ^{131}I-labelled myoglobin in human beings. Clin Chim Acta 17: 339–350
Llach F, Felsenfeld AJ, Hausler MR (1981) The pathophysiology of altered calcium metabolism in rhabdomyolysis induced acute renal failure. N Engl J Med 305: 117–123
McCarron D, Elliot WC, Rose JS, Bennett WM (1979) Severe mixed metabolic acidosis secondary to rhabdomyolysis. Am J Med 67: 905–910
Meroney WH, Arney GK, Segar WE, Black WH (1957) The acute calcification of traumatized muscle with particular reference to acute post-traumatic renal insufficiency. J Clin Invest 36: 825–832
Pham DH, Ash JM, Gilday DL, Arbus G (1987) Acute tubular necrosis secondary to rhabdomyolysis with complete absence of renal perfusion. Clin Nucl Med 12: 445–447
Reis ND, Michaelson M (1986) Crush injury to the lower limbs. J Bone Joint Surg 68A: 414–418
Ron D, Taitelman U, Michaelson M, Bar-Joseph G, Bursztein S, Better OS (1984) Prevention of acute renal failure in traumatic rhabdomyolysis. Arch Intern Med 144: 277–280
Schulze VE (1962) Rhabdomyolysis causing acute renal failure. Postgraduate Med 72: 145–150
Siegel AJ, Silverman LM, Evans WJ (1983) Elevated skeletal muscle creatine kinase MB isoenzyme levels in marathon runners. JAMA 250: 2835–2837
Ward MM (1988) Factors predictive of acute renal failure in rhabdomyolysis. Arch Intern Med 148: 1553–1557

Discussion

Dr Better was asked whether he had used hypertonic saline in the resuscitation of patients with crush injury. He had not done so, but Dr Arieff had been consulted on a number of occasions concerning the development of hypernatraemia following resuscitation with hypertonic saline. Dr Arieff was concerned that severe hypernatraemia and hyperosmolality could produce permanent brain damage and more muscle destruction. In general, he felt the use of hypertonic solutions in resuscitation should be discouraged. Dr Arieff then asked whether the hypocalcaemia associated with rhabdomyolysis in the early phase was related to the deposition of calcium within the damaged muscles. He was also concerned that hyperkalaemia could be made worse by leaving the damaged limb intact and not excising the muscle, or carrying out an amputation. Dr Better replied that the rehabilitation of people with an intact limb was much easier than when an amputation or debridement of the necrotic muscle was carried out. Furthermore, leaving the limb intact cut down the risk of infection. He emphasized this point because he had had many painful experiences of "lost limbs and lost souls". He confirmed that in his patients, the muscle appeared to absorb enormous quantities of calcium. He had not measured the uric acid levels in his patients, but in most reported cases this also was very high. Professor Cameron mentioned the problems of giving adequate analgesia to patients with rhabdomyolysis. He also commented that the development of compartmental syndromes seemed more common in his population of patients who had so-called non-traumatic rhabdomyolysis associated with narcotics and alcohol abuse.

Finally, the value of bicarbonate was discussed in the management of this condition. Professor Kleinknecht pointed out that many patients with non-traumatic rhabdomyolysis are hypokalaemic due to gastrointestinal losses, or for other reasons. Indeed, hypokalaemia appeared to be a risk factor for the development of rhabdomyolysis. Bicarbonate may not be required in these patients. Dr Bihari wondered whether a simple forced diuresis was as good as a forced alkaline diuresis. Dr Better replied that whilst there were no controlled studies of the use of bicarbonate in the prevention of acute renal failure associated with rhabdomyolysis in humans, he could not recommend forsaking this component of therapy since his results were so good.

Chapter 19

Renal Function After Open Heart Surgery

H. M. Koning and J. A. Leusink

Renal impairment following surgery can have considerable consequences for the patient. Severe postoperative renal dysfunction has a mortality exceeding 50%. The need for frequent dialysis imposes a heavy burden, not only on the patient, but also on the intensive care unit and laboratory services. Although mortality remains high and therapy is expensive, patients who recover are generally restored to health and do not require continued medical care, thus making therapy worthwhile.

Most cases of acute renal failure (ARF) which occur in the general district hospital are related to surgery or trauma and its complications. During the last three decades the typical story of ARF developing in young patients after major trauma or obstetric complications, has changed to that of ARF arising in elderly patients following complicated (usually abdominal) surgery (Stott et al. 1972).

ARF following general surgery is particularly associated with complications arising during or following surgery (McMurray et al. 1978). The majority of cases of ARF following gastrointestinal operations might have been avoided had appropriate preventive steps been taken. Patients who develop ARF related to intra-abdominal infection do so usually because of a delay in the diagnosis of surgical disease, namely perforated viscus, appendicitis or a ruptured diverticulum.

Major abdominal aortic surgery carries a risk of ARF because of the possible involvement of the renal vessels. Other risk factors include the advanced age of these patients, increased incidence of hypertensive nephrosclerosis and an angiographic procedure before operation. Surgery of a ruptured aortic aneurysm presents an additional risk of renal complications due to hypovolaemic shock.

ARF following cardiac surgery is not so obviously related to surgical complications. Nowadays it seems to be related to patients of older age with pre-existent diminished renal function who are undergoing complex cardiac surgery. Management of patients during and after open heart surgery has been improved.

However, special attention to these patients is mandatory if ARF is to be avoided.

Acute Renal Failure Following Cardiac Surgery

In the postoperative period following open heart surgery there is a close correlation between the degree of renal impairment and the postoperative mortality rate (Table 19.1). Normal postoperative renal function is associated with a low mortality of 0.8% whereas the mortality increases to 89% when the postoperative serum creatinine concentration exceeds 440 µmol l^{-1} (Abel et al. 1976).

Table 19.1. Incidence and mortality of renal dysfunction after open heart surgery

Renal function	Incidence (%)	Mortality (%)
Serum creatinine less than 135 µmol l^{-1}	72	0.8
Serum creatinine 135–220 µmol l^{-1}	21	10.6
Serum creatinine 220–440 µmol l^{-1}	3.4	23.5
Serum creatinine exceeding 440 µmol l^{-1}	3.6	88.8

ARF is a distinct pathophysiological entity which can cause various degrees of impairment. It is therefore confusing to distinguish between "functional" (mild) and "organic" (serious) ARF. However, in the literature renal impairment following cardiac surgery is divided into two forms: mild and serious ARF. The criteria of mild and serious ARF are in almost every study different, making comparisons of incidence and mortality difficult.

To overcome this problem all patients undergoing cardiac surgery in a one month period in 1985 in our hospital were compared with the results of other studies using their criteria of ARF (Table 19.2). The incidence and mortality of mild ARF were considerably lower. The incidence of serious ARF was also reduced, but not to the same extent as with mild ARF. The mortality of serious ARF remained the same compared with two other studies in the literature (Yeboah et al. 1972; Hilberman et al. 1979) but was decreased compared with two others (Brunner et al. 1972; Abel et al. 1976).

Table 19.2. Comparison of incidence (I) and mortality (M) of renal complications of patients in 1985 with previous studies using their criteria

	Mild ARF Their study		Our study		Serious ARF Their study		Our study	
	I	M	I	M	I	M	I	M
Yeboah et al. (1972)	26%	38%	9%	17%	5%	70%	2%	67%
Brunner et al. (1972)					3%	77%	2%	50%
Abel et al. (1976)	21%	11%	14%	0%	7%	57%	4%	40%
Hilberman et al. (1979)	2.5%	17%	26%	0%	3%	65%	2%	67%

In the beginning of the 1970s an increase in the incidence of renal complications following cardiac surgery was reported (Krian 1976). However, this trend of increasing frequency has been reversed, and currently a lower incidence and mortality can be expected. The major concern continues to be the high mortality of serious ARF.

Mortality in Patients with ARF Following Cardiac Surgery

The mortality in patients suffering from ARF can be differentiated into early and late mortality. The early mortality is greatly influenced by the underlying illness which was responsible for the initial development of ARF. The late mortality is related to the complications of ARF. Despite intensive therapy, late mortality is high, and related to sepsis, gastrointestinal bleeding, hyperkalaemia and multiple organ failure.

The causes of death of all patients with ARF following open heart surgery were studied. Cardiac failure in the first four days following operation was responsible for 46% of the fatalities. Sepsis, which occurred more than 4 days after surgery, was responsible for death in 39% and hyperkalaemia accounted for the remaining 15%. Other studies have also confirmed cardiac failure and infection as major causes of death in patients with ARF following open heart surgery (Casali et al. 1975; Brunner et al. 1972).

Despite frequent dialysis, optimal nutrition, and aggressive treatment of infections, the mortality of serious ARF remains high, and there is little prospect for an early improvement. The more successful approach to the problem of ARF is to attempt to decrease its incidence. Prevention of ARF following open heart surgery begins with knowledge of the pathogenesis of renal complications of open heart surgery.

Identification of Patients with ARF Following Cardiac Surgery

It has been suggested that failure to affect the mortality of serious ARF may reflect a change in population rather than a lack of improvement in management expertise (McMurray et al. 1978). Certainly the pattern of patients with ARF following cardiac surgery has changed. The population undergoing open heart surgery is becoming increasingly more elderly, and patients undergo increasingly complex cardiac surgery when already in a precarious state.

Table 19.3 shows age, pre-operative blood urea nitrogen (BUN) and the duration of cardiopulmonary bypass in several studies for patients with and without postoperative renal complications. Even in patients without renal complications an increase in age and a rise in blood urea nitrogen is found

Table 19.3. The values of variables reported in patients with normal renal function and with acute renal failure following open heart surgery in several studies

	Age (years)		Pre-operative BUN (mg 100 ml blood^{-1})		Duration CPB (min)	
	N	ARF	N	ARF	N	ARF
Brunner et al. (1972)					75	127
Abel et al. (1974)	51 ± 11.4	56 ± 10.8	16 ± 5.4	24 ± 15.6		
Abel et al. (1976)	47 ± 17	58 ± 8.3	15 ± 4.9	39 ± 34.5		
Hilberman et al. (1979)	57 ± 12	64 ± 13	19 ± 8	32 ± 20	110 ± 40	159 ± 62
Koning et al. (1985)	57 ± 10.5	71 ± 4.8	18 ± 5.4	44 ± 31.8	96 ± 34.5	126 ± 39.3

Mean values and standard deviation.

compared with the studies of the 1970s. This reflects the change in the population currently presenting for open heart surgery.

In patients with postoperative renal complications the age was higher, the renal function more diminished and the duration of cardiopulmonary bypass (CPB) longer, compared with patients without renal complications.

One can conclude from the foregoing information that the management of renal function has improved considerably. The incidence and mortality of mild ARF has decreased. Furthermore, the incidence of serious ARF has also decreased, despite the more difficult population. Only the mortality of serious ARF remains high. To forestall this complication, special attention should nowadays be directed to patients with an age above 70 and an already compromised pre-operative renal function.

Pathogenesis of Acute Renal Failure

Low cardiac output is the major determinant of renal dysfunction after open heart surgery (Hilberman et al. 1979). Severe depression of postoperative cardiac function with resultant renal ischaemia, is invariably present in patients who develop postoperative renal dysfunction.

The pathogenesis of ARF following cardiac surgery was considered to be multifactorial, consisting of the superposition of additional renal insults upon ischaemic kidneys (Hilberman et al. 1979; Krian 1976). Many variables have been shown to influence renal function during and following open heart surgery. In such a case a multivariate statistical analysis is appropriate to investigate its multifactorial nature. The results of such analyses have indicated that the main factor causing serious ARF is critical circulatory compromise in the postoperative period (Koning et al. 1985). The other major factor to emerge is the age of the patient. An age over 70 years was invariably associated with an increased risk for serious ARF.

Postoperative Renal Function

From the literature it is clear that patients who maintain normal renal function following open heart surgery have a number of characteristics in common (Table

19.4) (Porter et al. 1966; Hilberman et al. 1979; Myers et al. 1980, 1981). In patients with normal renal function a cardiac index exceeding 2.5 l min^{-1} m^{-2} is found. Glomerular filtration is maintained by an increase in the postglomerular resistance within the kidney, despite the decreased renal plasma flow.

Table 19.4. Characteristics of patients with normal renal function following open heart surgery

	Porter et al. (1966) (mean)	Hilberman et al. (1979) (mean ± SD)	Myers et al. (1980) (mean ± SEM)	Myers et al. (1981) (mean ± SEM)
Cardiac index (l min^{-1} m^{-2})	2.78	2.6 ± 0.5	2.8 ± 0.1	2.8 ± 0.16
Creatinine cl. (ml min^{-1} m^{-2})	38	57 ± 17	49 ± 2	44 ± 3.5
ERPF (ml min^{-1} m^{-2})		221 ± 54		183 ± 18.5
GFR/ERPF		0.28 ± 0.07		0.25 ± 0.02
serum creatinine (μmol l^{-1})				106 ± 9
FE$_{Na}$ (%)		0.48 ± 0.7	1.1 ± 0.3	1.0 ± 0.3
U/P osmol ratio	2.9		1.94 ± 0.08	

SD, standard deviation; SEM, standard error of the mean; Creatinine cl., creatinine clearance; GFR, glomerular filtration rate; ERPF, effective renal plasma flow; FE$_{Na}$, fractional excretion of sodium.

In patients with renal complications following open heart surgery a depressed cardiac index is observed together with a decreased glomerular filtration rate and renal plasma flow (Myers et al. 1980; Hilberman et al. 1980). The outcome and subsequent changes in renal function are dependent, not only on the severity of the postoperative haemodynamic depression, but also on its duration (Hilberman et al. 1980). If the cardiac index improves by the second or third day postoperatively a mild form of renal dysfunction is found. However, if the cardiac index remains depressed severe dysfunction is provoked with a mortality of 80%.

Postoperative Cardiac Performance

Patients with diminished cardiac function require optimalization of their systemic haemodynamics in order to avoid a low cardiac output state. Knowledge of the haemodynamic changes which occur during open heart surgery can lead to better peri-operative management of impaired myocardial performance and to a lower mortality. Haemodynamic influences during and following cardiopulmonary bypass seem to be more important for the development of low cardiac output than the pre-operative cardiac function (Koning and Leusink 1987).

During the first 24 hours cardiac function is sensitive to changes in systemic vascular resistance. A high systemic vascular resistance is of critical importance in the pathogenesis of low cardiac output following cardiopulmonary bypass (Taylor et al. 1977). Cardiopulmonary bypass can elict a marked sympatho-adrenal response which is associated with an increase in systemic vascular resistance and deterioration of postoperative myocardial performance (Taylor et al. 1977; Hoar et al. 1980; Kim et al. 1981; Reves et al. 1982). The most important factor influencing vasoconstriction is the flow rate during cardiopulmonary bypass (Sanger et al. 1960). An inadequate flow leads to activation of vasoconstrictive mechanisms which continue to impede cardiac function postoperatively. The flow rate used during cardiopulmonary bypass can induce changes which hinder postoperative cardiac performance and thus also renal performance. Optimal management of pump flow rate during cardiopulmonary bypass is an effective means of preventing cardiac and renal dysfunction after open heart surgery.

Management During CPB to Prevent Renal Dysfunction

The basic function of cardiopulmonary bypass is to provide an adequate flow of oxygenated blood to tissues in need and to prevent damage to organs (Robiscek et al. 1983). One of the organs vulnerable to damage is the kidney. Renal function may be considered to be an important circulatory parameter.

The changes in serum creatinine induced by open heart surgery are shown in Fig. 19.1. Only 3% of the patients had the same postoperative as pre-operative serum creatinine value. An increased serum creatinine was seen in 48% of patients postoperatively, whereas 49% had a decreased serum creatinine. Thus the effect of cardiac surgery on renal function is not exclusively negative. The flow rate during cardiopulmonary bypass and the age of the patient determines largely the renal response to cardiac surgery.

An inadequate flow rate used during cardiopulmonary bypass can have severe adverse effects in the postoperative period, even when hypothermia is used. In general, an inadequate flow rate leads to the activation of various vasomotor mechanisms consisting of:

Intrinsic vasomotor activity in vessels leading to vasoconstriction and a raised systemic vascular resistance,

Activation of the sympathetic system with venous and arterial constriction leading to a decreased venous blood capacity and a raised systemic vascular resistance, and

Activation of hormonal systems (noradrenaline, adrenaline, renin, angiotensin, aldosterone, and vasopressin)

A higher flow employed after a period of inadequate flow will reverse the raised systemic vascular resistance (Sanger et al. 1960) and the decreased venous capacity for blood. The activated hormonal mechanism will persist because of the decreased metabolism (hypothermia, lack of pulmonary blood flow) and can still

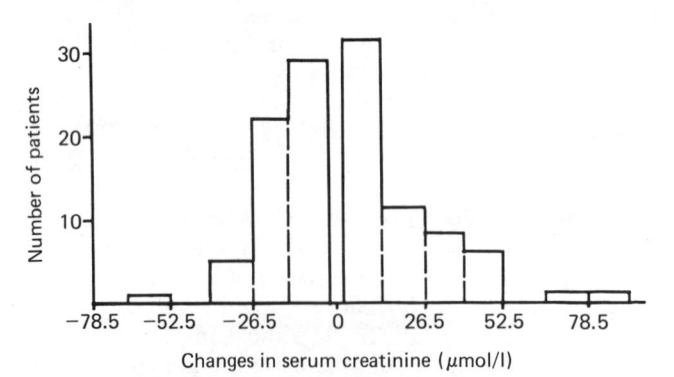

Fig. 19.1. Frequency distribution of changes in serum creatinine induced by open heart surgery. Adapted from Koning et al. (1987).

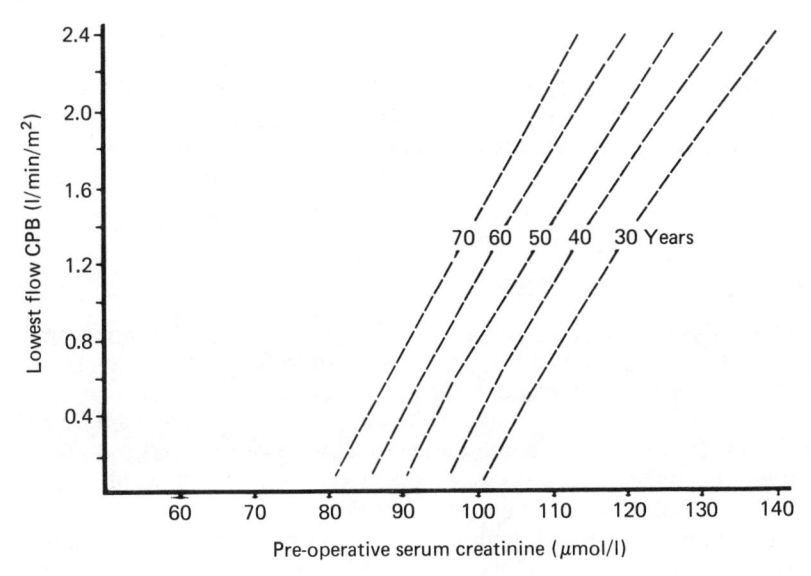

Fig. 19.2. Lowest blood flow for a desired postoperative serum creatinine of 110 μmol l^{-1}. Adapted from Koning et al. (1987).

adversely influence postoperative cardiac performance. All of these hormones are reported to be increased during the following cardiopulmonary bypass, although the extent of the increase is variable (Taylor et al. 1977; Hoar et al. 1980; Reves et al. 1982; Feddersen et al. 1985). The relationship between the flow rate used and the magnitude of hormonal activation during cardiopulmonary bypass in each study is not clear. The lowest blood flow is more important than the mean and the highest blood flow for the activation of vasomotor mechanisms, and this was not reported in the studies.

The renal response to cardiac surgery was used to determine the lowest acceptable flow rate during extra-corporeal circulation (Koning et al. 1987). Statistical analysis showed that changes in serum creatinine induced by cardiac surgery are influenced by a combination of lowest blood flow during cardiopulmonary bypass and the age of the patients. If renal complications are to be avoided adjustment of flow should take place according to the age and to the level of the pre-operative serum creatinine (Fig. 19.2).

Postoperative Cardiac Output Values for Optimal Renal Function

To prevent postoperative renal complications an optimal cardiac output should be present during the immediate postoperative period. In the postoperative period following open heart surgery a cardiac index of 2.4 l min^{-1} m^{-2} or more should result in an adequate renal blood flow (Koning et al. 1988).

Routine mechanical ventilation is advocated following open heart surgery (Sladen 1985). During artificial ventilation inferior vena cava haemodynamics have been implicated as a factor in kidney dysfunction in addition to changes in cardiac output (Marquez et al. 1979). Positive pressure ventilation impedes the venous return to the thorax due to the raised intrathoracic pressure. This leads to pooling of blood in the inferior vena cava and to an increase in renal venous pressure. Therefore, to achieve the same renal blood flow as during spontaneous ventilation a higher cardiac output is needed during the period of positive pressure ventilation. During the period of intermittent positive pressure ventilation a cardiac index of $2.9 \, l \, min^{-1} \, m^{-2}$ or more is recommended especially for the patients at risk for postoperative renal dysfunction (Koning et al. 1988).

Blood Trauma During Extra-corporeal Circulation

Haemolysis and activation of the complement system during cardiopulmonary bypass has been related to an increased risk for renal dysfunction following open heart surgery. Haemolysis alone is not sufficient to cause renal dysfunction and other serious complications are necessary, such as shock or severe acidosis (Krian 1976). There is direct evidence of complement activation during and following cardiopulmonary bypass, giving support to the hypothesis that a whole body inflammatory reaction of variable magnitude develops as a result of cardiopulmonary bypass and that a transient damaging effect, also on the kidney, results (Kirklin et al. 1983). However, this is not supported by the serum creatinine changes induced by cardiac surgery, since positive effects on the renal function are recorded in addition to the negative effects. Complement activation seems to be only of minor importance in the development of postoperative renal dysfunction.

Blood Pressure During Perfusion

The optimal or acceptable blood pressure during cardiopulmonary bypass is a matter of discussion. Experience has shown that the function and protection of vital organs depends on flow rather than on pressure, and the efficiency of perfusion is not assured by a seemingly adequate pressure alone. A minimal perfusion pressure of 35–40 mmHg is thought necessary to maintain capillary potency.

Some studies found a correlation between the duration of low blood pressure during extra-corporeal circulation and the incidence of postoperative renal dysfunction (Bhat et al. 1976; Yeboah et al. 1972). However, in another study the opposite finding was reported (Brunner et al. 1972). Also we could not find a statistical relation between blood pressure during extra-corporeal circulation and the development of impairment in renal function following open heart surgery (Koning et al. 1987) or acute renal failure in the postoperative period (Koning et al. 1985).

Summary and Conclusions

Open heart surgery is notorious for its renal complications even though an improvement in renal function is seen in almost half of the patients operated. Nevertheless acute renal failure is a frequent complication of open heart surgery, and is strongly related to the mortality in the immediate postoperative period.

However, the incidence and mortality of acute renal failure following open heart surgery seem to be decreasing, probably as a result of an improved general management. Still the mortality of serious acute renal failure remains high.

ARF following open heart surgery is associated with cardiac surgery in older patients with pre-existent diminished renal function. The impaired renal function is generally stable and can not explain the sudden loss of renal function during cardiac surgery, especially as other types of surgery (e.g. orthopaedics) rarely cause acute renal failure in the same population. The main differences between open heart surgery and other types of operation are:

The frequent occurrence of postoperative cardiac dysfunction and circulatory problems

The use of cardiopulmonary bypass during the operation

The use of postoperative artificial ventilation.

It is therefore possible that these features of open heart surgery contribute to the incidence of postoperative renal complications. Each of them can influence renal function and special attention should be directed to the prevention of a negative effect on renal function.

Good, intensive haemodynamic management during and following the operation seems essential for good results. The frequent occurrence of cardiac dysfunction following open heart surgery leads to a higher renal complication rate compared with other operations. The severity of the circulatory insufficiency associated with the occurrence of renal dysfunction determines the object of postoperative haemodynamic management. In the postoperative period of open heart surgery renal dysfunction is associated with a cardiac index of less than $2.5 \, l \, min^{-1} \, m^{-2}$. Hence, a cardiac index exceeding $2.5 \, l \, min^{-1} \, m^{-2}$ should be the main objective of haemodynamic management following open heart surgery.

Management during the period of extra-corporeal circulation determines the incidence of patients with low cardiac output following open heart surgery. The flow rate used during cardiopulmonary bypass has a pronounced influence on the postoperative cardiac performance. Low flow results in the development of postoperative vasoconstriction, with an increased risk of low cardiac output. The magnitude of the flow during CPB depends on the age of the patient and on the pre-operative renal function. In older patients and in patients with a pre-operative diminished renal function, a higher flow should be used.

Following cardiac surgery routine mechanical ventilation is advocated. During this period a selective impairment in renal perfusion can be provoked. In order to guarantee an optimal renal perfusion in this period a higher cardiac output is necessary. The period of postoperative mechanical ventilation should be as short as possible in order to prevent renal complications of open heart surgery.

References

Abel RM, Wick J, Beck CH, Buckley MJ, Austen WG (1974) Renal dysfunction following open heart operations. Arch Surg 102: 175–177

Abel RM, Buckley MJ, Austen WG, Barnett GO, Beck CH Jr, Fisher JE (1976) Etiology, incidence and prognosis of renal failure following cardiac operations. J Thorac Cardiovasc Surg 71: 323–333

Bhat JG, Gluck MC, Lowenstein J, Baldwin DS (1976) Renal failure after open heart surgery. Ann Intern Med 84: 677–682

Brunner L, Heisig B, Scheler F, Stapenhorst K, Tauschke D, Baumgarten C, Hoffmeister HE, Kirchhoff PG, Rastan H, Regensburger D, Stunkat R, de Vivie R, Koncz J (1972) Die Ursachen des akuten Nierenversagens nach Herz-Lungen-Maschinen-Operationen. Thoraxchirurgie 20: 26–37

Casali R, Simmons RL, Najarian JS, von Haritizsch B, Buselmeier TJ, Kjellstrand CM (1975) Acute renal insufficiency complicating major cardiovascular surgery. Ann Surg 181: 370–375

Feddersen K, Aurell M, Delin K, Haggendal J, Aren C, Radegran K (1985) Effects of cardiopulmonary bypass and prostacyclin on plasma catecholamines, angiotensin II and arginine-vasopressin. Acta Anaesthesiol Scand 29: 224–230

Hilberman M, Myers BD, Carrie BJ, Derby G, Jamison RL, Stinson EB (1979) Acute renal failure following cardiac surgery. J Thorac Cardiovasc Surg 77: 880–888

Hilberman M, Derby GC, Spencer RJ, Stinson EB (1980) Sequential pathophysiological changes characterizing the progression from the renal dysfunction to acute renal failure following cardiac operation. J Thorac Cardiovasc Surg 79: 838–844

Hoar PF, Stone JG, Faltas AN, Bendixen HH, Head RJ, Berkowitz BA (1980) Hemodynamic and adrenergic responses to anesthesia and operation for myocardial revascularisation. J Thorac Cardiovasc Surg 80: 242–248

Kim YD, Jones M, Hanowell ST, Koch JP, Lees DE, Weise V, Kopin IJ (1981) Changes in peripheral vascular and cardiac sympathetic activity before and after coronary artery bypass surgery: Interrelationships with hemodynamic alterations. Am Heart J 102: 972–979

Kirklin JK, Westaby S, Blackstone EH, Kirklin JW, Chenoweth DE, Pacifico AD (1983) Complement and the damaging effects of cardiopulmonary bypass. J Thorac Cardiovasc Surg 86: 845–857

Koning HM, Leusink JA (1987) Cardiac performance following open heart surgery. Thorac Cardiovasc Surg 35: 304–306

Koning HM, Koning AJ, Leusink JA (1985) Serious acute renal failure following open heart surgery. Thorac Cardiovasc Surg. 33: 283–287

Koning HM, Koning AJ, Defauw JJAM (1987) Optimal perfusion during extra-corporeal circulation. Scand J Thorac Cardiovasc Surg 21: 207–213

Koning HM, Leusink JA, Nas AA, van Scheijen EJ, van Urk P, Haas FJLM, Koning AJ (1988) Renal function following open heart surgery: The influence of postoperative artificial ventilation. Thorac Cardiovasc Surg. 36: 1–5

Krian A (1976) Incidence, prevention and treatment of acute renal failure following cardiopulmonary bypass. Int Anesthesiol Clin 14: 98–101

Marquez JM, Douglas ME, Downs JB, Wu WH, Mantini El, Kuck EJ, Calderwood HW (1979) Renal function and cardiovascular responses during positive airway pressure. Anesthesiology 50: 393–398

McMurray SD, Luft FC, Maxwell DR, Hamburger RJ, Futtey D, Szwed JJ, Lavelle KJ, Kleit SA (1978) Prevailing patterns and predictor variables in patients with acute tubular necrosis. Arch Intern Med 138: 950–955

Myers BD, Carrie BJ, Yee AR, Hilberman M, Michaels AS (1980) Pathophysiology of hemodynamically mediated acute renal failure in man. Kidney Int 18: 495–504

Myers BD, Hilberman M, Carrie BJ, Spencer RJ, Stinson EB, Robertson CR (1981) Dynamics of glomerular ultrafiltration following open heart surgery. Kidney Int 20: 366–374

Porter GA, Kloster FE, Herr RJ, Starr A, Griswold HE, Kimsey J, Lenertz H (1966) Relationship between alterations in renal hemodynamics during cardiopulmonary bypass and postoperative renal function. Circulation 34: 1005–1021

Reves JG, Karp RB, Buttner EE, Tosone S, Smith LR, Samuelson PN, Kreusch GR, Oparil S (1982) Neuronal and adrenomedullary catecholamine release in response to cardiopulmonary bypass in man. Circulation 66: 49–55

Robiscek F, Masters TN, Niesluchowski W, Yeager JC, Duncan GD (1983) Vasomotor activity during cardiopulmonary bypass. In: Utley JR (ed) Pathophysiology and techniques of cardiopulmonary bypass, vol II. Williams and Wilkins, Baltimore, pp 1–13

Sanger PW, Robiscek F, Taylor FH, Rees TT, Stam RE (1960) Vasomotor regulation during extracorporeal circulation and open-heart surgery. J Thorac Cardiovasc Surg 40: 355–374

Sladen RN (1985) Temperature and ventilation after hypothermic cardiopulmonary bypass. Anesth Analg 64: 816–820

Stott RB, Ogg CS, Cameron JS, Bewick M (1972) Why the persistently high mortality in acute renal failure? Lancet II: 75–78

Taylor KM, Morton IJ, Brown JJ, Bain WH, Caves PK (1977) Hypertension and the renin–angiotensin system following open-heart surgery. J Thorac Cardiovasc Surg 74: 840–845

Yeboah ED, Petrie A, Pead JL (1972) Acute renal failure and open heart surgery. Br Med J i: 415–418

Discussion

Dr Koning was questioned about the use of inotropes in his patients. Dopamine and mannitol were not used routinely during cardiopulmonary bypass and the only indication for dopamine in his patients following open heart surgery was the development of a low cardiac output. Dr Myers felt that the radionuclear method of measuring blood flow was not very accurate. He agreed that patients with chronic renal insufficiency required high pump flows during cardiopulmonary bypass, but he was unsure that the serum creatinine was a useful measure in such patients since they had a massive expansion of their whole body water. The volume of distribution of creatinine was greatly increased in such patients which probably reflects the volume loading that is common anaesthetic practice for patients undergoing cardiopulmonary bypass surgery. There then followed a general discussion concerning the various methods of measuring renal plasma flow that depend on radionuclear techniques. Essentially, all participants agreed that these were pretty inaccurate, and were only a qualitative guide rather than a means of obtaining quantitative data.

The discussion moved to the effects of mechanical ventilation on myocardial function. Dr Bihari pointed out that the effects of positive pressure are very different, depending on whether the patient is in heart failure or has a normal heart with a reduction in blood volume. He emphasized that there was a lot of interest these days in the way that positive pressure within the thorax can actually reduce left ventricular systolic peak wall tension and hence afterload in patients with left ventricular failure and dilated cardiomyopathy. He asked Dr Koning why they had wanted to reduce flow during bypass, since in most institutions flow was usually set somewhere between 2.2 and $2.4 \, l \, min^{-1} \, m^{-2}$. Dr Koning was also asked about pulsatile flow and whether this made a difference to end-organ function. Unfortunately, he had not studied it, but he thought that the main advantage of pulsatile flow appeared to be a reduction in the systemic vascular resistance following cardiopulmonary bypass. Dr Koning also maintained that in old patients with decreased renal function it was better to have an increase in blood flow, up to $3 \, l \, min^{-1} \, m^{-2}$, so as to preserve end-organ function.

The discussion moved on to the cerebral consequences of cardiopulmonary bypass and Dr Koning was asked whether these were seen in the same patients as those who developed renal dysfunction. Dr Koning pointed out that it was difficult to define neurological damage following cardiopulmonary bypass surgery since it may be minimal, in which case it appears to occur commonly, or significant, in which case it is fairly rare. All agreed that this was an important problem and may reflect similar end-organ damage as that seen in the kidney.

Chapter 20

Acute Renal Failure Following Heart and Heart–Lung Transplantation

M. E. Rogerson, G. H. Neild and F. D. Thompson

Introduction

The outcome of cardiac transplantation has improved and its application has been extended during the past 7 years. Similarly, combined heart and lung transplantation has been used for the management of an increasing number of end-stage pulmonary diseases with increasingly good results. One-year cardiac allograft survival of 80% is now commonplace (Schroeder and Hunt 1986) and 85% of these recipients are fully rehabilitated (Solis and Kaye 1986). The success of these techniques is due to a combination of improved surgical techniques and aftercare, and the use of cyclosporin (CS). Most heart transplant centres now use cyclosporin in combination with either low-dose steroids or azathioprine, thus reducing the impact of infection and steroid-related side effects.

In earlier years of cardiac transplantation, potential recipients were commonly moribund, cachectic and had established multi-organ failure, including renal failure, secondary to their low cardiac output. Now, since the technique has become more widely available and accepted, patients are being referred for assessment at an earlier stage of their disease and are being transplanted in a better general condition. Patients of older age and with systemic diseases are also referred, thus increasing again the complications which may develop. In such patients the stress of the transplant procedure and its associated fluid and metabolic changes, and the added risks of immunosuppression predispose to several complications including infection and renal failure.

Acute renal failure in this context may have many causes, and pre-existing prerenal failure, difficult fluid balance control in the peri-operative period and nephrotoxicity from cyclosporin (Moran et al. 1985) may all play a role. The incidence of acute renal failure in the heart and heart–lung recipients at Harefield Hospital was about 12% in 1986.

When cyclosporin was first used for cardiac transplantation, both daily doses and trough blood levels were considerably higher than are now used. This is reflected by the progressively lower incidence of acute renal failure, and improvement in renal function seen at all time intervals in healthy recipients (Martin et al. 1987). Some centres now avoid cyclosporin when there is evidence of renal impairment and doses are adjusted according to blood levels and in some cases renal function. Chronic cyclosporin nephrotoxicity has progressed in a few cases to end-stage renal failure (Myers et al. 1985).

This chapter reviews our experience in the management of acute renal failure following heart and heart–lung transplantation referred by a single centre.

Patients Studied

Between November 1984 and May 1988, 370 heart and 152 heart–lung transplants were performed at Harefield Hospital. During the same period 20 patients were transferred to St Paul's Hospital with acute renal failure following heart (12) or heart–lung (8) transplantation, including one heterotopic heart and three "Domino" heart transplants, donated from living donors who were themselves the recipients of heart–lung grafts. Other patients who developed renal failure in the immediate postoperative period were either too unstable to transfer or were managed by continuous haemofiltration in the transplant centre.

There were twelve males and eight females, mean age 38 (range 21–60) years, and indications for their operations were cardiomyopathy (8), ischaemic heart disease (4), right-to-left shunt (6), alpha-1-antitrypsin deficiency (1) and idiopathic pulmonary hypertension (1). Their management and outcome is described.

Renal Failure

Pre-operative assessment revealed renal impairment in 11, with mean plasma creatinine for all patients of 185 µmol l^{-1} (range 134–300 µmol l^{-1}), urea 16 (range 10.2–24) mmol l^{-1} (data for one patient unavailable). Two patients were on peritoneal dialysis at the time of transplantation.

Hepatic dysfunction was present in six of eight patients in whom information was available, with a mean plasma bilirubin 68.7 µmol l^{-1} (range 16–159, normal <17 µmol l^{-1}), alkaline phosphatase 213 IU l^{-1} (range 75–537, normal <200 IU l^{-1}), aspartate transaminase 35 IU l^{-1} (range 16–52, normal <40 IU l^{-1}).

Renal failure developed 2–60 days (median 7) after transplantation; the recipient of the heterotopic heart experienced immediate haemodynamic instability and oliguria; three patients were initially non-oliguric, one becoming anuric later. Treatment was initiated at the transplant centre in most cases and patients were transferred to the renal intensive care unit when sufficiently stable. In seven patients renal replacement was continued by intermittent haemodialysis, daily or on alternate days, three patients received high-volume haemofiltration because of cardiac instability, and in the remaining patients, daily low volume haemofiltration was carried out, with intermittent haemodialysis as necessary. One patient remained non-oliguric and did not require renal replacement therapy.

Vascular access, in the first instance, was achieved by double-lumen subclavian or left internal jugular catheter in 17, and femoral cannulae in two; these were replaced as necessary and arterio-venous shunts were substituted in 12 cases. Renal biopsy was contra-indicated by thrombocytopenia in the early part of the illness.

One patient who had required intra-aortic balloon pumping, high-dose adrenaline support, and peritoneal dialysis pre-operatively, had prolonged anuria despite otherwise good progress, and therefore underwent renal biopsy. This showed acute tubular necrosis and the patient recovered renal function after a period of 50 days. The other patient requiring peritoneal dialysis pre-operatively was shown to have cortical necrosis at post-mortem. Other post-mortem renal histology showed only acute tubular necrosis.

Cardio-respiratory Support

Post-operative management routinely includes the use of dopamine or dobutamine for the first few days; these had been continued or restarted in seven patients at the time of transfer, and two required additional high-dose adrenaline support. Inotropes were discontinued in five cases within 48 hours of arrival, one patient died after 36 hours of support and another required support until his death after 60 days.

Eight patients were artificially ventilated on arrival, three continued throughout (2, 4 and 24 days) and eight more became hypoxic requiring ventilation at a later stage. This was due to infection in seven and graft rejection in one; only three of these patients subsequently regained spontaneous ventilation.

Immunosuppression

Immediately following the operation, patients were given azathioprine 75–125 mg daily and CS 5–10 mg kg^{-1} day^{-1}. CS levels, at Harefield Hospital, were monitored daily by radio-immunoassay (RIA) of plasma samples taken pre-dose, and doses were adjusted according to daily levels and renal function. Graft rejection was diagnosed clinically with the help of external cardiac monitoring, daily ECG recordings and weekly endocardial biopsies.

The highest plasma CS level recorded in each patient was in the range 154–1463 ng ml^{-1}, mean 648 ng ml^{-1} (therapeutic range 150–300 ng ml^{-1}). Whole blood cyclosporin levels were measured in our unit by RIA (polyclonal antibody, Sandoz) and at the time of arrival, the mean pre-dose level was 537 ng ml^{-1}, range 75–2000 (therapeutic range 200–800 ng ml^{-1}). The drug had already been withdrawn in six patients and was stopped in one more, nevertheless, in each case the CS level remained greater than 200 ng ml^{-1} for more than seven days.

Azathioprine was continued at a dose dictated by the white blood cell count and prednisolone was introduced in those patients who were no longer receiving CS. In the five patients in whom CS was continued, the whole blood, trough level was maintained in the range 200–400 ng ml^{-1}, mean dose 4.9 mg kg^{-1} day^{-1} (range 2.5–10).

Rejection was diagnosed on seven occasions in six patients (3 heart, 3 heart–lung) by clinical criteria (pulmonary infiltrates or dysrhythmia) in four cases and after endocardial biopsy in three. Treatment was with pulses of methylprednisolone with or without antithymocyte globulin. All resolved satisfactorily by histological criteria.

Nutrition

Three patients remained well enough throughout to continue oral feeding. The majority however required intensive support with nasogastric feeds in four and full parenteral regimens with appropriate dialysis/filtration schedules in the others. Intralipid was not used in the heart–lung recipients.

Microbiology

Routine specimens were taken regularly to isolate pathogens and establish sensitivity patterns early where possible. Infection became evident in all patients, at some stage, with fever or haemodynamic instability. Pathogens were (a) *Pseudomonas* species commonly, colonizing seven patients in either chest or peritoneum, (b) other Gram-negative organisms (three cases), (c) *Candida* was a significant infection in four and probably non-invasive in three others; two of the former cases succumbed despite antifungal treatment and were found at post-mortem to have disseminated cytomegalovirus infection in addition to *Candida*, the third also died. Staphylococci caused lung abscesses in one case and *aspergillus* species were isolated from a pleural effusion, other clinical episodes of infection were culture negative.

Neurology

The level of consciousness deteriorated in nine patients to the point of coma. Three patients convulsed; one of whom was in respiratory failure, thrombocytopenic and with evidence of hepatocellular dysfunction. This patient's plasma CS level was 55 ng ml^{-1} at the time of fitting. The other two patients fitted at a time of high whole blood CS levels (680 and 500 ng ml^{-1} 3 days after stopping the drug), both were hyponatraemic (119 and 120 mmol l^{-1}) and had abnormal clotting tests. There were no localizing neurological signs. CAT scans and EEGs were not performed in the majority of cases. Convulsions were readily controlled with benzodiazepines.

Postoperative Laboratory Data

Hyponatraemia occurred in the postoperative phase in 15 of the patients. The lowest plasma sodium level recorded ranged from 118 to 134 mmol l^{-1} (mean 126.7) and was noted within the first week in 8 of these; in four it occurred later at the time of development of renal impairment. Six patients were hyponatraemic on arrival, mean 130.8 (119–142) mmol l^{-1}.

Abnormalities of liver function tests were noted in all patients at some time. Mean bilirubin level on arrival was 173 µmol l^{-1} (range 42–427 µmol l^{-1}), AST 45 (range 8–104) IU l^{-1} and alkaline phosphatase 371 (range 200–556) IU l^{-1}. All of these parameters deteriorated.

Eight patients had abnormal haemostasis on arrival (prothrombin time (PT) greater than 18 s and/or kaolin cephalin thromboplastin time greater than 42 s). This also deteriorated to a maximum mean PT of 21.5 (16–35) s, KCTT 58 (35–114) s, thrombin time 15 (12–24) s. Mean platelet count on arrival was 144 (range 32–412) $\times 10^9$ l^{-1} and was less than 100×10^9 l^{-1} in six patients.).

Outcome

All patients deteriorated initially, despite full support. Nine patients survived (45%). Mean age of the survivors was 34 years and mean time on dialysis was 21 (2–50) days compared with 41 years and 28 (1–90) days, respectively in the non-survivors. Four of the survivors had normal pre-operative renal function and only two required inotrope support after the immediate postsurgical period. Three of the eight patients who were ventilated at the time of transfer and only one of those who required later respiratory support survived. Coma was a poor prognostic sign since 7 of the 10 affected subsequently died; however two of the three patients who fitted lived despite the other, concurrent metabolic abnormalities described above.

Liver function tests were more abnormal in the non-survivors with prominent intrahepatic cholestasis.

Cause of death was established by post-mortem examination in seven of the ten who died. One other patient was transferred to his country of origin whilst still on dialysis but died shortly afterwards. Graft failure was the major cause of death in three: one (heterotopic heart recipient) had early pump failure, one overwhelming rejection – which predominantly involved the lungs – and a third had intractable dysrhythmias. Two patients had bronchopneumonia and hepatic failure and were found at post-mortem to have widespread cytomegalic intracellular inclusions in several organs. Sepsis and hepatic failure were prominent in four other cases.

Conclusions

Acute renal failure (ARF) in the recipients of heart and heart–lung transplantation is multifactorial. As in other series of "surgical" ARF ((Wheeler et al. 1986), the prerenal factors – hypotension and hypovolaemia – are prominent (14 cases) with established renal impairment in 11. However, CS is nephrotoxic and may potentiate other, particularly ischaemic, causes of renal impairment in these patients. CS may also contribute to coma and convulsions (Gross et al. 1985; Beaman et al. 1984) and to a syndrome similar to thrombotic thrombocytopenic purpura (Shulman et al. 1981). The outcome for patients who develop acute renal failure and its complications is poor, but may be more favourable in the younger recipients without pre-existing multi-system impairment.

In order to minimize CS toxicity care should be taken to monitor renal function and urine electrolytes carefully. Episodes of hypotension, the concomitant use of other nephrotoxic drugs and hepatic dysfunction will all increase the likelihood of ARF. The dose of CS should be reduced when either blood levels are hhigh or when creatinine rises. However, renal failure requiring dialysis is not a contraindication to cardiac transplantation.

References

Beaman M, Parvin S, Veitch PS, Walls J (1984) Convulsions associated with cyclosporin A in renal transplant recipients. Br Med J 290: 139–140
Gross MLP, Pearson RM, Sweny RB, Moorhead JF (1985) Convulsions associated with cyclosporine A in renal transplant recipients. Br Med J 290: 555
Martin M, Kingswood JC, Packham D, Cairns H, Khagani A, Thompson FD, Yacoub MH (1987) Determinants of cyclosporin nephrotoxicity following cardiac transplantation. Transplant Proc 19: 2516–2517
Moran M, Tomlanovitch S, Myers BD (1985) Cyclosporine-induced chronic nephropathy in human recipients of cardiac allografts. Transplant Proc: 17 (supp 1): 185–190
Myers BD, Ross J, Newton L, Leutscher J, Perloth M (1985) Cyclosporin-associated chronic nephropathy. N Engl J Med. 311: 699–705
Schroeder JS, Hunt SA (1986) Cardiac transplantation: Where are we? N Engl J Med 315: 961–963
Shulman N, Striker G, Deeg HJ, Kennedy M, Storb R, Thomas ED (1981) Nephrotoxicity of cyclosporin A after allogeneic marrow transplantation: glomerular thromboses and tubular injury. N Engl J Med 305: 1392–1395
Solis E, Kaye MP (1986) The registry of the international society for heart transplantation: third official report. J Heart Transplant 5: 2–5
Wheeler DC, Feehaly J, Walls J (1986) High risk acute renal failure. Q J Med 61: 977–984

Discussion

Dr Neild was asked why his patients had become hyponatraemic. He could not answer this question but confirmed that they had received large volumes of crystalloid. Dr Arieff and Dr Weston wondered whether these patients were not whole-body potassium depleted. Dr Ledingham thought that this was a difficult measurement to make and it was also difficult to know what to relate it to, since the body mass is greatly reduced in many cases.

Dr Neild accepted that sepsis was obviously an important factor in the death of some of his patients. Gram-negative organisms seemed to have caused a number of pneumonic infections. A number of participants thought that this was most probably related to the extensive immunosuppression that the patients had received. Dr Neild agreed that immunosuppression was a major problem, but the introduction of cyclosporin had eased the situation. Nevertheless, immunosuppression remained an art rather than a science, and many of the patients who develop renal failure had the so-called "sepsis syndrome", a clinical septicaemia with negative blood cultures. Dr Bion mentioned that Birmingham had become a large liver transplant centre and their surgeons had participated in the first United Kingdom triple transplant – liver, heart and lungs. It was interesting to see that this particular patient who developed five organ failure was markedly dehydrated. This emphasized one of the greatest problems in intensive care, that is the assessment of the circulating blood volume. As far as the adverse predicted factors for renal failure associated with liver transplantation were concerned, Dr Bion thought the three most important were pre-existing infection, prolonged or complicated surgery and hypovolaemia occurring at some point during the perioperative period. A similar clinical situation was seen in severe cardiac cachexia, preceding cardiac transplantation and in other patients who require massive surgery. He thought that one could generalize across the board to all surgical patients who require extensive and complicated surgery. Finally, Dr Bion mentioned again the problem of the ischaemic gut, which might be the source of endotoxin and endotoxaemia, the basis of the "sepsis syndrome".

Dr Myers mentioned the Stanford experience reporting the incidence of postoperative acute renal failure in the heart transplant programme as being only 1%, a little less than that seen in the general cardiac surgical cases. With the introduction of cyclosporin, the incidence of acute renal failure rose to 16% in the first two years, but is now back down to less than 10% since familiarity with the drug and drug levels had increased. Nevertheless, Dr Myers emphasized that cyclosporin nephrotoxicity in the setting of an ischaemic kidney appears to be a particularly lethal injury. He had noted massive interstitial fibrosis with a huge ischaemic loss of nephrons in kidneys treated this way. It clearly becomes an irreversible process even if the patient survives their low cardiac output state. Only recently had it been possible to pursuade the surgeons to cut back the cyclosporin dose in the setting of acute renal failure associated with cardiac transplantation. Presently 4 mg kg^{-1} day^{-1} of cyclosporin was used as a maintenance dose in such patients titrating it by the blood level.

Chapter 21

Bleeding in Acute Renal Failure

K. Andrassy

A bleeding tendency, associated with renal failure, has been recognized since the eighteenth century (Riesman 1907), but its pathogenesis has only recently been elucidated. The availability of dialysis has reduced the incidence of bleeding episodes, and the early use of dialysis in acute and chronic renal failure has been particularly effective in this respect. There certainly exists a difference in the severity of bleeding between patients suffering from acute renal failure compared with those with chronic renal failure. The bleeding tendency in chronic renal failure is usually mild; it is restricted to mucocutaneous sites, being manifest as epistaxis, petechiae and increased bleeding from wounds. This is different from severe haemorrhage, which may occur in patients with acute renal failure; severe bleeding may also occur in patients with end-stage renal failure when they are dialysed for the first time. The additional effects of drugs, required for the adequate treatment of patients suffering from renal failure, may further contribute to any bleeding tendency, as will be discussed. For the sake of clarity, the bleeding tendency caused by chronic renal failure, acute renal failure and dialysis will be considered separately.

Defect of Haemostasis in Chronic Renal Failure

The haemorrhagic diathesis of chronic renal failure is primarily a consequence of a platelet defect. The latter is not due to thrombocytopenia, although the platelet count is usually in the low normal range, but rather, it is caused by platelet dysfunction. Several lines of evidence support this statement. The most important clinical indicator of qualitative platelet defects is an increased bleeding time. This test is the most sensitive parameter of impaired platelet function; it usually becomes abnormal at a serum creatinine concentration greater than 440–530 µmol l^{-1} corresponding to a creatinine clearance of less than 15 ml min^{-1}. There is a significant correlation between the prolongation of bleeding time and the impairment of collagen-induced platelet aggregation (Steiner et al. 1979). In addition, other platelet abnormalities have been identified which worsen progressively with the severity of renal failure (Table 21.1). Thus reduced platelet aggregation after exposure to ADP, adrenaline, thrombin, arachidonic acid and occasionally ristocetin has also been described (Andrassy and Ritz 1985). The following provide further evidence of qualitative platelet defects in uraemia: defective platelet adhesion to subendothelial structures or foreign bodies (Castillo et al. 1986), decreased availability of platelet factor 3 and impaired clot retraction. Finally, biochemical analyses have revealed an abnormal content of nucleotides in platelets and a diminution of intraplatelet constituents, such as β-thromboglobulin, platelet factor 4, serotonin and of thromboxane generation in uraemia (Eknoyan and Brown 1981).

Table 21.1. Platelet abnormalities in uraemia

Impaired platelet aggregation with collagen, adrenaline, ADP, thrombin
Defective platelet adhesion on vessel subendothelium
Decreased platelet factor 3 availability
Diminished platelet content of ADP, ATP, ATP-ase, serotonin, β-thromboglobulin, platelet-factor 4
Diminished production of TXB$_2$ in response to thrombin
Increased activity of adenylate cyclase
Increased content of cAMP

Pathogenesis of Platelet Defects in Renal Failure

Since it was found that dialysis improves or even corrects several uraemic platelet abnormalities it has been suggested that substances accumulating in uraemia are responsible for platelet dysfunction. Indeed, when normal platelets are incubated in uraemic plasma they show an impaired aggregation (Stewart and Castaldi 1967) and, conversely, when platelets of uraemic patients are incubated with normal plasma they show improved aggregation. However, complete normalization does not occur. Urea, creatinine, phenols and guanidinosuccinic acid have been incriminated for this persisting defect. Some evidence argues for a role of urea in the genesis of the platelet defect. Thus at high concentrations (>33 mmol l^{-1}), urea is known to diminish thrombocyte adhesion (Eknoyan et al. 1969) and ADP-induced platelet aggregation. However, these effects of urea do not imitate the effects of uraemia perfectly, since urea but not uraemia increases thrombin-mediated platelet aggregation in vitro. On the other hand when urea concentrations in serum are raised by addition of urea to the dialysate, bleeding episodes and more-severe platelet dysfunction are observed. It has been reported that the ingestion of urea by healthy volunteers causes prolonged bleeding times and diminished platelet adhesion.

Impaired Relationship Between Endothelial and Platelet Function in Renal Failure

Von Willebrand Factor

One potentially relevant factor in thrombocyte dysfunction of uraemia – implicating capillary dysfunction – is von Willebrand factor (f VIII /vWf). An abnormality of vWf was assumed because of the therapeutic success of using cryoprecipitate or DDAVP to increase high-molecular-weight multimers of vWf. FVIII/vWf is synthesized by endothelial cells and megakaryocytes. It circulates in the form of high-molecular-weight multimers together with low-molecular-weight oligomers. vWf-defective platelets do not function normally in situations of high shear stress; this may be caused by platelets sticking to the subendothelium, to glass beads or to each other. It is thought that high-molecular-weight multimers of vWf interact with a number of specific platelet membrane receptors, (Deykin 1983) (glycoprotein Ib and IIb/IIIa) thus enabling platelets to adhere and aggregate. In addition plasma multimers of vWf serve as transport proteins of factor VIII. A selective deficiency of larger f VIII/vWf multimers results in clinical bleeding. In uraemic patients a diminished concentration of vWf multimers has been described by some (Remuzzi and Pusineri 1988), but not confirmed by other investigators. Therefore it remains to be proven that a deficiency of vWf multimers accounts for the haemostatic disorder in uraemia. On the basis of our own recent work we would like to offer a different explanation. It is concerned with vWf binding to receptors on platelets. In uraemia we have observed reduced binding of f VIII/vWf to the platelet receptor glycoprotein 1b. The platelet membrane glycoproteins were analysed using isoelectric focusing, two-dimensional gel electrophoresis, Western blot, incubation with biotinylated lectins and staining with silver and peroxidase. Furthermore a decreased binding of lectins to glycoprotein IIb/IIIa has been noted in uraemics but not in controls (Fig. 21.1) (Andrassy et al. 1988). This was further confirmed by incubation of platelet membranes with monospecific (receptor) glycoprotein antibodies. These latter studies revealed faint staining of glycoprotein Ib – the vWF receptor – and reduced staining of glycoproteins IIb/IIIa – the receptors for vWf and of collagen and thrombin (George et al. 1984). It is interesting that in Bernard–Soulier syndrome platelets lack a specific membrane receptor (glycoprotein Ib), that binds f VIII/vWf. Since uraemics lack the same receptor, the haemostatic disorder in uraemia may be regarded as an acquired Bernard–Soulier syndrome although it is uncertain whether the abnormal binding of vWf is due to a defect or the result of an interaction with the binding sites. The cause of the abnormal binding of vWf in uraemia is unknown. But the finding that platelet membrane phospholipids are modified in uraemia suggests that similar changes affecting glycoproteins might alter platelet receptors.

Prostaglandin I_2

Capillary wall function has been the least-studied aspect of abnormal haemostasis in uraemia. It is of note that several authors found increased prostaglandin I_2 (PGI_2) production in vessels of uraemic animals as well as of patients (Remuzzi et al. 1977). PGI_2 is the most active anti-aggregatory and vasodilating prostaglandin

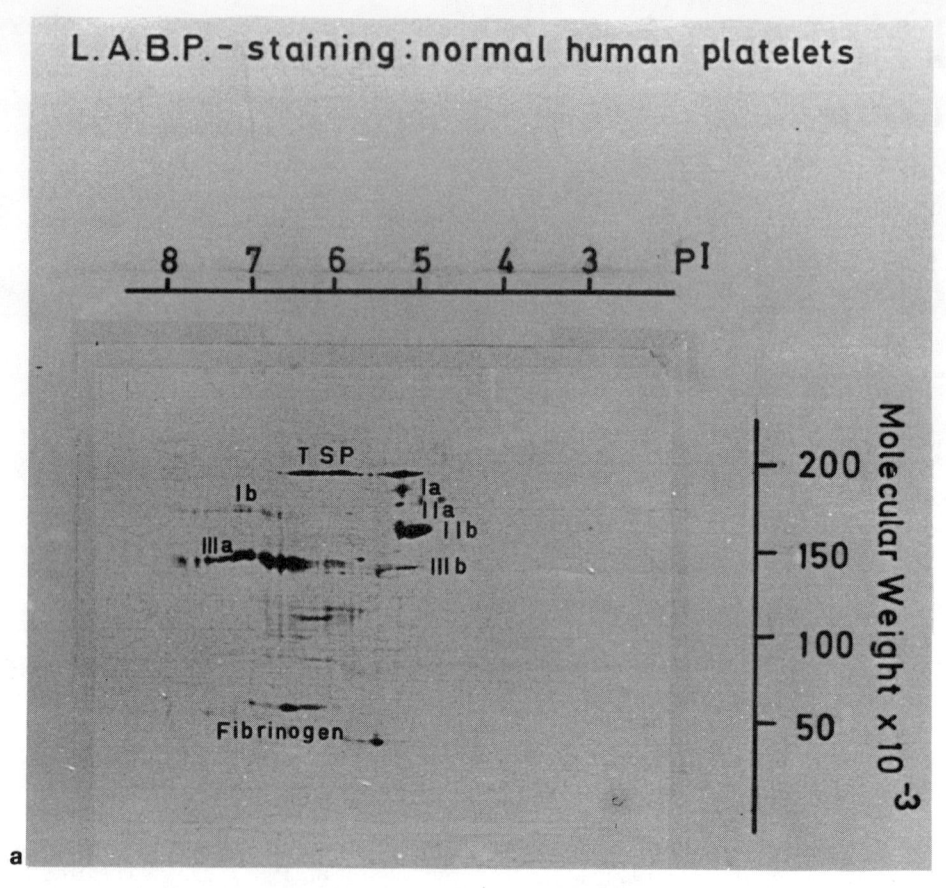

Fig. 21.1. Platelet membrane glycoproteins in patients with severe uraemia. Note absent staining of glycoproteins Ib and IIa and diminished staining of thrombospondin, glycoprotein Ia, IIb and IIIa.

derivative. In uraemic patients the baseline PGI_2 production is increased and plasma half-life is prolonged. Moreover endothelial PGI_2 synthesis and release are both stimulated by uraemic plasma. The active plasma constituents responsible for this effect have not yet been elucidated.

Other Factors Contributing to Uraemic Bleeding

One hypothesis links platelet dysfunction to increased parathyroid hormone (PTH) concentrations (Remuzzi et al. 1981). PTH accounts for many metabolic disturbances in uraemia and is thought by some to be the major uraemic toxin (Massry and Goldstein 1979). Bovine PTH extracts, when added to platelet-rich plasma, reduce platelet aggregation in response to ADP, collagen, thrombin and arachidonic acid. In uraemia the intracellular cyclic adenosine monophosphate content of platelets is unchanged; nonetheless the inhibitory effect of PTH on

L.A.B.P.- staining : uremic platelets

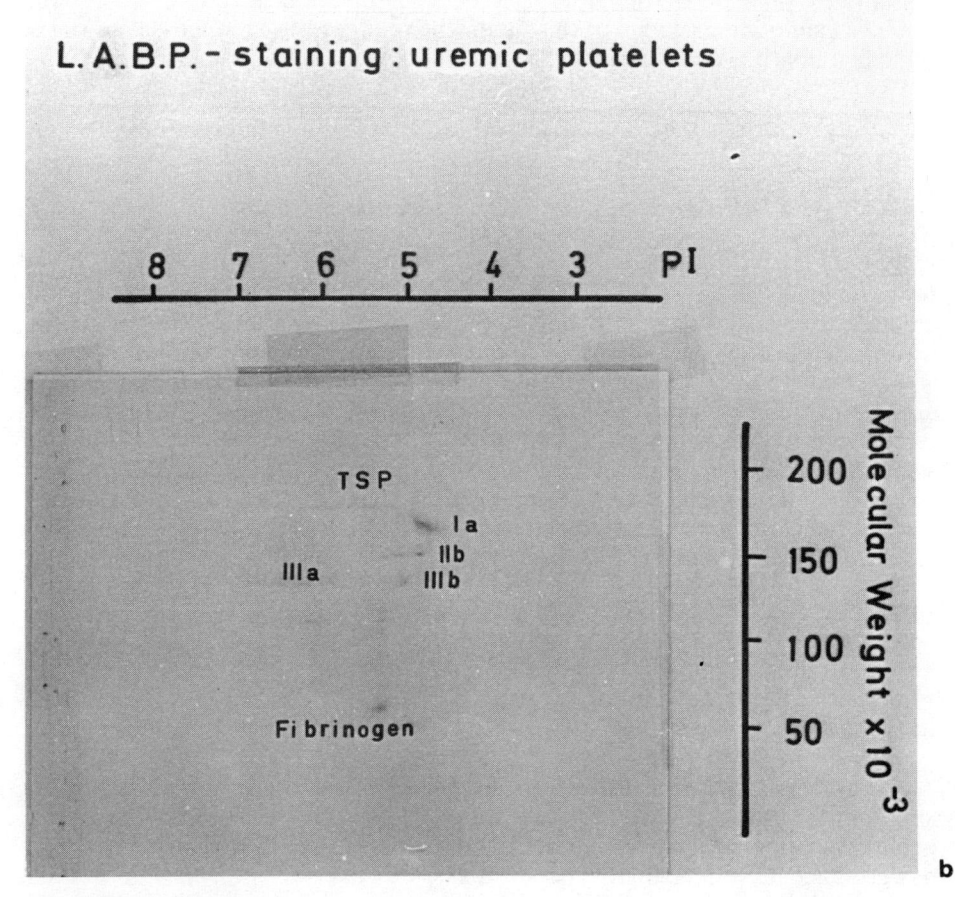

Fig. 21.1. (continued)

platelets is potentiated by theophylline. In addition, studies by Gura et al. (1982) demonstrated PTH-induced changes in platelet calcium content. However, Docci et al. (1986) were unable to demonstrate an association between platelet dysfunction and (secondary) hyperparathyroidism in chronic renal failure. Furthermore, treatment with 1,25-dihydroxycholecalciferol did not improve platelet dysfunction although intraplatelet calcium content was normalized. On the other hand it may be relevant that we have been unable to document abnormal bleeding time and platelet aggregation in distinct cases of severe (primary) hyperparathyroidism. Thus this subject needs more clarification.

Besides uraemic toxins the haematocrit may be an important determinant of bleeding time and platelet aggregation. A relationship between bleeding time and haematocrit is well documented in non-uraemic individuals; and more recently a similar relationship has also been demonstrated in uraemic subjects (Livio et al. 1982). There may be several ways in which red cells contribute to haemostasis. Altered rheology and modified ADP availability are primarily discussed. The haemostatic role of red blood cells is also well supported by recent observations that correction of anaemia by treatment with synthetic erythropoietin (rHuEPO) ameliorates platelet dysfunction. However, a direct effect of rHuEPO on platelets cannot be excluded at this time. The relationship between haemostasis and haematocrit is an important aspect of therapy as will be discussed below.

Defect of Haemostasis in Acute Renal Failure

In acute renal failure additional haemostatic defects may be superimposed on uraemic coagulation defects which have been described above. One important issue is the effect of selected drugs. This applies to beta-lactam antibiotics and to non-steroidal anti-inflammatory drugs (NSAIDS); other potentially interfering drugs, e.g. lipid-lowering drugs, should also be borne in mind (Andrassy and Ritz 1985). In addition acute renal failure may be caused by diseases which are associated with thrombocytopenia; this, on its own, carries an increased risk of bleeding. Such thrombocytopenia may either result from increased peripheral platelet destruction in the general circulation or from platelet consumption in the kidney due to an abnormal renal vessel wall platelet reaction. Examples include acute renal failure associated with disseminated intravascular coagulation, the haemolytic–uraemic syndrome and disseminated lupus erythematosus.

Beta-Lactam Antibiotics

Acute renal failure is frequently associated with bacterial infections. Therefore, antibiotic treatment may be required. Beta-lactam antibiotics, i.e. semisynthetic penicillins and cephalosporins, are frequently given to such patients. These are powerful agents with negligible nephrotoxic side effects. Beta-lactam antibiotics (with the exception of isoxazolyl penicillins) are mainly excreted by the renal route. When administered in regular doses they accumulate in uraemic patients. Penicillin G and ureidopenicillins (Andrassy et al. 1976a) are known to have potent inhibitory effects on platelet function if administered in high doses to patients with normal renal function (>15 g day^{-1}). The mechanism of this inhibition has been clarified to some extent. Reduced accessibility of adrenergic receptors to adrenaline, increased baseline and PGE$_1$-stimulated cyclic AMP concentrations and diminished TXB$_2$-generation in platelets following stimulation by ADP or adrenaline have all been demonstrated (Andrassy and Ritz 1977). It is of note that this penicillin-induced thrombocyte dysfunction is additive to the defect of uraemia *per se*. In addition high serum penicillin levels may occur from excessive doses given to patients with normal renal function; alternatively they may be found in uraemic patients given doses which are inappropriate for their level of renal function. Such patients exhibit a marked prolongation of bleeding time, diminished ADP-induced platelet aggregation and a high prevalence of bleeding episodes (Andrassy and Ritz 1977). Extremely high serum concentrations of penicillin produce a heparin-like coagulation defect in plasma (Andrassy et al. 1976b), which is characterized by prolongation of thrombin-reptilase and thrombin-coagulase times. Several authors have also observed bleeding episodes in patients with impaired renal function who had been given high doses of third-generation cephalosporins, i.e. latamoxef or cefoperazone. Latamoxef and cefoperazone have been shown to interfere with platelet function. This may occur in the presence of high serum trough concentrations in normal individuals and in patients with impaired renal function. More importantly a plasma coagulation defect (reflected in the prolongation of prothrombin time) may also occur. It is caused by the N-methyl-thiotetrazole (NMTT) side chain of the relevant cephalosporins (Lipsky 1983). Recent studies in our laboratory clarified the mechanism involved (Shearer et al. 1988). We detected the transient appearance of vitamin K_1 2,3-epoxide. This indicates a block of (hepatic) reductive regeneration of vitamin K_1, mediated by inhibition of vitamin K epoxide reductase. Such coumarin-like action is specifically observed with all NMTT-cephalosporins. Finally malnourished patients, patients on total parenteral nutrition and renal patients may also get hypoprothrombinaemia because of low initial vitamin K_1 stores (Shearer et al. 1988).

Non-steroidal Anti-inflammatory Drugs

Acetylsalicylic acid is used to prevent thrombosis of av-fistulas (Andrassy et al. 1974) in uraemic patients on chronic haemodialysis. It is also used to improve dialysis by inhibiting platelet deposits on dialysis membranes (Lindsay et al. 1972). Gaspari et al. (1987) demonstrated an effect of aspirin on platelet function which was specific for uraemia. Aspirin ordinarily has dual effects both on bleeding time and on platelet prostaglandin metabolism. In uraemics the bleeding time is prolonged more than in normal controls but this effect which is related to the presence of aspirin in blood is only transitory. On the other hand aspirin inhibits platelet thromboxane synthesis during the entire life span of the platelets. This might have implications for therapy with aspirin. Whether other non-steroidal anti-inflammatory drugs have similar effects in chronic renal failure has to be clarified in the future.

Disseminated Intravascular Coagulation (DIC)

When a DIC is followed by acute renal failure there is frequently an associated release of endotoxin (lipopolysaccharides). Endotoxin release may occur during infections with Gram-negative and Gram-positive bacteria (Weinstein and Klainer 1966). Other diseases potentially causing DIC and intrarenal coagulation are haemolysis, massive cell destruction (rhabdomyolysis), malignancies, obstetric complications and different types of shock. DIC is usually diagnosed on the basis of abnormal plasma coagulation tests. In the compensated form of DIC increased synthesis of clotting factors compensates for their consumption. Diagnostic findings include circulating fibrin monomers, recognized in the ethanol gelation test, an increase of fibrin degradation products and an elevated fibrinogen concentration. In decompensated DIC the consumption of coagulation factors and platelets results in decreased concentration of coagulation factors, such as decreased fibrinogen concentration, a reduced number of platelets and a prolonged prothrombin time; all of these may contribute to clinical bleeding (Colman et al. 1972).

Haemolytic–Uraemic Syndrome (HUS) and Thrombotic–Thrombocytopenic Purpura (TTP)

Haemolytic–uraemic syndrome is an important cause of acute renal failure in children. It is defined as the triad of azotaemia, thrombocytopenia and microangiopathic haemolytic anaemia. Clinical, epidemiological and pathological studies have suggested at least two subgroups, a typical (epidemic) and an atypical (sporadic) form. The typical form usually follows a prodrome of acute non-febrile gastroenteritis and presents acutely. The atypical form has an insidious onset; it may follow an upper respiratory tract infection or one of several other diseases. This is the form usually seen in adults; it may be associated with systemic diseases, the postpartum state or with the contraceptive pill. In some cases there is a family history of this illness. An association with several other drugs has also been described. These include cyclosporin A and several cytotoxic, anti-neoplastic drugs such as mitomycin C or 5-fluorouracil (Goldstein et al. 1979). In general HUS/TTP has proved to be much more heterogeneous than was believed in the past. HUS/TTP may result from a variety of different disease processes. Whatever the cause, the final result is extensive endothelial injury of the renal microvasculature (Editorial 1987). The haematological features of HUS are believed to be a consequence of the process. In TTP, which is a closely related syndrome vascular injury is similar. It occurs in many organs besides the kidneys; the resulting lesions and the associated haematological findings are more severe. In contrast to DIC, plasmatic coagulation is not so much affected. Thus prothrombin time, aPTT and fibrinogen are usually normal. Thrombocytopenia and signs of haemolysis (schistocytes) as well as impaired renal function are the hallmarks of these syndromes.

Defect of Haemostasis During Haemodialysis

Clotting and anticoagulation are the Achilles heel of haemodialysis (Andrassy et al. 1987). The necessity for heparin treatment during dialysis illustrates that dialysis membranes do not as yet possess the antithrombogenic properties of non-clottable (endothelial like) surfaces. The anticoagulation by heparin, the platelet dysfunction of uraemia and the platelet changes induced by the dialysis procedure itself (platelet activation by dialysis membranes) are all responsible for potential bleeding during haemodialysis. This is most significant at the very beginning of dialysis since it is at this time that uraemic platelet dysfunction has not been corrected by dialysis. The addition of heparin aggravates the platelet defect further because of its antiplatelet activity. If thrombocytopenia also happens to be present and if the dose of heparin is not adapted to the low platelet count, severe bleeding complications may occur. Many reports from the literature strongly emphasize this chain of events (Jaques 1980). In order to prevent bleeding complications in patients at risk several strategies have been recommended which are discussed below.

Therapeutic Possibilities

To reduce the bleeding tendency of uraemia frequent dialysis of adequate efficiency remains the standard procedure. It must be kept in mind, however, that dialysis does not completely correct the uraemic platelet defect. Thus different interventions are possible to improve bleeding abnormality in patients who manifest bleeding or in high-risk patients (Table 21.2). Because of the dependence of bleeding on haematocrit, the transfusion of blood will ameliorate the bleeding tendency within a short time. A haematocrit >30% should be achieved. Erythropoietin (rHuEPO) (150–450 U kg^{-1} $week^{-1}$) may also be used. It is a long-acting substance and any effect of treatment will not be obvious before the fourth to sixth week of treatment (Moia et al. 1987). Cryoprecipitate, desmopressin (DDAVP) and possibly conjugated oestrogens may also correct the uraemic bleeding tendency. Their mechanism of action involves the f VIII/vWf, yet the effects last for different periods of time. Cryoprecipitate (10 bags) has its maximal effect between 1 and 12 h after treatment; its effect disappears at 24–36 h after administration but repeated doses are equally effective (Janson et al. 1980). Desmopressin (DDAVP) (0.4 µg kg^{-1} i.v.) is effective for 4–24 h after administration but its action disappears with repeated application (Watson and Keogh 1982). A more long-lasting effect on bleeding tendency is obtained with the use of conjugated oestrogens (Premarin). It has been shown (Livio et al. 1986) that this compound has to be administered intravenously for several days (5 days; 3 mg kg^{-1}) to have an effect. Like cryoprecipitate or DDAVP the therapeutic response to conjugated oestrogens occurs within hours and an effect can be observed for up to 30 days after administration. But side effects of this therapy (hypertension, liver failure) have to be considered. In patients at a high risk of bleeding requiring dialysis it is possible to dialyse without anticoagulation for some time (Caruana et al. 1988). As an alternative approach, anticoagulation may be performed with prostacyclin or citrate (Smith et al. 1982; Pinnick et al. 1983) instead of heparin, but side effects limit their use. The modern concept of treatment of DIC consists of the supply of proteinase inhibitors (antithrombin III, fresh-frozen plasma) with small doses of heparin (5000–10 000 IU day^{-1}) depending on the bleeding risk of the patient; in addition, eradication of the underlying cause of DIC is essential (Andrassy 1985).

Table 21.2. Therapeutic strategies for the management of bleeding associated with renal failure

---

Blood transfusion (HKT >30%)
rHu-erythropoietin (120–450 U kg^{-1} $week^{-1}$ i.v.)
Cryoprecipitate (10 bags)
Desmopressin (0.4 µg kg^{-1} i.v. twice daily) or 3 µg kg^{-1} intranasally
Conjugated oestrogens (3 mg kg^{-1} i.v. for 5 days)

A variety of therapies has been suggested for HUS/TTP. Lack of controlled studies makes any recommendations concerning therapy difficult. In acute renal failure early dialysis is mandatory. Since HUS/TTP in childhood has a good prognosis no further treatment may be required. Plasma infusion seems to be of benefit in adult HUS/TTP with regard to a haematological remission. Whether patient survival or long-term renal function is favourably influenced remains to be seen (Remuzzi 1987). Antiplatelet agents have been of some value in adult HUS/TTP. Other drugs like vitamin E or PGI_2 have been tried but results have been variable. Thus treatment of adult HUS/TTP needs further evaluation.

References

Andrassy K (1985) Antithrombin III. Urban & Schwarzenberg, München
Andrassy K, Ritz E (1977) Penicillin and haemostasis. Cardiovasc Med 2: 604–608
Andrassy K, Ritz E (1985) Uremia as a cause of bleeding. Am J Nephrol 5: 313–319
Andrassy K, Malluche H. Bornefeld H, Comberg M, Ritz E, Jesdinsky H, Möhring K (1974) Prevention of p.o. clotting of av. Cimino fistulae with acetylsalicylic acid. Results of a prospective double blind study. Klin Wochenschr 52: 348–349
Andrassy K, Ritz E, Hasper P, Scherz M, Walter E, Storch H, Vömel W (1976a) Penicillin-induced coagulation disorder. Lancet II: 1039–1041
Andrassy K, Weisschedel E, Ritz E, Andrassy T (1976b) Bleeding in uraemic patients after carbenicillin. Thromb Haemost 36: 115–126
Andrassy K, Ritz E, Bommer J (1987) Effects of hemodialysis on platelets. Contrib Nephrol 59: 26–34
Andrassy K, Koderisch J, Lamminger C (1988) Defective platelet membrane receptors as a cause of uraemic bleeding. Blut 53: 243
Caruana RJ, Raja RM, Bush JV, Kramer MS, Goldstein SJ (1988) Heparin free dialysis: comparative data and results in high risk patients. Kidney Int 31: 1351–1355
Castillo R, Lozano T, Escolar G, Revert L (1986) Defective platelet adhesion on vessel subendothelium in uremic patients. Blood 68: 337–342
Colman RW, Robboy SJ, Minna JD (1972) Disseminated intravascular coagulation: an approach. Am J Med 52: 679–689
Deykin D (1983) Uremic bleeding. Kidney Int 24: 698–705
Docci D, Turci F, Delvecchio C, Gollini C, Baldrati L, Pistocchi E (1986) Lack of evidence for the role of secondary hyperparathyroidism in the pathogenesis of uremic thrombocytopathy. Nephron 43: 28–32
Editorial (1987) Unravelling HUS. Lancet II: 1437–1439
Eknoyan G, Brown CH (1981) Biochemical abnormalities of platelets in renal failure. Am J Nephrol 1: 17–23
Eknoyan G, Wacksman S, Glueck H, Will J (1969) Platelet function in renal failure. N Engl J Med 280: 677–681
Gaspari F, Vigano G, Orisio S, Bonati M, Livio M, Remuzzi G (1987) Aspirin prolongs bleeding time in uremia by a mechanism distinct from platelet cyclooxygenase inhibition. J Clin Invest 79: 1788–1797
George JN, Nurden AT, Phillips DR (1984) Molecular defects in interactions of platelets with the vessel wall. N Engl J Med 311: 1084–1098
Goldstein MH, Churg J, Strauss L, Gribetz D (1979) Hemolytic–uremic syndrome. Nephron 23: 263–272
Gura V, Creter D, Levi J (1982) Elevated thrombocyte calcium in uremia and its correction by 1a (OH) vitamin D treatment. Nephron 30: 237–239
Janson PA, Jubelirer SJ, Weinstein MJ, Deykin D (1980) Treatment of the bleeding tendency in uremia with cryoprecipitate. N Engl J Med 303: 1318–1322
Jaques LB (1980) Heparins:anionic polyelectrolyte drugs. Pharmacol Rev 31: 99–166
Lindsay RM, Ferguson D, Prentice CRM, Burton JA, McNicol GP (1972) Reduction of thrombus formation on dialyser membranes by aspirin and RA 233. Lancet I: 1287–1290

Lipsky JJ (1983) N-Methyl-thio-tetrazole inhibition of the gamma carboxylation of glutamic acid:possible mechanism for antibiotic-associated hypoprothrombinaemia. Lancet II: 192–193

Livio M, Gotti E, Marchesi E, Mecca G, Remuzzi G, De Gaetano G (1982) Uraemic bleeding: role of anaemia and beneficial effect of red cell transfusions. Lancet II: 1013–1015

Livio M, Mannucci PM, Vigano G, Mingardi G, Lombardi R, Mecca G, Remuzzi G (1986) Conjugated estrogens for the management of bleeding associated with renal failure. N Engl J Med 315: 731–735

Massry SG, Goldstein DA (1979) The search for uremic toxin(s) X × X = PTH. Clin Nephrol 11: 181–189

Moia M, Mannucci PM, Vizzotto L, Casati S, Cattaneo M, Ponticelli C (1987) Improvement in the haemostatic defect of uraemia after treatment with recombinant human erythropoetin. Lancet II: 1227–1229

Pinnick RV, Wiegmann TB, Diederich DA (1983) Regional citrate anticoagulation for hemodialysis in the patient at high risk for bleeding. N Engl J Med 308: 258–261

Remuzzi G (1987) HUS and TTP: variable expression of a single entity. Kidney Int 32: 292–308

Remuzzi G, Pusineri F (1988) Coagulation defects in uremia. Kidney Int 33 (Suppl 24): S13–S17

Remuzzi G, Cavenaghi A, Mecca G, Donati M (1977) Prostacyclin-like activity and bleeding in renal failure. Lancet II: 1195–1197

Remuzzi G, Benigni A, Dodesini P, Schiepatti A (1981) Parathyroid hormone inhibits human platelet function. Lancet II: 1321–1323

Riesman D (1907) Hemorrhages in the course of Bright's disease with especial reference to the occurrence of a hemorrhagic diathesis of nephrotic origin. Am J Sci 134: 709–716

Shearer MJ, Bechtold H, Andrassy K, Koderisch J, McCarthy PT, Trenk D, Jähnchen E, Ritz E (1988) Mechanism of cephalosporin-induced hypoprothrombinemia:relation to cephalosporin side chain, vitamin K metabolism, and vitamin K status. J Clin Pharmacol 28: 88–95

Smith MC, Crow JW, Cato AE, Park GD, Hassid A, Dunn MJ (1982) Prostacyclin substitution for heparin in long-term hemodialysis. Am J Med 73: 669–678

Steiner R, Coggins C, Carvalho A (1979) Bleeding time in uraemia: a useful test to assess clinical bleeding. Am J Haematol 7: 101–117

Stewart J, Castaldi P (1967) Uremic bleeding: a reversible platelet defect corrected by dialysis. Q J Med 36: 409–423

Watson AJS, Keogh JAB (1982) Effect off 1-deamino-8-D-arginine vasopressin on the prolonged bleeding time in chronic renal failure. Nephron 32: 49–52

Weinstein L, Klainer AS (1966) Septic shock – pathogenesis and treatment. N Engl J Med 274: 950–953

Discussion

Dr Weston opened the discussion by reporting some work that he had done concerning an inhibitor of ristocetin-mediated platelet aggregation in uraemic patients. He agreed with Dr Andrassy that parathormone seemed to inhibit platelet aggregation and that in some uraemic patients this hormone might account for their bleeding defect. Dr Weston thought that sulphinpyrazone was more likely to reduce platelet losses in the haemodialyser, while having little effect on the integrity of the gastrointestinal mucosa. Dr Andrassy replied that intravenous aspirin seemed to work very well in patients who required some sort of prosthetic graft. The aspirin appeared to reduce platelet deposition on these grafts and prolong patency. He thought aspirin was more efficacious than sulphinpyrazone.

Dr Neild asked Dr Andrassy about his work concerning the glycoproteins on the platelet membrane. Dr Neild was not clear whether the German group had found this defect in all uraemic patients or whether it was a subgroup with a severe bleeding tendency. Dr Neild spoke of a very small minority of uraemic patients who had a bleeding tendency, the origin of which was difficult to identify. Such cases had a very prolonged bleeding time, which could usually be shortened by giving DDAVP. Dr Andrassy replied that most of his work had been in patients with chronic renal failure who had very severe platelet defects before going on to haemodialysis treatment. All discussants agreed that this was a very complex problem, but DDAVP seemed to be useful in preventing or reducing bleeding in uraemics who haemorrhaged. Moreover, the prostacyclin users emphasized that this compound could be administered to anticoagulate uraemic patients and given its short in vivo half-life, could be withdrawn rapidly at times of crisis.

Chapter 22

Mechanisms of Uraemic Encephalopathy

A. I. Arieff and C. L. Fraser

Introduction

New techniques of both pharmacological and dietary therapy have the potential to decrease the incidence of acute and chronic end-stage renal disease (Brenner et al. 1982; Klahr et al. 1983). Acute renal failure is a major complication among patients being treated in the intensive therapy unit (ITU), and among patients with either acute or chronic renal failure, nervous system dysfunction remains a major cause of disability. Such patients will manifest a variety of neurological disorders (Raskin and Fishman 1976; Teschan and Arieff 1985; Teschan et al. 1979). Even after the institution of adequate dialysis therapy, patients with acute renal failure (ARF) may continue to manifest subtle nervous system dysfunction, such as impaired mental activity, generalized weakness, sexual dysfunction and peripheral neuropathy (Raskin and Fishman 1976; Teschan and Arieff 1985; Teschan et al. 1979; Said et al. 1983). Patients with chronic renal failure who have not yet received dialytic therapy may develop symptoms ranging from mild sensorial clouding to delirium and coma (Raskin and Fishman 1976; Teschan and Arieff 1985). The dialytic treatment of end-stage renal disease has itself been associated with at least three distinct disorders of the central nervous system. These include dialysis disequilibrium syndrome, progressive intellectual dysfunction and dialysis dementia (Fraser and Arieff 1988b). Dialysis disequilibrium syndrome occurs in a small number of patients and is a consequence of the initiation of dialysis therapy. Dialysis dementia is a progressive and generally fatal encephalopathy which can affect patients on chronic haemodialysis as well as children with chronic renal failure who have not been treated with dialysis (Baluarate et al. 1977; Andreoli et al. 1984). It is generally not a problem in patients in the ITU, nor is progressive intellectual dysfunction, which may also occur in many patients who are being treated with maintenance dialysis therapy (Osberg et al. 1982).

Besides those neurological disorders which are specifically related to uraemia and/or dialysis, a number of other neurological entities occur with increased frequency in patients with end-stage renal disease who are being treated with dialysis (Raskin and Fishman 1976; Teschan and Arieff 1985). Additionally, patients with end-stage kidney disease are also at risk of developing any of the structural brain lesions or metabolic encephalopathies which might affect the general population (Teschan and Arieff 1985). Therefore, when a patient with renal failure presents with altered mental status, a thorough and complete evaluation is necessary to establish the proper diagnosis.

The entire problem of the effects of acute and chronic renal failure on the central nervous system, as well as the biochemical abnormalities, testing procedures, structural abnormalities and effects of therapy will be found in two recent review articles (Fraser and Arieff 1988a,b).

Uraemic Encephalopathy

Uraemic encephalopathy may occur in patients with either acute or chronic renal failure when glomerular filtration rate falls below approximately 10% of normal (Teschan and Arieff 1985). It is very common in patients being treated with intensive therapy. As with other organic brain syndromes these patients display variable disorders of consciousness that can affect psychomotor behaviour, thinking, memory, speech, perception and emotion (Teschan and Arieff 1985; Teschan et al. 1979). The severity and rate of progression of symptoms vary directly with the rate at which renal dysfunction develops. In patients with acute renal failure, uraemic symptoms are generally more severe and progress more rapidly than in patients with chronic renal failure (Cooper et al. 1978; Locke et al. 1961; Arieff 1985). In progressive chronic renal failure, the number and severity of symptoms may vary cyclically, with intervals of well-being in an otherwise inexorable downhill course. The symptoms are usually ameliorated by dialysis and are generally relieved almost entirely after successful renal transplantation (Raskin and Fishman 1976; Teschan and Arieff 1985; Brenner et al. 1982).

Differential Diagnosis of Uraemic Encephalopathy

Uraemic encephalopathy should be suspected in patients with renal failure if there are clinical signs and symptoms consistent with central nervous system deterioration. Patients in the ITU often have multiple organ failure and the presenting symptoms of uraemic encephalopathy may be similar to those of other metabolic encephalopathies (Teschan and Arieff 1985; Arieff 1985), so that there is some risk of misdiagnosis and mistreatment. The problem of differential diagnosis is made more complex by the fact that patients with renal failure may also develop other intercurrent illnesses which may induce encephalopathy. If a patient with renal insufficiency is taking a drug with potential central nervous system toxicity that is excreted or metabolized primarily by the kidney, the ensuing central nervous system symptoms may be due either to the drug which has reached toxic levels at ordinary dose rates or to uraemia (Teschan and Arieff

1985). In patients with both advanced liver and renal diseases, it is often difficult to determine whether the encephalopathy is due to either hepatic or renal causes or both (Losowsky and Scott 1973). In such patients the blood urea nitrogen and serum creatinine do not always adequately reflect the degree of functional renal impairment (Papadakis and Arieff 1987). Thus, many patients with cirrhosis, ascites, normal blood urea nitrogen and creatinine may in fact have a glomerular filtration rate which is below 30 ml min^{-1} (Papadakis and Arieff 1987). In patients with normal liver function protein and amino acids in the gastrointestinal tract are metabolized by bacteria and mucosal enzymes in the colon to form ammonia. The ammonia then enters the liver through the portal circulation where most of it participates in the urea cycle to form urea (Fraser and Arief 1985). The majority of the urea so produced is excreted in the urine and the remainder enters the colon via hepatoenteric recirculation (Losowsky and Scott 1973). However, in patients with renal failure the major route for the elimination of urea is not available, thus, there is a rapid and sustained increase in blood urea nitrogen (BUN). Because of the elevated blood urea nitrogen, the amount of urea which enters the colon by recirculation is increased. In uraemic subjects, the additional urea in the gut is again acted on by bacteria and mucosal enzymes, resulting in further increased ammonia production. This may then lead to an increase in both plasma ammonia concentration and brain uptake of ammonia (Deferrari et al. 1981; Lieber and Lefevere 1959), resulting in an increased risk of developing encephalopathy in patients with both kidney and liver failure.

Central Nervous System Consequences Resulting from Acute Renal Failure

Abnormalities of the mental state are early and sensitive indices indicating the development of neurological disorders in patients with acute renal failure. In the ITU, the initial presentation of patients with acute renal failure may include signs of toxic psychosis, abnormal mental status, lassitude and lethargy, with evidence of disorientation and confusion appearing later. Physical findings may include cranial nerve signs, nystagmus, dysarthria, abnormal gait and various abnormalities of skeletal muscles, such as weakness, fasciculations and asymmetrical variation in deep tendon reflexes. These findings may progress to include asterixis and hyperreflexia with unsustained clonus at the ankle. If uraemia is left untreated and allowed to progress, seizures and coma often supervene (Raskin and Fishman 1976; Teschan and Arief 1985).

Electroencephalograms in patients with acute renal failure are generally grossly abnormal when the diagnosis of acute renal failure is first made (Cooper et al. 1978). In most instances, the percentage of electroencephalogram power less than either 5 Hz or 7 Hz is 20 times greater than the normal value. The abnormal percentages of electroencephalogram frequencies both above 9 Hz and below 5 Hz are not usually improved by dialysis within the first eight weeks of treatment, although they may return to normal with recovery of renal function. If renal failure continues, the electroencephalogram may transiently worsen both during and after haemodialysis and this pattern may continue for up to six months after the initiation of dialysis therapy (Cooper et al. 1978; Locke et al. 1961; Guisado et al. 1975; Kiley et al. 1976; Hughes 1980).

Central Nervous System Consequences Resulting from Chronic Renal Failure

At this time, patients with chronic renal failure are often treated aggressively for other medical and surgical conditions which would have been contraindications to therapy in the recent past. Thus, it is worthwhile to review the numerous neurological manifestations of chronic renal failure. The electroencephalogram findings in patients with chronic renal failure are usually not as severe as those reported in patients with acute renal failure. In general there is good correlation between the percentage of electroencephalogram frequencies and power below 7 Hz and the decline of renal function as estimated by serum creatinine (Teschan et al. 1979; Kiley et al. 1976). After the initiation of dialysis there may be an initial period of clinical stabilization during which time the electroencephalogram continues to deteriorate. However, after approximately 6 months of dialysis treatment the electroencephalogram tends to normalize. Normal values may not be reached, however, unless the patient receives a kidney transplant (Teschan et al. 1979; Kiley et al. 1976; Hughes 1980). In patients with chronic renal failure certain cognitive functions are also impaired. These include attention span, speed of decision-making, short-term memory and mental manipulation of symbols (Souheaver et al. 1982).

Psychological Testing in Renal Failure

Generally, patients with acute renal failure are too sick to undergo psychological testing, although several different types of psychological tests have been used to evaluate patients with chronic renal failure. These tests were designed to evaluate the effects of either dialysis, renal transplantation or parathyroidectomy on central nervous system symptoms in patients with renal failure (Teschan and Arieff 1985; Arieff 1985; Souheaver et al. 1982; Cogan et al. 1978). The possible effects of parathyroid hormone on psychological function have also been evaluated in patients who were being treated with dialysis (Cogan et al. 1978).

Effects of Uraemia on the Brain

Biochemical Changes in Brain in Uraemia

To determine the possible causes of the electroencephalogram abnormalities and the clinical manifestations observed in patients with renal failure, biochemical studies have been carried out in the brains of both patients and laboratory animals (Goldstein and Massry 1978; Arieff et al. 1973, 1977; Perry et al. 1985). In patients with acute renal failure, the brain content of water, potassium and magnesium is normal, that of sodium and aluminium are slightly elevated (Arieff et al. 1973; Alfrey et al. 1976), while that of calcium is almost twice the normal value (Cooper et al. 1978; Cogan et al. 1978). Similar results have also been reported in dogs with acute renal failure (Goldstein and Massry 1978; Arieff et al. 1973; Arieff and Massry 1974). It has also been reported that the permeability of uraemic rat brain to certain inert molecules such as inulin and sucrose is increased, while permeability to weak acids such as sulphate, penicillin, and dimethadione is normal to low (Arieff 1985; Arieff et al. 1973, 1977). In the brain of rats with acute renal failure, creatinine phosphate, ATP, and glucose are increased while AMP, ADP, and lactate are decreased. Thus the uraemic brain appears to utilize less ATP and produce less ADP, AMP and lactate. These changes are also associated with a decrease in both brain metabolic rate and cerebral oxygen consumption (Van den Noort et al. 1968; Scheinberg 1954; Mahoney et al. 1984) and are consistent with a generalized decrease in brain energy utilization.

In animals with either acute or chronic renal failure, both urea concentration and osmolality are similar in brain, cerebrospinal fluid, and plasma (Arieff et al. 1973; Mahoney and Arieff 1983). There is an increase in brain osmolality in acute renal failure due to an increase in the brain urea concentration (Arieff et al. 1973). However, contrary to observations in acute renal failure, in animals with chronic renal failure, approximately half the increase in brain osmolality is thought to be due to the presence of undetermined solute (idiogenic osmoles) and most of the remainder is due to an increase in urea concentration (Perry et al. 1985; Mahoney and Arieff 1983). Also, in both human and laboratory animals with renal failure, the pH of cerebrospinal fluid and intracellular pH in brain are both normal (Arieff 1985; Arieff et al. 1973; Mahoney and Arieff 1983). In general, therefore, studies in brains of both animals and patients with renal failure have revealed several biochemical changes which are associated with the uraemic state. However, such investigations have revealed only limited information about the fundamental mechanisms which might induce the clinical symptoms of uraemic encephalopathy.

Subcellular Studies in Brain

In several studies, investigators have attempted to evaluate the effects of uraemia on the central nervous system by using subcellular analysis. In two early studies the Na,K-ATPase activity in crude brain preparations were found to be normal to low (Van den Noort et al. 1968; Minkoff et al. 1972). More recently, studies carried out in metabolically active and highly purified brain synaptosomes (vesicles isolated from the presynaptic area in brain) (Fraser et al. 1985a), have shown that both the Na,K-ATP pump and several calcium pumps are altered in uraemic rats (Fraser et al. 1985a, b), although water and urea permeabilities were not affected by uraemia (Verkman and Fraser 1986). The alterations in the calcium pumps are felt to be due largely to parathyroid hormone acting through cyclic AMP-independent pathways (Fraser and Sarnacki 1988a), as well as to the uraemic environment *per se* (Fraser and Sarnacki 1988b). Since the calcium pumps at the nerve terminals mediate neurotransmitter release in the central nervous system, the abnormalities in uraemia may affect information processing in the uraemic state.

Pathology

There are no distinct pathological lesions in brains of patients with ARF. Pathological studies of the brains of patients who have died with chronic renal failure (Teschan et al. 1979; Arieff 1985; Burks et al. 1976) have shown that there is evidence of necrosis of the granular layer of the cerebral cortex, small intracerebral haemorrhages and necrotic foci. Subdural haemorrhage, which was once a common finding in uraemic patients, is now infrequently observed and cerebral oedema is not generally present in either uraemic patients or laboratory animals (Cogan et al. 1978; Arieff et al. 1973; Perry et al. 1985; Arieff and Massry 1974). In general, pathological changes in brains of patients who have died with either acute or chronic renal failure are non-specific and may relate to other concomitant underlying disease states (Burks et al. 1976; Rotter and Roettger 1974; Hagstam 1971).

Parathyroid Hormone as a Possible Central Nervous System Uraemic Toxin

Although there are many factors which may contribute to uraemic encephalopathy, most investigators have shown no correlation between the degree of encephalopathy and any of the commonly measured blood chemistries associated with renal dysfunction, such as blood urea nitrogen, creatinine, bicarbonate or pH (Hughes 1980; Massry 1985). However, in recent years, there has been considerable discussion about the role of parathyroid hormone as a possible uraemic toxin, and there is a substantial amount of evidence suggesting that parathyroid hormone may in fact exert adverse effects on the central nervous system in uraemia (Cooper et al. 1978; Cogan et al. 1978; Goldstein and Massry, 1978; Fraser et al. 1985a,b; Fraser and Sarnacki 1988a,b; Massry 1985).

In uraemic dogs, both the electroencephalogram and brain calcium abnormalities discussed earlier can be prevented by parathyroidectomy (Guisado et al. 1975; Arieff and Massry 1974; Akmal et al. 1984). Conversely, many of the central nervous system abnormalities observed in uraemia, such as the electroencephalogram abnormalities, can be reproduced by administering parathyroid hormone to normal animals, while maintaining calcium and phosphate in the normal range. Thus, parathyroid hormone appears to produce certain of the central nervous system changes of uraemia in normal dogs (Guisado et al. 1975; Minkoff et al. 1972; Slatopolsky et al. 1980; Heath et al. 1980). Similarly, in humans parathyroid hormone has been shown to produce central nervous system effects even in the absence of impaired renal function (Cogan et al. 1978). Neuropsychiatric symptoms have been reported to be among the most common manifestations of primary hyperparathyroidism (Slatopolsky et al. 1980; Heath et al. 1980; Crammer 1977; Gatewood et al. 1975). Patients with primary or secondary hyperparathyroidism have electroencephalogram changes similar to those observed in patients with acute renal failure (Cogan et al. 1978; Goldstein and Massry 1978; Goldstein et al. 1980), and one common denominator between these two groups appears to be the increased plasma level of parathyroid hormone.

As demonstrated in laboratory animals (Guisado et al. 1975; Goldstein and Massry 1978), parathyroidectomy in patients with primary hyperparathyroidism results in improvement of both the electroencephalogram and psychological testing, suggesting a direct effect of parathyroid hormone on the central nervous system (Cogan et al. 1978). In uraemic patients, both the electroencephalogram changes and abnormalities of psychological testing are also improved by either parathyroidectomy or medical suppression of parathyroid hormone (Cogan et al. 1978; Goldstein et al. 1980). The mechanisms by which parathyroid hormone might impair central nervous system function are not completely understood. However, calcium is an essential mediator of neurotransmitter release and also plays an important role in a large number of intracellular activities. Thus, it is possible that alteration of brain calcium may disrupt cerebral function by interfering with any of these processes (Williamson et al. 1985; Rasmussen 1986). Overall, it appears that parathyroid hormone itself has direct toxic effects on the central nervous system. In other systems, parathyroid hormone has a reported association with decreased survival of red blood cells, impaired myocardial contractility, impotence, pruritis and bone disease (Massry 1985; Akmal et al. 1984, 1985; Slatopolsky et al. 1980; Hampers et al. 1968; Coburn 1985; Arnaud 1973). Except for the effects on bone, these additional proposed toxicities require more data before the existence of such effects can be considered confirmed.

Neurological Complications of the Therapy of Uraemia

Dialysis Disequilibrium Syndrome

In patients with renal failure, there are several central nervous system disorders which may occur as a consequence of dialytic therapy. Patients in the ITU who develop acute renal failure belong to one of the risk categories apt to experience dialysis disequilibrium syndrome, which can occur in patients being treated with haemodialysis (Kennedy et al. 1962). The syndrome may include symptoms such as headache, nausea, emesis, blurring of vision, muscular twitching, disorientation, hypertension, tremors and seizures (Arieff 1982; Kennedy et al. 1963; Rodrigo et al. 1977). More recently, the syndrome of dialysis disequilibrium syndrome has been expanded to include milder symptoms, such as muscle cramps, anorexia, restlessness and dizziness (Pagel et al. 1982; Grushkin et al. 1972). Although it was originally thought that the electroencephalogram findings were abnormal in dialysis disequilibrium syndrome (Rodrigo et al. 1977), recent studies have suggested that the electroencephalogram is in fact normal (Teschan et al. 1979; Kiley et al. 1976; Hughes 1980). Dialysis disequilibrium syndrome has been reported among patients of all age groups; however it occurs most commonly among elderly and paediatric patients (Porte et al. 1973). The syndrome is generally associated with rapid haemodialysis of patients with acute renal failure, although it has been reported following routine maintenance haemodialysis in patients with chronic renal failure (Kennedy et al. 1963; Pappius and Dossetor 1967).

The pathogenesis of dialysis disequilibrium syndrome has been extensively investigated in animal models of renal failure (Arieff et al. 1973; Kennedy et al. 1964). It was first postulated that dialysis disequilibrium syndrome was probably due to the "reverse urea effect", where it was hypothesized that urea was cleared less rapidly from the brain than from the blood, resulting in an osmotic gradient between the blood and brain. This osmotic gradient would then lead to a net movement of water into the brain, resulting in cerebral oedema (Arieff et al. 1978). It has since been shown that during dialysis, urea is cleared from brain at the same rate as it is from blood (Arieff et al. 1973; Kennedy et al. 1964), so there is no blood to brain osmotic gradient based on the movement of urea alone. However, rapid haemodialysis of dogs with acute renal failure does result in an increase of brain osmolality, and cerebral oedema. It is now felt that the cerebral oedema may be due to a decrease in the intracellular pH of the cerebral cortex as a consequence of increased production of organic acids (Arieff et al. 1977). It was subsequently demonstrated that decreasing the rate and increasing the frequency of dialysis as part of the initial therapy of acute renal failure led to amelioration of both the symptoms and biochemical derangements of dialysis disequilibrium syndrome (Arieff et al. 1973, 1977; Kennedy et al. 1963; Pagel et al. 1982).

The symptoms of dialysis disequilibrium syndrome are usually self limited but recovery may take several days. New approaches to dialysis treatment may have also helped to ameliorate the clinical picture of dialysis disequilibrium syndrome (Rouby et al. 1980), as most reports of seizures, coma, and death were only reported prior to 1970. Within the last decade the reported symptoms have generally been milder, consisting of nausea, weakness, headache, fatigue, and muscle cramps. The diagnosis of dialysis disequilibrium syndrome must be differentiated from a number of disorders which may affect the central nervous system in dialysis patients (Table 22.1) and thus, should be one of exclusion (Arieff 1985).

Table 22.1. Dialysis dementia subgroups

I. Sporadic endemic
   1. No clear relation to aluminium
   2. Worldwide distribution
   3. No known therapy

II. Epidemic
   1. Geographical clusters
   2. Often related to aluminium in dialysis water
   3. Epidemic usually stops with treatment of water supply
   4. Probably related to other trace elements in water (Sn, Mn, Co, Mg, Fe)

III. Childhood
   1. May be due to non-specific effect of uraemia on immature brain
   2. No clear association with aluminium

Dialysis Encephalopathy

Dialysis encephalopathy is a progressive, frequently fatal neurological disease which is seen almost exclusively in patients being treated with chronic haemodialysis. Although early studies focused on the distinctive neurological findings of this disorder (Alfrey et al. 1972; Mahurkar et al. 1973), recent reports have suggested that some forms of dialysis encephalopathy may often be part of a multi-system disease which includes encephalopathy, osteomalacic bone disease, proximal myopathy and anaemia (Ward et al. 1978; Pierides et al. 1980; Prior et al. 1982; Dunea et al. 1978). The aetiology of dialysis encephalopathy remains controversial, but it most likely represents a symptom complex which is the final common pathway for a variety of processes. Dialysis encephalopathy occurs uncommonly in the setting of the ITU, and will thus be only briefly discussed here. However, patients with dialysis encephalopathy may be misdiagnosed as having other disorders of the central nervous system, and thus physicians in the ITU must be aware of it.

Dialysis encephalopathy can be subdivided into at least three forms: (a) an epidemic form; (b) encephalopathy associated with childhood renal disease; and (c) an endemic form (Alfrey et al. 1972; Mahurkar et al. 1973; Baluarate et al. 1977; Rotundo et al. 1982; Cartier et al. 1978). The initial reports of dialysis encephalopathy were all of the endemic form and usually occurred in patients who had been on chronic haemodialysis for over two years (Alfrey et al. 1972; Mahurkar et al. 1973). The initial symptoms include dysarthria, apraxia, slurring of speech with stuttering and hesitancy. The patients may also develop personality changes, psychosis, dementia, myoceonus, and seizures. The initial symptoms are usually intermittent and often worsen during dialysis. In most cases, the disease progressed to death within six months (Alfrey et al. 1976). Recent reports of the epidemic form of dialysis encephalopathy have suggested that it is due to contamination of the dialysate water with trace metals, such as aluminium (Ward et al. 1978; Dunea et al. 1978; Berkseth and Shapiro 1980; Arieff et al. 1979; Rivera-V'azquez et al. 1980).

The electroencephalogram in patients with dialysis encephalopathy has been described elsewhere (Cooper et al. 1978; Arieff et al. 1979; Nadel and Wilson 1976), but these electroencephalogram changes may precede overt clinical symptoms by 6 months. The diagnosis depends on the presence of the typical clinical picture, the characteristic electroencephalogram pattern, and most important, exclusion of other causes of central nervous system dysfunction (Dunea et al. 1978; Rotundo et al. 1982; Berkseth and Shapiro 1980; Rivera-V'azquez et al. 1980).

Intellectual Impairment

Intellectual impairment is another frequently recognized complication in many patients with renal failure who are being treated with dialysis (English et al. 1978; Osberg et al. 1982). However, the syndrome is not as well defined as is dialysis encephalopathy, there is no anatomical lesion which can be correlated with intellectual deterioration and there are no associated neurological abnormalities. Although some studies suggest that the overall intellectual level in chronic renal failure patients does not differ significantly from normal (Treischmann and Sand 1971), most studies have suggested that the Weschler Adult Intelligence Scale full-scale IQ in dialysis patients is below that of the general population. There also appears to be impairment of intellectual level as represented by the Weschler deterioration quotient. The data on verbal learning obtained with the Walton–Black Modified Word Learning Test and performance learning obtained with the Block Design Learning Test did not indicate any gross learning abnormality. Based on psychological testing, the general consensus is that chronic renal failure is often associated with organic-like loss of intellectual function, particularly information processing capacities, but the aetiology is unclear (English et al. 1978; Osberg et al. 1982; Treischmann et al. 1971; McDaniel 1971).

Acknowledgement. Supported by the Research Service of the Veterans Administration Medical Center, San Francisco, CA.

References

Akmal M, Goldstein DA, Multani S, Massry SG (1984) Role of uremia, brain calcium, and parathyroid hormone on changes in electroencephalogram in chronic renal failure. Am J Physiol 246: F575–F579

Akmal M, Telfer N, Ansari AN, Massry SG (1985) Erythrocyte survival in chronic renal failure: Role of secondary hyperparathyroidism. J Clin Invest 76: 1695–1698

Alfrey AC, Mishell JM, Burks J, Contigugmlia SR, Rudolph H, Lewin E, Holmes JH (1972) Syndrome of dyspraxia and multifocal seizures associated with chronic hemodialysis. Trans Am Soc Artif Intern Organs 18: 257–261

Alfrey AC, LeGendre GR, Kaehney WD (1976) The dialysis encephalopathy syndrome: Possible aluminum intoxication N Engl J Med 294: 184–188

Andreoli SP, Bergstein JM, Sherrard DJ (1984) Aluminum intoxication from aluminum containing phosphate binders in children with azotemia not undergoing dialysis. N Engl J Med 310: 1079–1084

Arieff AI (1982) Dialysis disequilibrium syndrome: Current concepts on pathogenesis. In: Schreiner GE, Winchester JF (eds) Controversies in nephrology, vol IV. Georgetown University Press, Washington DC, pp 367–376

Arieff AI (1985) Effects of water, electrolyte and acid base disorders on the central nervous system. In: Arieff AI, DeFronzo RA (eds) Fluid, electrolyte and acid base disorders. Churchill Livingstone, New York, pp 969–1040

Arieff AI, Massry SG (1974) Calcium metabolism of brain in acute renal failure. Effects of uremia, hemodialysis and parathyroid hormone. J Clin Invest 53: 387–392

Arieff AI, Massry SG, Barrientos A, Kleeman CR (1973) Brain water and electrolyte metabolism in uremia: effects of slow and rapid hemodialysis. Kidney Int 4: 177–187

Arieff AI, Guisado R, Massry SG, Lazarowitz VC (1977) Central nervous system pH in uremia and the effects of hemodialysis. J Clin Invest 58: 306–311

Arieff AI, Lazarowitz VC, Guisado R (1978) Experimental dialysis disequilibrium syndrome: prevention with glycerol. Kidney Int 14: 270–278

Arieff AI, Cooper JD, Armstrong D, Lazarowitz VC (1979) Dementia renal failure and brain aluminum. Ann Intern Med 90: 741–747

Arnaud CD (1973) Hyperparathyroidism and renal failure. Kidney Int 4: 89–95

Baluarate HR, Gruskin AB, Hiner LB, Foley CM, Grover WD (1977) Encephalopathy in children with chronic renal failure. Clin Dial Transplant Forum 7: 95–98

Berkseth RO, Shapiro FL (1980) An epidemic of dialysis encephalopathy and exposure to high aluminum dialysate. In: Schreener GE, Winchester JF (eds) Controversies in nephrology, vol II. Georgetown University Press, Washington, DC, pp 42–51

Brenner BM, Meyer TW, Hostetter TH (1982) Dietary protein intake and progressive nature of kidney disease: the role of hemodynamically mediated glomerular injury in the pathogenesis of progressive glomerular sclerosis in aging, renal ablation and intrinsic renal disease. N Engl J Med 307: 652–659

Burks JS, Alfrey AC, Huddlestone J, Norenberg MD, Lewin E (1976) A fatal encephalopathy in chronic hemodialysis patients. Lancet I: 764–768

Cartier F, Allain P, Gary J, Chatel M, Peckers S (1978) Progressive myoclonic encephalopathy in dialysis patients. Nouv Presse Med 7: 97–102

Coburn JW (1985) Renal osteodystrophy. In: Arieff AI, DeFronzo RA (eds) Fluid, electrolyte and acid–base disorders. Churchill Livingstone, New York, pp 729–776

Cogan M, Covey C, Arieff AI, Wisniewski A, Clark O, Lazarowitz VC, Leach W (1978) Central nervous system manifestations of hyperparathyroidism. Am J Med 65: 963–970

Cooper JD, Lazarowitz VC, Arieff AI (1978) Neurodiagnostic abnormalities in patients with acute renal failure: evidence for neurotoxicity of parathyroid hormone. J Clin Invest 61: 1448–1455
Crammer JL (1977) Calcium metabolism and mental disorder. Psychol Med 7: 557–560
Deferrari G, Garibotto G, Robaudo C, Ghigerri GM, Tizianello A (1981) Brain metabolism of amino acids and ammonia in patients with chronic renal insufficiency. Kidney Int 20: 505–510
Dunea G, Mahurkar SD, Mamdami B, Smith EC (1978) Role of aluminum in dialysis dementia. Ann Intern Med 88: 502–504
English A, Savage RD, Britton PG, Ward MK, Kerr DNS (1978) Intellectual impairment in chronic renal failure. Br Med J i: 888–890
Fraser CL, Arieff AI (1985) Hepatic encephalopathy. N Engl J Med 313: 865–873
Fraser CL, Arieff AI (1988a) Nervous system complications of the uraemic state. Ann Intern Med 108: 143–153
Fraser CL, Arieff AI (1988b) Neurological complications of uraemia. In: Schrier RW, Gottschalk CW (eds) Diseases of the kidney, 4th edn. Little, Brown, Boston MA, pp 3063–3092
Fraser CL, Sarnacki P (1988a) Evidence that parathyroid hormone mediated calcium transport in rat brain synaptosomes is independent of cAMP. J Clin Invest 81: 982–988
Fraser CL, Sarnacki P (1988b) Parathyroid hormone mediates changes in calcium transport in uraemic rat brain synaptosomes. Am J Physiol 254: F837–F844
Fraser CL, Sarnacki P, Arieff AI (1985a) Abnormal sodium transport in synaptosomes from brain of uraemic rats. J Clin Invest 75: 2014–2023
Fraser CL, Sarnacki P, Arieff AI (1985b) Calcium transport abnormality in uraemic rat brain synaptosomes. J Clin Invest 76: 1789–1795
Gatewood JW, Organ CH, Mead BT (1975) Mental changes associated with hyperparathyroidism. Am J Psychiatr 123: 129–132
Goldstein DA, Massry SG (1978) Effect of parathyroid hormone and its withdrawal on brain calcium and electroencephalogram. Miner Electrolyte Metab 1: 84–91
Goldstein DA, Feinstein EI, Chiu LA, Pattabhiraman R, Massry SG (1980) The relationship between the abnormalities in EEG and blood levels of parathyroid hormone in dialysis patients. J Clin Endocrinol Metab 51: 130–134
Grushkin CM, Korsch B, Fine RN (1972) Hemodialysis in small children. JAMA 221: 869–871
Guisado R, Arieff AI, Massry SG (1975) Changes in the electroencephalogram in acute uremia: Effects of parathyroid hormone and brain electrolytes. J Clin Invest 55: 738–745
Hagstam KE (1971) EEG frequency content related to chemical blood parameters in chronic uremia. Scand J Urol Nephrol 7(Suppl 1): 1–56
Hampers CL, Katz AI, Wilson RE, Merrill JP (1968) Disappearance of uraemic itching after subtotal parathyroidectomy. N Engl J Med 279: 695–697
Heath H, Hodgson SF, Kennedy MA (1980) Primary hyperparathyroidism. N Engl J Med 303: 189–194
Hughes JR (1980) Correlation between EEG and chemical changes in uremia. Electroencephalogr Clin Neurophysiol 48: 583–594
Kennedy AC, Linton AL, Eaton JC (1962) Urea levels in cerebrospinal fluid after hemodialysis. Lancet I: 410–411
Kennedy AC, Linton AL, Luke RG, Renfrew S (1963) Electroencephalographic changes during hemodialysis. Lancet I: 408–411
Kennedy AC, Linton AI, Renfrew S, Luke RG, Dinwoodie A (1964) The pathogenesis and prevention of cerebral dysfunction during dialysis. Lancet I: 790–793
Kiley JE, Woodruff MW, Pratt KL (1976) Evaluation of encephalopathy by EEG frequency analysis in chronic dialysis patients. Clin Nephrol 5: 245–250
Klahr S, Buerkert J, Purkerson ML (1983) Role of dietary factors in the progression of chronic renal disease. Kidney Int 24: 579–587
Lieber CS, Lefevere A (1959) Ammonia as a source of gastric hypoacidity in patients with uremia. J Clin Invest 38: 1271–1277
Locke SJ, Merrill JP, Tyler HR (1961) Neurological complications of acute uremia. Arch Intern Med 108: 75–86
Losowsky MS, Scott BB (1973) Hepatic encephalopathy. Br Med J iii: 279–281
Mahoney CA, Arieff AI (1983) Central and peripheral nervous system effects of chronic renal failure. Kidney Int 24: 170–177
Mahoney CA, Sarnacki P, Arieff AI (1984) Uremic encephalopathy: Role of brain energy metabolism. Am J Physiol 247: F527–F532
Mahurkar SD, Dhar SK, Salta R, Meyers L, Smith EC, Dunea G (1973) Dialysis dementia. Lancet I: 1412–1415

Massry SG (1985) Current status of the role of parathyroid hormone in uraemic toxicity. Contrib Nephrol 49: 1–11
McDaniel JW (1971) Metabolic and central nervous system correlates of congnative dysfunction with renal failure. Psychophysiology 8: 704–713
McLachlan DRC (1989) Aluminum and Alzheimer's disease. Neurobiology of aging (in press).
Minkoff L, Gertner G, Darawb M, Mercier C, Levin ML (1972) Inhibition of brain sodium–potassium ATPase in uraemic rats. J Lab Clin Med 80: 71–78
Nadel AM, Wilson WP (1976) Dialysis encephalopathy: a possible seizure disorder. Neurology 26: 1130–1134
Osberg JW, Meares GJ, McKee DC, Burnett GB (1982) Intellectual functioning in renal failure and chronic dialysis. J Chron Dis 35: 445–457
Pagel MD, Ahmad S, Vizzo JE, Scribner BH (1982) Acetate and bicarbonate fluctuations and acetate intolerance during dialysis. Kidney Int 21: 513–518
Papadakis MA, Arieff AI (1987) Unpredictability of clinical evaluation of renal function in cirrhosis: a prospective study. Am J Med 82: 945–952
Pappius HM, Dossetor JB (1967) The effects of rapid hemodialysis on brain tissues and cerebrospinal fluid of dogs. Can J Physiol Pharmacol 45: 129–147
Perry TL, Yong VW, Kish SJ, Ito M, Foulks JG, Godolphin WJ, Sweeney VP (1985) Neurochemical abnormalities in brains of renal failure patients treated by repeated hemodialysis. J Neurochem 45: 1043–1048
Pierides AM, Edwards WG, Cullum UX, McCall JT, Ellis HA (1980) Hemodialysis encephalopathy with osteomalacic fractures and muscle weakness. Kidney Int 18: 115–124
Porte FK, Johnson WJ, Klass DW (1973) Prevention of dialysis disequilibrium syndrome by use of high sodium concentration in the dialysate. Kidney Int 3: 327–333
Prior JC, Cameron EC, Knickerbocker WJ, Sweeney VP, Suchowersky O (1982) Dialysis encephalopathy and osteomalacic bone disease. Am J Med 72: 33–42
Raskin NH, Fishman RA (1976) Neurologic disorders in renal failure. N Engl J Med 294: 143–148, 204–210
Rasmussen H (1986) The calcium messenger system. N Engl J Med 314: 1094–1101; 1164–1170
Rivera-V'azquez AB, Noriega-S'anchez A, Ramirez-Gonzalez R, Martinez-Maldonado M (1980) Acute hypercalcemia in hemodialysis patients: distinction from dialysis dementia. Nephron 25: 243–246
Rodrigo F, Shideman J, McHugh R, Busemeier T, Kjellstrand C (1977) Osmolality changes during hemodialysis. Ann Intern Med 86: 554–561
Rotter W, Roettger P (1974) Comparative pathologic–anatomic study of cases of chronic renal insufficiency with and without hemodialysis. Clin Nephrol 1: 257–265
Rotundo A, Nevins TE, Lipton M, Lockman LA, Mauer SM, Michael AF (1982) Progressive encephalopathy in children with chronic renal insufficiency in infancy. Kidney Int 21: 486–491
Rouby JJ, Rottenbourg J, Durande JP (1980) Hemodynamic changes induced by regular hemodialysis and sequential ultrafiltration hemodialysis: A comparative study. Kidney Int 17: 801–810
Said G, Boudier L, Selva J, Zingraff J, Drueke T (1983) Different patterns of uremic polyneuropathy: a clinicopathologic study. Neurology 33: 567–574
Scheinberg D (1954) Effects of uremia on cerebral blood flow and metabolism. Neurology 4: 101–105
Slatopolsky E, Martin K, Hruska K (1980) Parathyroid hormone metabolism and its potential as a uraemic toxin. Am J Physiol 238: F1–F12
Souheaver GT, Ryan JJ, DeWolfe AS (1982) Neuropsychological patterns in uremia. J Clin Psychol 38: 490–496
Teschan PE, Arieff AI (1985) Uremic and dialysis encephalopathies. In: McCandless DW (ed.) Cerebral energy metabolism and metabolic encephalopathy. Plenum, New York, pp 263–286
Teschan PE, Ginn HE, Bourne JR, Ward JW, Hamel B, Nunally JHC, Musso M, Vaughn WK (1979) Quantitative indices of clinical uremia. Kidney Int 15: 676–697
Treischmann RB, Sand PI (1971) WAIs and MMPI correlates of increasing renal failure in adult medical patients. Psychol Rep 29: 1251–1262
Van den Noort S, Eckel RE, Brine K, Hrdlicka JT (1968) Brain metabolism in uraemic and adenosine-infused rats. J Clin Invest 47: 2133–2142
Verkman AS, Fraser CL (1986) Water and non-electrolyte permeability in brain synaptosomes isolated from normal and uraemic rats. Am J Physiol 250: R306–R312
Ward MK, Feest TG, Ellis HA, Parkinson IS, Kerr DS (1978) Osteomalacic dialysis osteodystrophy: evidence for a water-borne aetiological agent probably aluminium. Lancet I: 841–845
Williamson JR, Cooper RH, Joseph SK, Thomas AP (1985) Inositol triphosphate and diacylglycerol as intracellular second messengers in liver. Am J Physiol 248: C203–C216

Discussion

Dr Macias opened the discussion by emphasizing that the elderly who develop acute renal failure have tremendous behavioural alterations, such that very often and early on in their illness, cognitive function was greatly reduced. This clinical change in cerebral function was observed early in the absence of any change in the EEG. He thought that the environmental factor was important in the development of confusion and this might well reflect the so called "white wall" syndrome; this was a known cause of confusion and psychosis in the ICU in the absence of any other organ disturbance. Dr Arieff emphasized that abnormalities in the EEG could persist despite dialysis, until renal function had recovered. Most of the other participants thought that environmental factors in the ICU were very important and Dr Schrier mentioned that there had been reports concerning the treatment of cardiac arrhythmias which were unresponsive to all drug therapy until the patients were removed from the ICU. Stress syndromes in the ICU are greatly underemphasized concluded Dr Bihari.

Dr Arieff was asked whether sodium, potassium-ATPase inhibition as demonstrated in the synaptosome model, would lead to cytotoxic cerebral oedema in patients with acute renal failure. He thought that this would be the case, but the distribution of inhibition of Na,K-ATPase in the brain might be patchy so that oedema would not be generalized, nor detectable by CT scanning, nor cause problems in terms of raised intracranial pressure. However, Dr Arieff emphasized that there was no major alteration in the blood–brain barrier permeability in uraemic states, but he reminded all participants that dialysis had the tendency to increase brain osmolality, lower pH and cause cerebral oedema of a transitory nature. Dr Solez referred to the abnormal EEG associated with cyclosporin administration in the rat. Apparently, at a dose of 10–20 mg kg^{-1} a disturbed EEG is seen and a lethal seizure disorder can occur at higher doses. Certainly seizures have been reported in cyclosporin-treated patients, but Dr Arieff had not investigated this problem.

Chapter 23

Measuring Severity of Illness

J. Bion

Scientific advance is dependent on the capacity to measure; and measurement requires the development of suitable instruments. Caring for the critically ill is an area of high-technology medicine where measurement forms an essential part of clinical management, and yet until recently there have been relatively few developments in measuring the single factor common to all critically ill patients: severity of illness. Without such a method, assessment of these patients requires an analysis of disparate factors and depends upon the experience and powers of observation of the clinician involved, a process which is frequently subjective and may be prone to error. Severity scoring can provide an objective measure which may be useful in the stratification of patients for therapeutic trials, for audit of clinical performance, and in the prediction of outcome.

The ideal measure should be appropriate to the population it is intended to describe. It should be independent both of the observer and of therapy, and its accuracy should be verifiable against clearly defined outcomes which do not form part of the criteria employed to construct the system. It should be reasonably easy to use, and applicable to as wide a population as possible, not limited to a particular diagnostic group. The results must be reproducible in a new population. The system should be useful, and must therefore have an impact on clinical practice.

Scoring systems can be devised using two main methods: the attribution of weights based on clinical experience, or the use of data-search techniques. In the first method, weights are attached to various factors considered important by consensus between clinicians, as exemplified by the Glasgow Coma Scale (Teasdale and Jennett 1974), the Trauma Score (Champion et al. 1981), and the APACHE score (Knaus et al. 1985), or by using linear analogue scales as in the Sepsis Score (Elebute and Stonor 1983). The second method employs multivariate analysis using linear or logistic regression, discriminant analysis (Afifi and Azen 1979), or recursive partitioning (Friedman 1977); these complex statistical techniques require a defined outcome, and then seek for those factors in the data

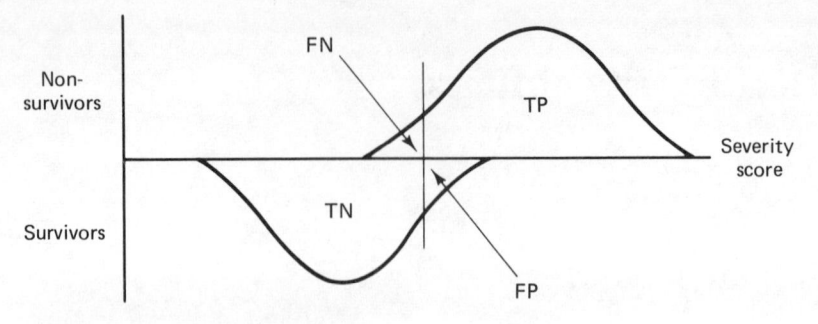

Fig. 23.1. Choosing the cut-off point.

presented to them which predispose to that outcome. Weights are then assigned to each factor and a formula derived for the whole group. Clinical examples using data-search techniques include the prediction of outcome from non-traumatic coma (Levy et al. 1985), head injury (Murray 1986), and critical illness (Teres et al. 1987). In both methods, the sum of the weights is an expression of risk of the defined outcome. The clinical method requires the establishment of an hypothesis (the weighting system) which can then be validated in the same way that a new treatment is assessed. Data-search methods derive their results from training populations which must then be validated on second external populations ("test" groups) in order to exclude the possibility that results are a consequence of quirks in the data.

The accuracy of scoring systems is assessed by their capacity to predict a certain outcome or event. This is satisfactory when the defined outcome is not amenable to interference (for example, the measurement of time and the earth's rotation). However, in the assessment of critical illness, it is death or survival which are most commonly chosen as outcome events; and it is precisely these events which we most want to influence in our management of patients. This dilemma is most clearly exemplified by Knaus and colleagues (Wagner et al. 1986) who showed that whereas in patients admitted to intensive care with sepsis there was a linear relationship between admission APACHE II score and risk of death, in patients with diabetic ketoacidotic coma there was no such relationship; they attributed this to the possession of a specific therapeutic agent (insulin) for the latter group. Had the APACHE system been tested only on diabetics, it would have been discarded as useless. This confusion between prediction and measurement is reflected in the attitude of clinicians who regard severity scoring as a threat to clinical judgement.

Severity scoring is a method of reducing a number of variables to a single value expressing severity of illness, and it is therefore a form of measurement identical to any other clinical test. Using death or survival as the outcome events, assessment of accuracy therefore requires an analysis of the proportion of patients correctly predicted to die or survive, expressed as a proportion of the total. To do this it is necessary to examine a population in which the outcome event is known (or will become known), and to define the value at which death is predicted to occur. This value is known as the cut-off point, and is equivalent to the value at which a test can be described as positive. The cut-off point can either be selected from the raw data to give the best overall estimate of outcome (Fig. 23.1), or it can be predetermined according to the value attached to a particular outcome. For example, since the cost of incorrectly predicting death might be the premature cessation of treatment in a patient who would otherwise have survived, the cut-off point can be set at a severity score value above that of any known survivor; the penalty of this approach is the prediction of survival for many patients who subsequently die. Fig. 23.1 provides a graphical example of the terms employed in the construction of the 2×2 table (Table 23.1) from which sensitivity and specificity can be calculated.

Table 23.1. Classification of test results in a study population in which the outcome is known, using a 2×2 table

Disease status ("actual outcome")	D+ (Died)	D− (Survived)	Total
Test result ("predicted outcome")			
T+ (Non-survivor)	TP	FP	TP+FP = total +ve
T− (Survivor)	FN	TN	FN+TN = total −ve
Total	TP+FN (Total deaths)	FP+TN (Total survivors)	Total in study population

TP, true positives (predicted to die, died).
FP, false positives (predicted to die, survived).
FN, false negatives (predicted to survive, died).
TN, true negatives (predicted to survive, survived).

Sensitivity = True positive rate = TP/TP+FN × 100.
Specificity = True negative rate = TN/TN+FP × 100.

The Acute Physiology and Chronic Health Evaluation (APACHE) System

The most widely validated form of severity scoring for general intensive care is the APACHE II score (Knaus et al. 1985). This system was constructed by consensus between clinicians, and has been refined using multivariate analysis. It is based on the principle that outcome from acute illness is most likely to be affected by the extent of homeostatic disturbance, and the state of health of the individual before the acute disease supervened. It incorporates twelve physiological variables together with additional weighting for age and a past history of chronic disease. Based on a study population of over 5000 patients, logistic regression has been used to calculate further weights for specific diagnostic categories in order to improve predictive power; using a cut-off point for risk of death of 50%, the system has a sensitivity of 47%, a specificity of 95%, and an overall correct classification rate of 85.5%. In addition to its use for the prediction of outcome for groups of patients, the APACHE II system has been used to assess quality of care in different intensive care units (ICUs) (Knaus et al. 1986;

Zimmerman et al. 1988), to examine the use of "do not resuscitate" orders (Zimmerman et al. 1986), in the audit of ambulance transport of critically ill patients (Bion et al. 1985, 1988a), to review the provision of parenteral nutrition services (Chang et al. 1986), and to stratify patients in controlled therapeutic trials (Knaus et al. 1984; Ledingham et al. 1988).

There are three points about the APACHE system which need further consideration. These are the collection of data, the use of the Glasgow Coma Scale, and diagnostic weighting.

The data used in the APACHE system are the "worst values" recorded for each variable in every 24 hour period. This approach maximizes the severity of physiological instability. It requires that the data collector be experienced in the use of the system, and adds to the work required for its completion. This may be a problem in ICUs without research staff where the nurses are asked to complete the forms. The alternative approach is to use a single time-point; this simplifies the collection of data, but may result in unrepresentative values being recorded. It provides a "snapshot" view of physiology. In practice, it seems to make no difference to the accuracy of the system using either method (Bion et al. 1985).

The Glasgow Coma Scale (GCS) is the sole measure of neurological function in the APACHE system, and is, therefore, heavily weighted to a maximum of 12 points. It is particularly difficult to interpret in patients with metabolic cerebral disorders who are undergoing controlled ventilation, but is easier to assess in other patients provided that care is taken in the use of sedative agents. Current practice is to use the best value obtainable within any 24 hour period; in the absence of known cerebral disease, and in the presence of sedative drugs, it is reasonable to assume that the GCS is normal.

Diagnostic weighting was introduced in order to improve predictive power; as described above, patients with diseases which are amenable to specific treatments, such as diabetic coma and insulin, may not demonstrate a close relationship between admission APACHE score and outcome. The problem is that the weights attached to each diagnosis will need to be reviewed as new and more specific therapies are introduced. An alternative is to examine the degree of reversibility of physiological disturbance, and to incorporate this as a measure of outcome. This can be done by recording the proportional change in score from admission, and using this technique for day 4 of ICU stay a sensitivity of 75% and specificity of 87% has been obtained for a cut-off point of 50% for risk of death (Bion et al. 1988b). This compares well with data from other studies, and is a method which does not require updating as therapeutic skills improve.

The science of prediction is still at an early stage of development, and it is important to realize that severity scoring is primarily a form of measurement with prediction only one of its many potential uses. Outcome need not be restricted to death or survival, and as predictive capacity improves we will need to look at quality of survival as a separate outcome. Considerable refinements are required to improve predictive power, and there is no system available which could be used to determine the fate of individual patients. Indeed, the concept that a completely infallible predictive system could be devised is naïve, and carries with it the implication that future medical advances will not alter outcome from critical illness. At present, severity scoring is best used for audit, and for stratification in medical research; if used in the assessment of individual patients, it must be remembered that these methods are guides, not substitutes, for experienced clinical judgement.

References

Afifi AA, Azen SP (1979) Statistical analyses: a computer-orientated approach, 2nd edn. Academic Press, New York
Bion JF, Edlin SA, Ramsay G, McAbe S, Ledingham IMcA (1985) Validation of a prognostic score in critically ill patients undergoing transport. Br Med J 291: 432–434
Bion JF, Wilson IH, Taylor PA (1988a) Non-specialist transport of the critically ill: audit by sickness scoring. Br Med J 296: 170
Bion JF, Aitchison TC, Edlin SA, Ledingham IMcA (1988b) Sickness scoring and response to treatment as predictors of outcome from critical illness. Intensive Care Med 14: 167–172
Champion HR, Sacco WJ, Carnazzo AJ, Copes W, Fouty WJ (1981) Trauma score. Crit Care Med 9: 672–676
Chang RWS, Jacobs S, Lee B. (1986) Use of APACHE II severity of disease classification to identify intensive-care-unit patients who would not benefit from total parenteral nutrition. Lancet I: 1483–1487
Elebute EA, Stonor HB (1983) The grading of sepsis. Br J Surg 70: 29–31
Friedman JH (1977) A recursive partitioning decision rule for non-parametric classification. IEEE Trans Comput 16: 404–408
Knaus WA, Wagner DP, Draper EA (1984) The value of measuring severity of disease in clinical research on acutely ill patients. J Chron Dis 37: 455–463
Knaus WA, Draper EA, Wagner DP, Zimmerman JE (1985) APACHE II: a severity of disease classification system. Crit Care Med 10: 818–829
Knaus WA, Draper EA, Wagner DP, Zimmerman JE (1986) An evaluation of outcome from intensive care in major medical centres. Ann Intern Med 104: 410–418
Ledingham IMcA, Alcock SR, Eastway AT, McDonald JC, McKay IC, Ramsay G (1988) Triple regimen of selective decontamination of the digestive tract, systemic cefotaxime, and microbiological surveillance for prevention of acquired infection in intensive care. Lancet I: 786–790
Levy DE, Caronna J, Singer BH, Lapinski RH, Frydman H, Plum F (1985) Predicting outcome from hypoxic-ischaemic coma. JAMA 253: 1420–1426
Murray GD (1986) Use of an international data bank to compare outcome following severe head injury in different centres. Stat Med 5: 103–112
Teasdale G, Jennett B (1974) Assessment of coma and impaired consciousness. A practical scale. Lancet II: 81–84
Teres D, Lemeshow S, Avrunin JS, Pastides H (1987) Validation of the mortality prediction model for ICU patients. Crit Care Med 15: 208–213
Wagner DP, Knaus WA, Draper EA (1986) Physiologic abnormalities and outcome from acute disease. Evidence for a predictable relationship. Arch Intern Med 146: 1389–1396
Zimmerman JE, Knaus WA, Sharpe SM, Anderson AS, Draper EA, Wagner DP (1986) The use and implications of Do Not Resuscitate orders in intensive care units. JAMA 255: 351–356
Zimmerman JE, Knaus WA, Judson JA, Havill JH, Trubuhovich RV, Draper EA, Wagner DP (1988) Patient selection for intensive care: A comparison of New Zealand and United States hospitals. Crit Care Med 16: 318–325

Discussion

Professor Cameron initiated the discussion by describing a small number of patients with acute renal failure who had been studied at Guy's Hospital. APACHE II scoring had been used on admission and on a daily basis to follow the course of these patients, and, as others had found, the patients who survived tended to demonstrate a fall in APACHE II score whilst those who died, did not. Professor Cameron and Dr Bihari both emphasized that it was impossible to use this form of prognostication to define individual patients who should not receive treatment. All participants agreed that APACHE II scoring could not be used to limit the application of expensive medical care to individual patients. Nevertheless, Dr Bihari was quite insistent that APACHE II scoring should become a routine procedure in general intensive care since he felt that it should be impossible to publish controlled clinical trials involving intensive care patients unless some sort of scoring of the severity of illness was included in the study. Dr Bihari then commented that although there was a large database of patients who had undergone APACHE II scoring in the United States and formed the core around which William Knaus had built his system, a similar database was required in the various European countries in order to validate the scoring system in a different environment of health care. Professor Cameron agreed and stated that two phases were essential; first the generation of the data in terms of documenting the admission of patients to intensive care with some score of the severity of their illness; and then their application to a particular population at risk with an analysis of severity scoring carried out in a prospective fashion. Dr Parsons drew attention to a concern that surrounds the distinction between dying in intensive care in contrast to the withdrawal of treatment. Dr Bion agreed that severity scores can become self-justifying prophecies since some doctors confused measurement with prediction. He emphasized the difference between the measurement of severity of illness compared with the prediction of outcome. Obviously these two are linked and one leads to the other in a large population of patients. Yet, in the individual case, prediction of outcome cannot be made from the severity of illness score alone. This was absolutely fundamental.

The discussion turned to whether the APACHE II scoring system was the appropriate system to use in general intensive care units. Dr Kleinknecht pointed to the wide application of the acute physiology score of Jean-Roger Le-Gall. Indeed, Dr Bion had modified the APACHE II system to produce his own Sickness Score. Everyone thought that the Glasgow Coma Scale component of the APACHE II scoring system formed a particularly difficult area. The acute physiology scoring system as used in France is similar to the APACHE II system, but it gives a score of 3 points to a patient receiving mechanical ventilation with PEEP.

Dr Bion said he used the ratio of the inspired concentration to the arterial oxygen tension, rather than the alveolar-arterial oxygen tension gradient, in his system as it was simpler and had been shown to give a more accurate value for pulmonary shunt. Dr Bihari preferred the use of the APACHE II scoring system as had been developed by the Washington Group purely in so far as it was in widespread use in North America, and it allowed a certain comparison of results of intensive care between units.

The discussion then turned to iatrogenic disease in the intensive care unit. Dr Arieff pointed out that a number of measures which are thought of as therapy in fact may often worsen the prognosis of the patient. As examples he suggested the use of noradrenaline for the treatment of hypotension associated with cardiogenic shock, the administration of bicarbonate for metabolic acidosis, the prescribing of high-dose steroids for septic shock, the use of repeated episodes of haemodialysis which often decrease renal perfusion in the management of acute renal failure, the administration of drugs with toxic side effects, and the development of hypernatraemia associated with hyperalimentation. He wondered how the various scoring systems could separate out this iatrogenic component which clearly contributed to the ultimate prognosis of the patient. Dr Bion had no answer to this other than to emphasize that the severity of illness of the patient should be assessed as soon as that patient is admitted to intensive care, rather than waiting for the application of therapy. Dr Lazarus emphasized the inadequacy of mortality as an end point. He thought it was appalling that there was a large number of patients who struggled through an illness within the intensive care unit and survived, but then went on to be discharged to a nursing home in the community and continue their existence at enormous cost to society; perhaps they lived for another couple of months, often attended by a nurse who was disinterested in their care, and subsequently died. Their quality of life during this period although difficult to judge, appears extremely poor. Surely, some other measure must be included in an assessment of outcome from intensive care other than survival. All participants agreed with this view and Dr Bion revealed that a quality of life measure in the community was now being included in the various epidemiological studies of survival following a period of intensive care.

Dr Better remembered that many years ago Max Harry Weil and others had proposed that lactic acid concentration in the blood and the temperature of the big toe are the most important prognostic factors in the assessment of a patient with acute circulatory failure. Similarly, in patients with congestive heart failure the serum sodium was apparently the best predictor of death in such cases. He wondered whether the scoring systems were becoming too complex in an attempt to predict the outcome of some disease. Dr Bion re-emphasized the simple principle that outcome prediction was quite different from the measurement of severity of illness. He maintained that it was important to measure the severity of illness so that intensive care physicians knew what they were dealing with. If intensive care physicians then wanted to use the measurement of severity of illness to predict outcome, that was up to the individual physician concerned. At this point the discussion was terminated.

Section V
Strategies in Management of Acute Renal Failure

Chapter 24

Prophylaxis of Acute Renal Failure in the Intensive Care Unit

J. M. Lazarus

Introduction

The term prophylaxis is defined as measures designed to guard from, ward off or prevent disease. Prevention of a disease depends largely on the ability of the physician to *predict* when the disease may occur, to know what factors cause the disease, and to identify the susceptible patient. Thus, the keys to successful prophylaxis of acute renal failure (ARF) in the intensive care unit (ICU) revolve around identification of those patients susceptible to ARF and the clinical situations during which ARF is likely to occur. Obviously, prophylactic treatment can only be provided in those instances where the onset of a potential insult can be identified. Prophylactic care is not a possibility in those patients who have ARF due to trauma or catastrophic events outside of the hospital. There are no figures available on the incidence or prevalence of ARF. Considering the tremendous number of patients admitted to ICU facilities around the world, ARF is not a common complication (Fig. 24.1). Thus, the practical application of prophylaxis in ARF is more difficult than one would first think. Prophylactic treatment of *all* patients in ICUs is not medically or economically practical. Despite the low incidence, prevention and/or reversal of ARF is important because of its persistently high morbidity and mortality.

In this chapter, I will not consider those aetiologies of ARF related to acute glomerulonephritis or acute interstitial disease (except drug induced). Although the extracellular fluid volume status (ECV) of the patient is the major issue in this discussion, the group of patients who have "prerenal" azotaemia *per se* as the cause of ARF will not be considered. Obviously, if such patients do not receive appropriate therapy (i.e. volume replacement) they may progress to acute tubular necrosis (ATN). Likewise, "post-renal" ARF will not be discussed, although obstruction is certainly one of the major causes of reversible ARF. Suffice it to say that, in this day and age, any patient with ARF should be evaluated by renal ultrasound for even the remote possibility of obstruction.

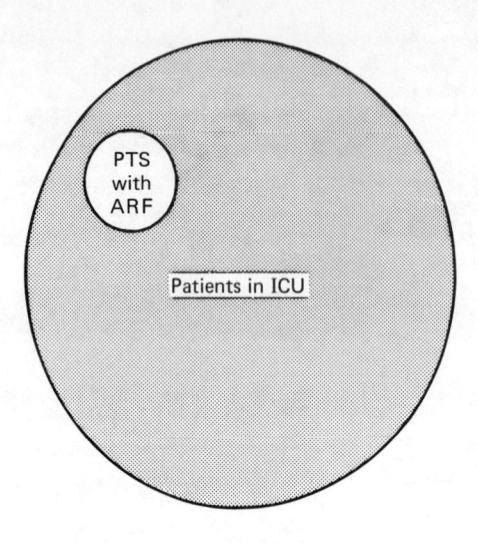

Fig. 24.1. The number of patients with ARF as a complication in relation to the number of patients admitted to ICU facilities around the world.

There are some patients in whom the aetiology of ARF is so obvious that ultrasound is not necessary. However, it is a benign study and potentially important in ruling out a major cause of ARF. The primary emphasis of the discussion will be directed to prevention of ARF due to ATN and/or acute interstitial nephritis related to drug nephrotoxicity.

Because of the difficulty of identifying patients prior to an unexpected catastrophic event and initiating preventive or prophylactic treatment, most research and published information concerns reversal of diagnosed ARF. There is no reason to assume that treatment modalities which have been studied in patients with established or early ARF are useful in a prophylactic or preventive approach. However, there is likewise no reason to preclude their consideration in such a setting. Because of the limited number of treatment options for purely prophylactic treatment, I will discuss a number of therapies which have been suggested for early ARF, considering their use in a preventive or prophylactic manner.

The topic of preventive or prophylactic treatment of ARF has been reviewed in a number of publications (Luke and Kennedy 1967; Tiller and Mudge 1980; Mandal et al. 1983; Andreucci 1984; Puschett 1985; Brezis et al. 1986; Levinsky and Bernard 1988). The vast majority of data have been accumulated from experimental ARF in animal models which may or may not be appropriately related to human experience. There are some clinical studies in humans, but only a scarce handful have looked at preventive or prophylactic treatments in a prospective, controlled fashion and much of the available information is from anecdotal cases or small, uncontrolled studies.

Selection of Patients for Consideration for Prophylactic Treatment of ARF

In the thousands of patients admitted to ICUs, there are treatments we might initiate for some to prevent ARF, but would not offer to all patients in ICUs. Let me first discuss the treatment or standards of medical care that should be provided to *every* patient sufficiently ill that they require admission to an intensive care setting. Table 24.1 outlines the important general principles of preventive treatment in this group of patients. These are all obvious, basic, and generally accepted approaches to medical care. However, we have all seen patients in whom these basic principles are violated with the subsequent development of renal failure. Thus, the basis of ARF prevention is the application of good general medical care.

Table 24.1. Basic care of all ICU patients

1.	Establish level of renal function
2.	Maintain adequate extracellular fluid volume
3.	Avoid or minimize nephrotoxic exposure
4.	Avoid or minimize unnecessary procedures

Measurement of the Level of Renal Function

All patients in ICUs should undergo the studies outlined in Table 24.2 to establish the level of renal function early. The most obvious assessment of function is observation of urine output. The critically ill patient should have accurate measurement and documentation of fluid intake as well as urinary output. The patient's body weight, often helpful in verifying or interpreting intake and output, should be obtained daily and recorded. The urinalysis and sediment examination may be very helpful in establishing presence of prior renal disease. The ability of the kidney to concentrate urine will also give some clue as to renal function. Specific gravity of urine is not often measured routinely. We have become sufficiently sophisticated that measurements of serum and urine osmolarity are now obtained when concentration ability is to be measured. These studies are important measures in certain cases, but are not warranted in every patient admitted to an ICU. It would not seem unreasonable, however, that as part of the routine urinalysis, the specific gravity be included. The most used and relied upon measures of renal function are the serum creatinine and urea nitrogen and electrolytes. These laboratory tests are ordered in nearly every patient in the hospital and certainly should be obtained serially in the critically ill ICU patient. Serum creatinine is perhaps a better measure of glomerular filtration rate than is the urea nitrogen. The latter, however, may be a better measure of the uraemic milieu in advanced renal failure. Both these tests may vary greatly, depending

Table 24.2. Initial evaluation of renal function for all patients in an ICU setting

1.	Careful documentation of intake and output and body weight
2.	Urinalysis with sediment examination and specific gravity
3.	Serum creatinine and urea nitrogen and electrolytes
4.	Renal ultrasound?

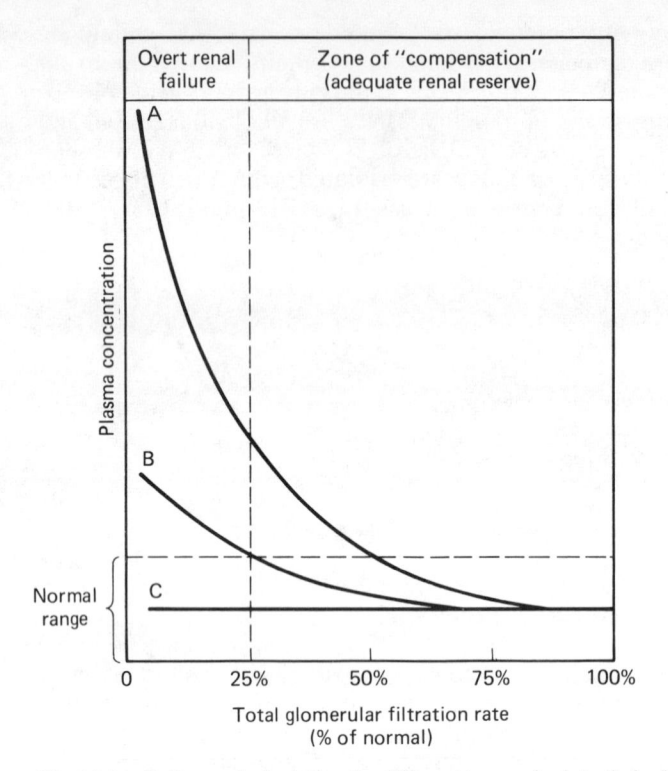

Fig. 24.2. Patterns of adaptation for different types of solutes in body fluids in chronic renal failure. Curve A describes the pattern seen with substances such as creatinine and urea. Curve B reflects the pattern of substances such as phosphate, urate, potassium and hydrogen ions. Curve C reflects the pattern of solutes such as sodium and chloride. (From Brenner et al. 1987).

upon body mass, degree of hydration, protein intake, blood in the intestine and a number of other factors. More importantly, because of tubular absorption of creatinine and urea, the serum values of creatinine and urea nitrogen may not become elevated out of the normal range until GFR is reduced by as much as 50% (Fig. 24.2). Thus, these most relied on standards for measurement of renal function offer only a crude estimation of true glomerular filtration rate. As will be discussed later, one of the principle factors in susceptibility to ARF is pre-existing renal insufficiency. Thus, accurate measurement of function is no small issue. Usually, it is not sufficiently important that *all* patients being admitted to ICUs have a creatinine clearance or a more exact test such as the iothalamate or ytterbium DTPA clearance. In certain situations, the physician may be suspicious of a decrease in glomerular filtration rate and desire more specific measurement. Thus, these tests may be indicated in such patients at risk (see below). In the general population in ICUs, however, the mainstay of renal function measurement will probably continue to be the serum creatinine and urea nitrogen together with urine output. It is important that these studies be performed, however it is equally important that the physician appreciates that these studies may not reflect *exact* renal function. Ultrasound studies are now generally available, are easy to perform and non-invasive. Not every patient in an ICU requires renal ultrasound, but, at the first sign of problems with renal function, one should be obtained. Also, if an abdominal ultrasound is obtained on any patient the radiologist should make note of renal size and the collecting system as a baseline.

Establishment and Maintenance of Adequate Intravascular Fluid Volume

The establishment and maintenance of adequate extracellular or intravascular fluid volume is essential in all patients in the ICU. If the patient arrives in the ICU in a volume-depleted state, one of the first therapies is to replace appropriate volume in the form of blood products or crystalloid. This should *always* occur before institution of pressor agents or "prophylactic" drug treatment. Estimation of extracellular fluid volume is not always easy, particularly in severely and acutely ill patients. The usual measures which we utilize are listed in Table 24.3. However, many of these may be difficult to measure in the patient in the ICU. For instance, patients may be too ill to assume an upright position for measurement of postural blood pressure or pulse change. Skin turgor in the elderly or severely ill patient is often difficult to assess. Elderly patients may have venous sclerosis or may have multiple venous lines in place which makes estimation of venous distension difficult. Laboured mouth breathing will obviate the oral mucous membrane as a measure of hydration. Patients may have findings such as oedema, hepatomegaly and pulmonary rales from other organ system disease such as liver disease, pneumonia and low serum albumin which may give conflicting clues. Large third space fluid losses may not be appreciated. Most importantly, many of these patients may have severe left and/or right heart failure with subsequent clouding of the usual measures of volume status. Placement of a central venous or pulmonary capillary wedge pressure line may be necessary. Not *all* patients in the ICU should have a central venous line or wedged pulmonary capillary catheter and it would seem inappropriate to go to these extremes simply to measure intravascular volume in all patients. However, in those patients with renal compromise in which prerenal azotaemia and ATN cannot be distinguished, the use of such measures is very useful (see below). One other measure of adequacy of intravascular volume is a trial of rapidly administered fluid to increase urinary output. Often the cardiologist, pulmonary specialist or intensivist will be

Table 24.3. Clinical evaluation of ECV

1.	History of intake and output
2.	Postural blood pressure and pulse
3.	Jugular venous pressure
4.	Skin turgor
5.	Mucous membrane moisture
6.	Occular pressure
7.	Oedema, hepatomegaly, rales, third space fluid
8.	Urine chemistries
9.	Central venous pressure
10.	Pulmonary wedge pressure
11.	Trial fluid push

concerned with achieving minimal extracellular fluid volume while the nephrologist pushes for high levels of intravascular volume. This difference of opinion in fluid management is particularly obvious in the patient with heart failure and decreasing renal function in whom the cardiac failure is possibly the cause of decreased renal perfusion. In most major medical centres dialysis (peritoneal, haemodialysis, or ultrafiltration) is readily available and can be performed promptly to reverse the effect of previously administered fluid if the patient responds adversely.

Avoidance of Nephrotoxins and Procedures

Avoidance of nephrotoxic drugs and marginally necessary surgical and diagnostic procedures in the patient with renal insufficiency is obviously important and is discussed later. How vigorous should the physician be in avoiding potentially nephrotoxic drugs, radiocontrast procedures or other procedures in patients in the ICU who do not have prior renal disease or insufficiency? One must weight the risks and benefits of each individual drug or procedure. If renal function is normal, there is no pre-existing renal disease, and intravascular volume is appropriate, the potential benefit of most drugs and procedures is generally greater than the risk. Multiple physicians from different subspecialty disciplines, making isolated decisions may lead to problems. It is important that the patient in the ICU has a single physician aware of the patient's overall condition, mindful of the potential risk and benefit of drug treatment and procedures, who will consider the recommendations of other physicians involved in the case, resolve any differences of opinion and determine the course of action.

Susceptible Patients or Patients at Increased Risk of ARF

The foregoing recommendations have been suggested for all patients that enter ICUs. There are more specific preventive or prophylactic regimens for patients susceptible to ARF. There are two subgroups of "at risk" or susceptible patients to be considered. The first is that group of patients who undergo a treatment modality that specifically causes renal injury independent of other factors. Such patients are those with malignancies who undergo treatment with chemotherapeutic agents, such as methotrexate, cysplatinum or others in which there is direct toxic effect on the kidney or damage related to severe hyperuricaemia due to cell breakdown (Garnick et al. 1988). An increased flow of alkaline urine has been demonstrated to be important in preventing ARF in some of these patients (Tiller and Mudge 1980; Gonzales-Vitale et al. 1977; Hayes et al. 1977; Pitman et al. 1977). The benefits of increased urine flow, with either volume or diuretics, in preventing renal failure from other nephrotoxins, such as amphotericin B, is not clear (Olivero et al. 1975; Bullock et al. 1976). These types of patients who are not likely to be seen in the ICU, are not pertinent to the discussion, and will not be discussed further.

The other group of "at risk" patients are those more likely to have a precipitous decrease in renal function, with even a minor insult, because of underlying factors. Several studies have identified such susceptible patients (Abel et al. 1976; Rasmussen and Ibels 1982; Hou et al. 1983; Shusterman et al. 1987) and are summarized in Table 24.4. Patients with diabetes mellitus, multiple myeloma or obstructive jaundice may not be at risk in and of themselves, but when accompanied by mild renal insufficiency or volume depletion, the likelihood of ARF is substantial. Table 24.5 outlines those events which are most frequently associated with precipitation of acute tubular necrosis. The incidence of these precipitating insults causing ARF has been documented in a number of studies (Balslov and Jorgensen 1963; Swartz et al. 1978; McMurray et al. 1978; Bullock et al. 1985; Wheeler et al. 1986). Only a few of these events can be anticipated and are amenable to prophylactic treatments. In patients at increased risk and likely to encounter one of these insults, more aggressive measures of preventive treatment might be considered. First, the risk factor itself should be eliminated if possible. This is not possible with regard to the age of the patient, pre-existing renal failure, or accompanying diagnoses. However, vigorous maintenance of adequate extracellular or intravascular volume and control of blood pressure are the keystones to prevention of established renal failure in this at-risk group of patients in the ICU.

Table 24.4. Patients susceptible to acute renal failure

1.	Pre-existing decrease in renal function
2.	Decreased extracellular or intravascular volume
3.	Increased age
4.	History of significant hypertension
5.	History of diabetes mellitus with 1 and 2 above
6.	History of multiple myeloma with 1, 2 above and radiocontrast
7.	Obstructive jaundice in combination with 1 and 2 above

Table 24.5. Insults causing acute tubular necrosis

1.	Hypotension
	   Trauma and burns
	   Surgical
	   Sepsis
	   Cardiac event
	   Drugs
	   Profound and prolonged volume depletion

2.	Rhabdomyolysis with myoglobinuria or haemolysis with haemoglobinuria
3.	Nephrotoxins
4.	Sudden decrease in renal blood flow Cross-clamp of aorta or renal artery
5.	Renal artery embolus

Approach to the Patient at Increased Risk of ARF

Measurement of Renal Function

In patients with previously compromised renal function, more intensive and frequent monitoring of renal function is necessary (Table 24.6). Whereas it might not be appropriate to measure creatinine clearance in all patients in the intensive care setting, it is appropriate to consider a 4 h, 8 h or 24 h creatinine clearance or iothalomate or ytterbium clearance in patients with mild elevation of serum creatinine and urea where a more exact level of GFR would be informative. Decisions to initiate preventive therapy prior to a surgical procedure, e.g. reconstruction of the renal arteries or surgery on the aorta, are dependent on exact knowledge of renal function if the serum creatinine is between 1.2 and 2.0 mg dl^{-1} (0.1 and 0.18 mmol l^{-1}). Likewise, dosing of nephrotoxic drugs and use of radiocontrast agents are dependent on knowledge of exact renal function. If such measurements cannot be made, then assumption of the worst case scenario, i.e. assume the lowest possible GFR, for that level of serum creatinine or urea is appropriate in the prevention of ARF.

Table 24.6. Renal function evaluation for patients at increased risk of acute renal failure

1.	Careful documentation of fluid intake and output and body weight
2.	Urinalysis with sediment examination and serum and urine osmolarity
3.	Serial serum creatinine and serum urea nitrogen
4.	Renal ultrasound
5.	Creatinine clearance
6.	Iothalamate or ytterbium DTPA clearance?

Establishment and Maintenance of Extracellular or Intravascular Volume

For the most part, precipitating insults in the susceptible patients are not avoidable. As noted previously, the most important of the risk factors that one can affect is inadequate intravascular volume. In the patient with compromised renal function, volume depletion is more likely because of inability of the kidneys to concentrate urine in the face of fluid loss. In this group of patients, assurance of adequate intravascular extracellular volume is essential when they are to be exposed to radiocontrast studies, nephrotoxic drugs and potential hypotension-inducing procedures. Equally important is the avoidance of further fluid depletion during preparation for a procedure. For example, some radiological procedures require a clean bowel and the patient to be NPO prior to the procedure. This combination may well lead to volume depletion at a most inopportune time.

As indicated earlier, clinical estimation of volume status is difficult in the critically ill ICU patient. In patients at increased risk, more exact determination of intravascular volume is necessary. One is more inclined to place a central venous or pulmonary capillary wedge catheter for right and left pressure measurements. The physician faces a particular dilemma in the patient with compromised renal function in whom aggressive volume replacement is contemplated. If the patient, indeed, is in an early phase of ARF rather than experiencing prerenal azotaemia, then the vigorous fluid challenge may place the patient in pulmonary oedema. Assurance of adequate renal perfusion in the patient with heart disease and a propensity for pulmonary oedema is especially difficult. However, as mentioned earlier, the ready availability of procedures such as ultrafiltration, haemodialysis and peritoneal dialysis with which the fluid over-load can be reversed, makes this not an unreasonable approach. Willingness on the part of the nephrologist to "rescue" the patient should fluid be pushed too far, is essential in establishing an atmosphere where the major risk factor of volume depletion can be avoided.

Avoidance or Minimization of Nephrotoxicity.

There are numerous reports of nephrotoxic ARF, due to a variety of drugs. Most of these drugs are listed in Table 24.7. The mechanism of injury may be ATN, interstitial nephritis, glomerular damage, intratubular or ureteral obstruction, or by adversely affecting intrarenal haemodynamics. Many of the drugs listed have caused ARF in isolated cases and are felt to be related to idiosyncratic reactions. Some, however, such as aminoglycosides are truly nephrotoxic. Because aminoglycosides are excreted by the kidneys as well as being nephrotoxic, their use is extremely sensitive to underlying renal function. In general, avoidance of such drugs in the high-risk renal failure patient is preferable. There are many instances where aminoglycosides cannot be substituted; in such cases appropriate adjustment of the dosage level is mandatory. In patients with prior renal function compromise and volume depletion, the class of non-steroidal anti-inflammatory drugs (prostaglandin inhibitors) are much more hazardous than in the population at large.

Few physicians will recall all the drugs listed here or their route of excretion, degree of protein binding and volume distribution. Review of the pharmacological literature, in particular the route of excretion is important prior to use of a drug in patients with renal compromise. In instances where pharmacological information of potentially nephrotoxic drugs is not available, measurement of serum drug levels should be performed. In addition to the usual nephrotoxic drugs listed, patients with renal insufficiency may not tolerate vasoconstrictor or vasodilator drugs because of their potential adverse effect on blood pressure and/or renal haemodynamics.

As in patients without risk factors, avoidance of an unnecessary diagnostic and therapeutic procedure is important in decreasing the incidence of ARF. In these patients however, the risk/benefit ratio is much higher. Use of toxic contrast agents, nephrotoxic drugs or decisions about semi-elective surgery must be considered more cautiously. Often physicians not closely involved with the patient's care make decisions with regard to procedures. For instance, the decision to use a contrast agent with a CT scan may be made by the radiologist and not the physician who knows the patient and his renal function best. Sometimes patients undergo a series or combination of studies and procedures, e.g. contrast study immediately followed by vascular surgery, which is even more likely to precipitate worsening renal function. A delay between the investigative procedure and surgery, may allow time to assure maximum urinary flow and adequate intravascular volume between the procedures. If the patient's renal function is in a state of flux, particularly if it seems to be decreasing, the possibility of deferring or avoiding some therapeutic or diagnostic procedure might be considered. In patients at high risk, communication with the various physicians

Table 24.7. Drugs reported to cause alteration of renal function

Antineoplastic and/or immunosuppressive agents	*Analgesics*	*Diuretics*
Cis-platinum	Salicylates	Mannitol
Mitomycin	p-Amino salicylate	Thiazides
Methotrexate	Aminopyrine	Frusemide
Methyl CCNU	Phenacetin	Organic mercurials
Interferon	Methysergide	Chlorthalidone
Cyclosporin	Zoxazolamine	*Anaesthetic agents*
Radio-opaque contrast agents	Phenylbutazone	Chloroform
Diatrizoate meglumine	Indomethacin	Ethyl chloride
Diatrizoate sodium	Ibuprofen	Divinyl ether
Iothalamate sodium	Medofenamate	Halothane
Iopanoic acid	Metanamic acid	Fluroxene
Ipodate sodium	Diflunisal	Cyclopropane
Iodipamide	Sulindac	Methoxyflurane
Bunamiodyl sodium	Fenoprofen	*Antihypertensives*
	Naproxen	Hydralazine
	Tolmetin	Propranolol
	Piroxicam	Captopril
	Ibopamine	Nifedepine
	Zomepirac	Enalapril
	Antibiotics	
Sulphonamides	Puromycin	Gentamicin
Penicillins	Actinomycin	Tobramycin
Tetracycline	Pentamidine	Amikacin
Doxycycline	Piroxicam	Cephaloridin
Amphotericin	Bacitracin	Cephalothin
Vancomycin	Neomycin	Cephalexin
Rifampicin	Streptomycin	Acyclovir
Erythromycin	Colistin	Polymixin
Trimethaprim	Kanamycin	
	Miscellaneous	
Amphetamines	Tolbutamide	Demeclocycline
Diazepam	Urethane	Diphenylhydantoin
Amoxapine	Quinine	Allopurinol
Cimetidine	ε-Aminocaproic acid	Probenecid
Lithium	Hexadimethine br.	D-Penicillamine
Phenindione	Phenazopyridine	Gold
Trimethadione	EDTA	Dextran
Paramethadione	Methimazole	

involved with the patient's care is necessary to alter or avoid procedures important in preserving renal function. One physician must coordinate the various opinions for treatment in these patients.

Risks of Hyperalimentation in ARF

The role of hyperalimentation in ARF is controversial. Studies in the late 1960s and early 1970s suggested that intravenous hyperalimentation with amino acids not only increased patient survival but had a beneficial effect on recovery from ARF (Lee et al. 1967; Abel et al. 1973). Subsequent reviews have suggested that adequate calories and protein are important particularly in the malnourished patient with regard to survival, but a beneficial effect on renal function has not been demonstrated (Mitch and Wilmore 1988). It has been shown in experimental animals with decreased renal mass that glomerular hyperfiltration and increased glomerular pressure may be related to glomerulosclerosis and progressive renal insufficiency. These abnormalities can be affected beneficially by restriction of protein intake (Brenner et al. 1982). Studies in human subjects with ARF also suggest reduction in protein intake may have a beneficial effect on progression (Maschio et al. 1982; Rosman et al. 1984). Recent investigations on the effect of protein intake on renal function following an acute ischaemic insult in animal models has suggested that increased protein intake may not be helpful, but may in fact be detrimental (Andrews and Bates 1986; Andrews 1987; Feingold et al. 1987). Other investigators have reported intravenous amino acid administration in animal models of ischaemic ARF to cause worsening of renal function (Oken et al. 1980; Solez et al. 1982; Zager and Venkatachalam 1983). There may be a difference in response, depending on the particular amino acid used, with administration of lysine having a detrimental effect whereas administration of glycine, arginine and glutamic acid, during the course of another insult, produces no persistent functional impairment (Malis et al. 1984; Solez 1984). Others have reported in various models that glycine and glutathione (David et al. 1987; Nguyen et al. 1987) and polyaspartic acid (Bennett et al. 1987) may be protective. Many patients in ICUs now receive intravenous hyperalimentation to avoid malnutrition. It is possible that amino acid administration, if excessive, may have a detrimental effect, particularly if administered prior to an ischaemic or nephrotoxic insult. Epstein et al. (1987) have suggested that tubular cells of the medullary thick ascending limb are particularly vulnerable to anoxic damage related to increased metabolic demands. It is conceivable that increased protein intake could increase the workload of these cells requiring an increased energy expenditure, thus making an already delicate system more susceptible to injury. This is not to suggest that patients should not receive hyperalimentation with caloric and protein replacement. However, in those patients with renal compromise, the quantity and type of amino acids administered prior to a potential ischaemic insult, must be considered a factor and *excessive* protein loading should probably be avoided.

Drug Treatment

The foregoing comments concern a general approach to avoiding ARF in patients at increased risk. There are other specific treatments (i.e. drug administration) which have been suggested to prevent ARF. Many drugs have been suggested to be useful; however, it is not always clear that in the process of administering the drugs, correction of volume deficit was not part of the process and in retrospect, may have been as important as the drug effect. It is mandatory that adequate intravascular volume be established *before* institution of any of the drugs listed below. For the most part, drug treatment has been described in patients with "early" ARF. Of the drugs listed in Table 24.8, only mannitol and frusemide have been used in both animals and humans in a prophylactic or preventive manner, that is, before ischaemia or nephrotoxicity. The remainder have been used in "early" or "established" ARF. They will be discussed here in as much as they may be potentially useful if administered prior to an anticipated renal insult.

Table 24.8. Drugs used to prevent or reverse acute renal failure

Diuretics
  Mannitol
  Loop diuretics
Dopamine
Beta Blockers
Calcium channel blockers
Angiotensin I-converting enzyme inhibitors
Prostaglandins
Atrial natriuretic peptide
Thyroxine
Desferrioxamine
Papaverine
Bradykinin
Acetylcholine
Theophylline
Fructose-1,6-diphosphate
Anti-oxidants
ATP-$MgCl_2$

Diuretics

Diuretics, primarily mannitol and frusemide, have been extensively studied in animal models and in man in the treatment and prevention of ARF. The rationale for their use is outlined in Table 24.9. Previous investigators divided treatment into that intended for "early" or incipient ARF and "established" ARF (Barry and Malloy 1962; Eliahou and Bata 1965; Luke et al. 1970; Barry et al. 1961). Examination of an approach to diuretic use was further developed (Levinsky and Bernard 1988) and a third group was added consisting of patients in whom diuretic therapy was truly prophylactic. The animal studies of diuretic use in ARF have been extensively reviewed and summarized (Levinsky and Bernard 1988) (Table 24.10). I will concentrate on clinical studies and not the extensive experimental data in animals, despite the fact that the clinical studies have not been well controlled and are much smaller in number. The majority of the clinical

Table 24.9. Possible actions of diuretics in acute renal failure

1.	Mannitol has been suggested to reduce or limit cell swelling and thus decrease tubular cell injury
2.	Mannitol may cause increased extracellular volume expansion thus increase cardiac output, decrease blood viscosity and decrease systemic oncotic pressure causing increased glomerular filtration rate
3.	Mannitol and loop diuretics increase intratubular flow thus preventing obstruction
4.	Mannitol and loop diuretics may have a direct effect on smooth muscle causing vasodilatation of glomerular capillaries. They may also act by increasing prostaglandins or decreasing renin
5.	Loop diuretics may inhibit tubuloglomerular feedback thus increasing glomerular filtration rate
6.	Loop diuretics may produce an increase in cytochrome aa_3 oxidation consistent with a decrease in transport-related oxygen consumption

Table 24.10. Diuretics in experimental ARF

Model	Mannitol		Frusemide	
	Proph.[a]	Therap.	Proph.	Therap.
Prerenal[b]	+	+		−
Ischaemic[c]	+	+	+	−
Noradrenaline	+		+	+
Glycerol	+		−	−
Methaemoglobin	+	±	−	+
Mercuric chloride	+	+	±	−
Uranyl nitrate				−
Cephaloridine[d]			+	−
Amphotericin		+	+	−
Cis-platinum	+		+	
Folic acid			+	

[a] Proph., diuretic given prophylactically before induction of ARF; Therap., diuretic given at time of or after induction of ARF. +, diuretic improved renal function; −, no effect on renal function; ±, conflicting results.
[b] Prerenal, maintained partial arterial occlusion.
[c] Ischaemic, after total arterial occlusion.
[d] Cephaloridine was given alone or with other toxins.
From Levinsky and Bernard (1988).

studies were carried out in the 1960s and 1970s and several in the 1980s. I have been unable to find studies on the use of diuretics in clinical ARF since 1984. It is apparent from Table 24.11 which summarizes the reported clinical studies, that when used either prophylactically or therapeutically, in controlled or uncontrolled studies, diuretics do indeed increase urinary output. However, only a few of these studies demonstrate that diuretic therapy either protects or improves renal function. In some it was suggested that there is a decrease in the need for dialysis or a shortening of the duration of ARF. In only one study has survival been affected favourably. In the controlled studies in which diuretics were given prophylactically, an effect on the incidence of ARF is difficult to interpret because of the extremely low rate of ARF in controls. The studies of diuretic use in ARF are difficult to compare because of the different circumstances under which they were carried out, i.e. prophylactic vs therapeutic, controlled vs uncontrolled, the variety of causes of ARF, differences in doses of diuretic, differences in duration of treatment and differences in the manner in which the drug was evaluated, i.e. percentage response or a comparison of means. Some of the frusemide studies were carried out only in patients who had previously failed mannitol. Nonetheless, based on these clinical studies, and the controlled animal studies, it has been generally concluded that these agents may play a role in the protection of the patient with compromised renal function who has adequate extracellular volume, when he/she is to be subjected to an event in which renal blood flow may be compromised, e.g. repair of an aortic aneurysm or renal artery or any other procedure with a high likelihood of hypotension. Both mannitol and frusemide have been suggested to be more effective when used prophylactically in the patient with obstructive jaundice (Dawson 1965; Untura 1979) and when administered prior to radiocontrast studies (Oguagha et al. 1981; Anto et al. 1981). As mentioned earlier, some studies have suggested that diuretics may play a role if administered prior to administration of known nephrotoxins. The major

Table 24.11. Clinical studies of diuretics in ARF

Source	Study date	Drug	Treatment	Study	Cause of ARF	Results				
						Urine output	Renal function	Need for dialysis	Survival	Incidence of ARF
Baird et al. (1963)	1961	M	P	C	Vasc. surg.	↑	↑			±↓
Eliahou and Bata (1965)	1962	M	T	U	Misc.	↑				
Beall et al. (1963)	1963	M	P	C	Vasc. surg.	↑	↔			None
Smith et al. (1963)	1963	M	P	C	Vasc. surg., open heart	↑	↔			None
Glenn (1964)	1964	M	P	C	Vasc. surg., open heart	↑	↔			None
Powers et al. (1964)	1964	M	P	U	Cardio-pulm. bypass and open heart					±↓
Yeh et al. (1964)	1964	M	P, T	U	Vasc. surg. and trauma					±↓
Berman et al. (1964)	1964	M	P	U	Open heart surg.	↑				±↓
Eliahou (1964)	1964	M	P	C	CY surg. and cardio-pulm. bypass	↑	↔			↔
Etheredge et al. (1965)	1964	M	T	U	Surgery	↑				
Dawson (1965)	1965	M	P	U	Open heart	↑	↑			±↓
Kahn et al. (1965)	1965	M	P	C	Obst. jaundice and surg.	↑	↑			↓
Luke et al. (1965)	1965	M	P	C	Open heart	↑	↔			None
Scheer (1965)	1965	M	T	U	Misc. surg.	↑	↑		↔	
Luke et al. (1970)	1965	M	T	U	Misc. surg.	↑				
Fries et al. (1971)	1965	M	T	U	Misc. surg.	↑	±↑			
Barry et al. (1961)	1970	F	P	U	Misc. surg.	↑	↔		↔	
Cantarovich et al. (1971)	1971	F	T	U	Misc. surg.	↑	↔	±↓	↔	
Yeboah et al. (1972)	1971	F	T	C	Misc. surg.	↑	↑	↓	↔	
Baek et al. (1973)	1972	M, F	T	U	Open heart surg.	↑				
Kjellstrand (1972)	1972	F	P, T	U	Misc. surg.	±↑				
Stott et al. (1972)	1972	EA	T	U	Surg. and trauma	↑	↑	↓	↔	

Drug: M, mannitol; F, frusemide; EA, ethacrynic acid.
Treatment: P, preventive or prophylactic treatment; T, therapeutic.
Study: C, controlled; U, uncontrolled.
Results: ↑, increased; ↓, decreased; ↔, no effect; ±, equivocal or conclusion based on questionable data.

Table 24.11. (continued)

Source	Study date	Drug	Treatment	Study	Cause of ARF	Results				
						Urine output	Renal function	Need for dialysis	Survival	Incidence of ARF
Cantarovich et al. (1973)	1972	F	T	U	Misc. surg.	↑	↔	↓	↔	
Muth (1973)	1973	F	T	C	Misc. surg.	↔	↔	↓	↔	
Brown et al. (1973)	1973	F	T	U	Misc. surg.	↑	↔	↓	↔	
Brown et al. (1974)	1973	F	T	U	Misc. surg.	±↑	↔	±↓	↔	
Bradley et al. (1974)	1974	F	T	C	Misc. surg.	↑	↑			
Ray et al. (1974)	1974	F	T	U	Surg. and trauma	↑	↔			
Epstein et al. (1975)	1974	M, F	P, T	U	Surg.		↔		↔	↔
Chandra et al. (1975)	1975	F	T	U	Misc. surg.	↑	↔			
Minuth et al. (1976)	1975	F	T	C	Misc. surg.	↑	↑		↔	
Kleinknecht et al. (1976)	1976	F	P, T	C	Misc. surg.	±↑	↔	↓	↔	
Lucas et al. (1977)	1976	F	T	C	Misc. surg.	↑	↔	↔	↔	
Anderson et al. (1977)	1977	F	T	U	Misc. surg.	↑	↔			
Untura (1979)	1977	F	T	U	Misc. surg.	↑		↓	↓	
Nuutinen et al. (1978)	1978	M	P	C	Obst. jaundice and surg.		↑			
Valdes et al. (1979)	1978	F	P	C	Open heart surg.		↑			
Brown et al. (1981)	1979	M	T	U	Surg. and trauma	↑	↑			
Oguagha et al. (1981)	1981	F	T	C	Surg. and trauma	↑	↔	↔	↔	
Anto et al. (1981)	1981	F	P	U	Radio-contrast					↓
Fink (1982)	1981	M	T	U	Radio-contrast	↔	↑		↓	
Rigden et al. (1984)	1982	F	P						↓	
Anderson and Schrier (1987)	1984	M	P	C	Open heart surg.	↑			↔	

Drug: M, mannitol; F, frusemide; EA, ethacrynic acid.
Treatment: P, preventive or prophylactic treatment; T, therapeutic.
Study: C, controlled; U, uncontrolled.
Results: ↑, increased; ↓, decreased; ↔, no effect; ±, equivocal or conclusion based on questionable data.

point of contention in interpretation of these studies is whether the diuretics actually have an effect or whether extracellular volume was concomitantly increased and the latter was the cause of a beneficial effect. In any event, it appears reasonable that patients who are susceptible and who face risk of decreased renal blood flow, may benefit from 25 g of mannitol or 40–120 mg of frusemide intravenously prior to the procedure. There is little to suggest that, if the patient is volume repleted, these agents are harmful.

Dopamine

Dopamine has been advocated for treatment of ATN (Anderson and Schrier 1987). So-called, "renal dose" dopamine (1–3 µg kg $^{-1}$ min^{-1}) has a slight but positive effect on blood pressure; yet, causes intrarenal vasodilatation with presumed increase in urine output (Janada 1976; Pichler et al. 1976; Henderson et al. 1980; Davis et al. 1982). Some of these clinical studies suggest an improvement in renal function but suffer from the same deficiencies as the diuretic studies. Dopamine has been reported to be particularly useful in reversing early renal failure when combined with frusemide (Talley et al. 1970; Gerstner and Grunberger 1980; Lindner 1983; Graziani et al. 1984). These studies suggested an increase in urine output; however, the effect on renal function has been positive in only two of the studies (Gerstner and Grunberger 1980; Lindner 1983). In patients who are well hydrated, dopamine has rarely been effective in my experience except in those patients who are hypotensive and the positive effect of dopamine is due to increase in blood pressure. In those patients in whom dopamine has been administered and seemingly has had no effect, its continued use after the first several hours of treatment is not warranted. Dopamine has rarely been studied as a prophylactic agent. In one animal study of induced ARF, prophylactic dopamine combined with mannitol and loop diuretics cause an increase in urine output and function (Lindner et al. 1979). In another similar study, no effect on survival was noted (Mann et al. 1986). There has been only one clinical study of dopamine used to prevent renal impairment (Polson et al. 1987). In this small but controlled study, patients undergoing liver transplantation given dopamine before surgery had a significantly lower incidence of renal failure. It is conceivable that administration of dopamine prior to an insult may be more beneficial than when given after the insult. Further studies are warranted, however, before such treatment can be recommended.

Beta Blockers

The hypothesis that release of renal renin plays a role in the pathogenesis of ATN led to the use of beta blocker drugs to prevent renin release in animal models with ARF (Iaina et al. 1975; Eliahou et al. 1977; Stowe et al. 1978; Klein 1978; Orndorff et al. 1978). Other investigations suggested that beta blockers alleviated ischaemic ARF by a specific beta-adrenergic blockade effect on tubules (Iaina et al. 1980). A subsequent study utilizing several beta blockers in a pretreatment protocol, suggested that azotaemia was markedly reduced in $HgCl_2$-induced ARF (Gaal and Siklos 1982). The combination of propranolol and captopril, again in a prophylactic protocol in animal models, was shown to protect the kidney from ischaemic damage (Ishigami et al. 1985). There are no reported studies of beta blockers in human subjects with ARF used either prophylactically or after onset of ARF. These agents may well cause vasodilatation of the renal vasculature via a renin effect; however, they also cause peripheral vasodilatation and cardiac effects. Their use in critically ill patients, frequently suffering hypotension, would be difficult to envision. Whether administration intrarenally, prior to an anticipated insult, would have a positive effect is unknown. There is no evidence that patients who happen to be on beta blocker therapy for other reasons prior to admission to an ICU or prior to some catastrophic event have a lesser incidence of ARF. Maintenance of blood pressure would seem to be a more important issue than the theoretical benefit of beta blocker drug effect on renin release or tubular protection. Also, the use of beta blockade in patients with renal disease has been reported to worsen renal function (Warren et al. 1974; Snell and Wallace 1974) and to precipitate ARF when used in combination with non-steroidal anti-inflammatory drugs (James et al. 1982).

Calcium Channel Blockers

The majority of recent literature on drug treatment of ARF concerns the use of calcium channel blockers. Since 1983, multiple studies have been carried out with different animal models of ARF induced by various mechanisms (Burke and Schrier 1983; Goldfarb et al. 1983; Wait et al. 1983; Papadimitriou et al. 1983; Malis et al. 1983; Scriabine et al. 1984; Burke et al. 1984; Lee et al. 1985; Loutzenhiser et al. 1985; Wagner et al. 1986; Garthoff et al. 1987; Rose et al. 1987). In these studies, verapamil, diltiazem and nifedipine were the calcium channel blockers. Recent papers report other new calcium channel blocking agents. The drugs have been given both before and after an insult but the majority of studies have administered the drug intrarenally. All of these studies demonstrated a benefit when the drugs were given prior to induced ARF. Some of the studies have also suggested that there is benefit from calcium channel blockers when given after the insult (Burke and Schrier 1983; Wait et al. 1983; Burke et al. 1984; Lee et al. 1985; Wagner et al. 1986). Schrier et al. (1984) and Puschett (1987) have reviewed the pharmacology and protective effect of calcium channel blockers. Shrier et al. (1984) suggested that vasodilatation is, perhaps, not the primary benefit, but that calcium channel blockers protect against progression from ischaemia to cell death by reducing calcium transport and excessive calcium uptake in mitochondria. Investigators have recently used calcium channel blockers in renal transplantation models and shown benefit when the drugs are given prior to organ transplant (Shapiro et al. 1985; Agatstein et al. 1987; Eisinger et al. 1985). Two studies in human subjects demonstrated that verapamil (Duggan et al. 1985) and diltiazem (Wagner et al. 1987) led to improved urine output and renal function when administered prior to transplantation. It has been suggested that these drugs may also have a beneficial effect on cyclosporin nephrotoxicity in addition to their effect on the ischaemic component of renal failure (Iaina et al. 1986; Bunke and Wilder 1987). In addition to these few studies in renal transplant patients, there are two studies of calcium channel blockers in human ATN. In one controlled study of patients undergoing coronary arteriography, nifedipine given before the procedure was shown to exert a protective effect against radiocontrast nephrotoxicity (Pourrat and Douste-Blazy

1984). However, in this study there was only minimal change in renal function (13% increase in serum creatinine in the control group; 3% increase serum creatinine in the nifedipine group). In a second small study, patient's charts were retrospectively reviewed to determine if oral administration of calcium channel blockers prior to surgery had a beneficial effect on outcome (Hull and Hasbargen 1985). Preoperative administration of calcium channel blockers by mouth had no protective effect on renal function following surgery.

Because calcium channel blocking agents also cause a decrease in blood pressure, animal investigations have been principally using the intrarenal route to avoid peripheral systemic effects. It would seem that in the ICU setting intra-arterial administration would be the most effective approach. It is my understanding that clinical studies with intrarenal injections of calcium channel blockers in patients with "early" ARF are under way in several medical centres. Calcium channel blockers used in such a manner would seem reasonable if administered immediately after insult to the kidneys. Use of these drugs intra-arterially in a prophylactic approach is more problematic; invasion of the vascular system for intrarenal catheterization is not a minor procedure. However, administration of the drug prior to renal transplant or intrarenally immediately prior to interruption of renal blood flow during vascular surgery may be reasonable uses. One should keep in mind the possible risk of hypotension in this setting as well as isolated reports of diltiazem as a cause of ARF (TerWee et al. 1984; Shallcross et al. 1986). Although calcium channel blocker drugs seem to be potentially very useful, widespread use of these agents in ICU patients should appropriately await further studies.

Other Antihypertensive Agents

The value of vigorous treatment of malignant hypertension to reverse ARF has been debated. Although some have shown no benefit to ARF (Mattern et al. 1972), there are numerous reports of renal failure reversal with reduction of blood pressure with drug treatment (Woods and Blythe 1967; Mroczek et al. 1969; Sevitt et al. 1971; Eknoyan and Siegel 1971; Woods et al. 1974; Luft et al. 1978; Simon et al. 1979; Bennett 1979). In particular, the use of angiotensive converting enzyme inhibitors, captopril and enalapril, have been shown to be associated with reversal of renal failure in scleroderma renal crisis (Zawada et al. 1981; Barnett 1981; Chapman et al. 1986; Sorensen et al. 1983; Wasner et al. 1978; Milsom and Nicholls 1986; Rasmussen et al. 1983). Captopril and enalapril have also been reported to improve renal failure resulting from hypertension from other causes (Rasmussen et al. 1983; Mourad et al. 1985; Reams and Bauer 1986). Unfortunately, these drugs have been incriminated as *causes* of ARF, both as an idiosyncratic reaction (Luderer et al. 1981; Steinman and Silva 1983) and by adversely affecting renal haemodynamics in patients with renal vascular disease and sodium depletion (Farrow and Wilkinson 1979; Hricik et al. 1983; Fotino and Sporn 1983; Coulie et al. 1983; Hricik 1985; Brivet et al. 1985; Funck-Brentano et al. 1986; Schubiger et al. 1988). Therefore, these drugs must be used with great caution in this setting. In animal studies when given prophylactically, captopril has had mixed results. In postischaemic ARF, the drug was reported to be beneficial in reducing the severity of ARF (Scanu et al. 1987; Magnusson et al. 1983); however, in aminoglycoside-induced ARF it seemed to have little influence on the course (Luft et al. 1982). There are insufficient data at present to recommend the use of captopril or enalapril as prophylactic agents. Their use in malignant hypertension associated with renal failure is advocated as long as renal artery stenosis is not an accompanying problem and the patient is not sodium depleted. Oral clonidine has been reported to have a salutary effect on the course of mercuric chloride-induced ARF in animals (Eknoyan et al. 1983). In this study, the drug was given daily five days prior to the insult and would seem to have little practical value. No other antihypertensive agents have been described in the treatment or prevention of ARF. In summary, except in malignant hypertension and scleroderma, the use of antihypertensive agents would not seem warranted. In fact, they probably should be avoided because of the possibility of aggrevation of hypotension.

Prostaglandins

ARF may be due in part to derangements in normal prostaglandin metabolism – thromboxane overproduction and/or prostaglandin deficiency. Stoff and Clive (1986) have reviewed the literature on the pathophysiology of prostaglandins in ARF. Based on the finding that prostaglandins increase intrarenal blood flow, glomerular capillary ultrafiltration coefficient, tubular glomerular feedback and counteract vasoconstrictor hormones, many investigators suggested that they may have a beneficial effect on ARF. The role of prostaglandin in ARF is supported by animal investigators in which both intra-arterial and inravenous administration of PGE_2 (Mauk et al. 1977; Weub et al. 1978; Neumayer et al. 1985), PGE_1 (Moskowitz et al. 1975; Kaufman et al. 1987) and PGI_2 (Isenberg et al. 1981) prior to induction of various types of experimental ARF were shown to be protective. Use of the thromboxane synthesis inhibitor, imidazole, resulted in conflicting results with regard to protection of ARF (Watson et al. 1986; Papanicolaou et al. 1987). To date, there has been only one report of prostaglandins administered to humans with ARF (Vincenti and Goldberg 1978). In this study of patients with hepatorenal syndrome, administration of prostaglandin A_1 caused a decrease in arterial blood pressure. The combination of dopamine and prostaglandin A_1 maintained blood pressure, allowing larger doses of both agents to be administered. Significant improvement in renal function was not observed. There are no reports of prostaglandins being administered prior to exposure to a potential insult. On the other hand, a large number of experimental and clinical studies have indicated aggravation or precipitation of ARF by prostaglandin inhibitors (Stoff and Clive 1986). As suggested earlier, agents which interfere with or inhibit prostaglandins, i.e. the non-steroidal anti-inflammatory agents, should be avoided in patients in the ICU setting. Such drugs are positively contraindicated in those patients with modest renal insufficiency who may possibly be volume depleted.

Atrial Natriuretic Factor

Based on findings in normal animals that atrial natriuretic factor (atrial natriuretic peptide, atrial peptin III, ANF) reverses the action of vasoconstrictors and produces vasodilatation and increases glomerular filtration rate, this agent has been examined in animals with experimental ARF. In a variety of animal models including noradrenaline, glycerol, cyclosporin and gentamicin-induced ARF as well as ischaemic and hypotensive haemorrhage models, ANF was shown to reduce the incidence and severity of ARF (Schafferhans et al. 1986a,b, 1987; Heidbreder et al. 1986; Capasso et al. 1987a,b; Nakamoto et al. 1987; Shaw et al. 1987; Yasmineh et al. 1987; Neumayer et al. 1987). ANF was administered intrarenally and intravenously after an insult in most studies but in two investigations it was given prior to the insult (Schafferhans et al. 1986a,b, 1987). In all these studies, ANF was shown to ameliorate the frequency and degree of ARF. To date, use of ANF has not been reported in human subjects either before or after hypotensive ATN or exposure to nephrotoxins. Based on the animal data, there seems to be a role for intrarenal administration of ANF in ARF patients. Depending on the results in such studies, its use prior to a procedure in a prophylactic manner may also be indicated.

Thyroxine

Considering the fact that thyroxine increases energy turnover in most tissues, one would assume that increased thyroxine would be detrimental in the energy-susceptible thick ascending limb. However, based on investigations in animal studies suggesting that thyroxine was helpful in reducing the severity of ARF, Straub (1976) reported the use of oral thyroxine in paediatric patients with early ARF and noted a diuresis with prompt normalization of renal function. In subsequent studies in mercuric chloride-induced ATN in rats, thyroxine was demonstrated to act, not through a systemic effect but locally by accelerated reversal of an ATPase enzymatic defect (Schulte-Wissermann et al. 1977). Investigators from other centres indicated that administration of thyroxine resulted in enhanced recovery from acute toxic renal insults due to potassium dichromate injury and gentamicin nephrotoxicity (Siegel et al. 1984; Cronin and Newman 1985; Cronin et al. 1986, 1987; Mills et al. 1987) again by reversing an enzymatic abnormality, increasing Na,K-ATPase activity. Other than the initial study by Straub, thyroxine has not been used in patients with ARF and, in particular, has not been administered to patients prophylactically.

Desferrioxamine

The hydroxyl radical (OH^-) resulting from ischaemia is thought to be a major factor in tubular cell death. It has been suggested that chelation of the metal catalyst (Fe^{3+}) might be helpful in reducing hydroxyl radical formation. In an antiglomerular basement membrane animal model, desferrioxamine was administered in the acute phase of glomerular injury, to prevent neutrophil dependent immune renal injury, by interfering with neutrophil function through chelation of the hydroxyl radical (Boyce and Holdsworth 1986). The hydroxyl radical scavenger dimethylthiourea was also used in this study. Both of these drugs were shown to cause significant attenuation of renal injury. Desferrioxamine has also been used to reduce ischaemic cardiac injury based on the concept of iron chelation in the prevention of hydroxyl radical formation (Menasche et al. 1987). In the recent meetings of the American Society of Nephrology, two abstracts described the use of desferrioxamine and dimethylthiourea in ARF animal models. In a glycerol-injected model with myoglobinuria and haemoglobinuria, desferrioxamine was shown to prevent renal injury (Paller 1987). In the other study, both desferrioxamine and dimethylthiourea showed a beneficial effect in glycerol-induced ARF (Walker and Shah 1987). These drugs have not been used in human subjects, either before or at the time of renal injury. Desferrioxamine when given intravenously may cause hypotension. In addition, it has been reported as a cause of ARF in one case report (Batey et al. 1979). Thus, its use as a therapeutic agent demands further animal investigations. Because of the presumed method of action, hydroxyl ion chelation, it would seem not to be suited for prophylactic use.

Miscellaneous Agents

There have been isolated reports of other substances used in the treatment or prevention of ARF in animal models. Papaverine administered to experimental animals has been shown to increase diuresis and reduce the severity of ARF (Valido et al. 1977). Bradykinin and secretin, two renal vasodilators, were studied in a noradrenaline-induced ARF model. Bradykinin and secretin both increased renal blood flow; however, only bradykinin increased urine flow and solute excretion (Patak et al. 1979). In a subsequent study, bradykinin had no effect in an occlusive renal artery ischaemic model (Lewis et al. 1984). In 10 patients with nephrotoxicity acetylcholine was shown to cause a marked increase in cortical renal blood flow as measured by xenon-washout. However, no other beneficial effects were noted (Ladeforged 1977). In a noradrenaline-induced animal model, acetylcholine was found to increase renal blood flow but not improve inulin clearance because of persistence of intratubular deposits or obstruction (Conger et al. 1981). Based on the hypothesis that adenosine-mediated haemodynamic changes play a role in ischaemia-induced ARF, theophylline has been used in postischaemic animal models. In these studies, pretreatment with relatively high doses of intravenous theophylline, which acts as an adenosine receptor antagonist, has been shown to protect against a reduction in inulin clearance (Lin et al. 1986, 1988). Fructose-1,6-diphosphate has been used in experimental ischaemia and shock on the basis that it augments anaerobic carbohydrate utilization in ischaemic and hypoperfused tissue by restoring activity of glycolysis and by intervening in the Embden–Meyerhoff pathway, both as a metabolic regulator and a high energy substrate. This agent has been used in various models of hypoperfusion and ischaemia and has been shown to be protective of various organ systems (Markov et al. 1980; Webb 1985; Markov 1986). In one study of rats subjected to 30 minutes of renal artery occlusion, pretreatment with fructose-1,6-diphosphate protected inulin clearance and solute excretion rates (Didlake et al. 1985). There is one study describing the use of probucal, an antioxidant, in an ischaemic animal model. Improvement in single nephron GFR after antioxidant therapy was thought to be related to prevention of a decrease in plasma flow (Bird et al. 1987). The role of adenine nucleotide ATP-$MgCl_2$ in the treatment of acute renal failure has been extensively reviewed (Siegel and Gaudio 1988). All investigations with ATP-$MgCl_2$ have examined its use only as an agent for reversing injury.

In only one of the above studies of miscellaneous agents has the drug been used in human subjects. There are few data to support their use as clinical agents at the present time. Detrimental systemic effects due to hypotension are a major concern with most of these drugs. All may have some role to play, however, and further research is warranted. None of these agents can be advocated for clinical use as a prophylactic agent.

It seems that the most effective route of administration of drugs in the treatment of ARF would be directly into the renal artery to avoid systemic effects. In these critically ill patients in ICUs, however, invasion of the arterial vasculature to place a renal artery catheter is no small issue. Problems of vascular complications and sepsis together with unanticipated side effects of the drug, even though administered in small amounts and directed to the kidneys, must be considered. If ARF has been detected which is not related to prerenal or postrenal causes the benefit of reversal of ATN may be significant and worth the risks. Selection of patients who would undergo prophylactic intra-arterial infusion is a much more difficult decision. Such a decision and action will probably occur in the operating room and not in the ICU.

References

Abel RM, Beck CH Jr, Abbott WM, Ryan JA Jr, Barnett GO, Fischer JE (1973) Improved survival from acute renal failure after treatment with intravenous essential L-amino acids and glucose. Results of a prospective double-blind study. N Engl J Med 288: 695–699

Abel RM, Buckley MJ, Austen WG et al. (1976) Etiology, incidence, and prognosis of renal failure following cardiac operations. Results of a prospective analysis of 500 consecutive patients. J Thorac Cardiovasc Surg 71: 323–333

Agatstein EH, Farrer JH, Kaplan LM, Randazzo RF, Glassock RJ, Kaufman JJ (1987) The effect of verapamil in reducing the severity of acute tubular necrosis in canine renal autotransplants. Transplantation 44: 355–357

Anderson RJ, Schrier LW (1987) Acute renal failure. In: Braunwald E, Isselbacher KJ, Petersdorf RG, Wilson JD, Martin JB, Fauci AS (eds) Harrison's principles of internal medicine, 11th edn. McGraw-Hill, New York, p 1154

Anderson RJ, Linas SL, Berns AS et al. (1977) Nonoliguric acute renal failure. N Eng J Med 296: 1134–1138

Andreucci VE (1984) Prevention of ischemic/toxic acute renal failure in humans. In: Andreucci VE (ed) Acute renal failure: pathophysiology, prevention and treatment. Martinus Nijhoff, Boston, pp 119–143

Andrews PM (1987) Pathophysiology of acute renal failure and toxic nephropathy. Dietary protein restriction prior to renal ischemia can reduce postischemic uremic symptoms and cellular injury during ischemia. Am Soc Nephrology 20th Annual Meeting, p 205A (abstr)

Andrews PM, Bates SB (1986) Dietary protein prior to renal ischemia dramatically affects postischemic kidney function. Kidney Int 30: 299–303

Anto HR, Chou SY, Porush JG, Shapiro WB (1981) Infusion intravenous pyelography and renal function: Effects of hypertonic mannitol in patients with chronic renal insufficiency. Arch Intern Med 141: 1652–1656

Baek SM, Brown RS, Shoemaker WC (1973) Early prediction of acute renal failure and recovery: II. Renal function response to furosemide. Ann Surg 178: 605–608

Baird RJ, Firor WB, Barr HWK (1963) Protection of renal function during surgery of the abdominal aorta. Can Med Assoc J 89: 705–708

Balslov JT, Jorgensen HE (1963) Clinical studies: A survey of 499 patients with acute anuric renal insufficiency. Am J Med 34: 753–764

Barnett AJ (1981) Medical treatment of hypertension and renal failure in scleroderma. Aust NZ J Med 11: 411–415
Barry KG, Malloy JP (1962) Oliguric renal failure. JAMA 179: 510–513
Barry KG, Cohen A, Knochel JP, Whelan TJ, Beigel WR, Vargasch, LeBlanc PC (1961) Mannitol infusion II. The prevention of acute functional renal failure during resection of an aneurysm of the abdominal aorta. N Engl J Med 264: 967–972
Batey R, Scott J, Jain S, Sherlock S (1979) Acute renal insufficiency occurring during intravenous desferrioxamine therapy. Scand J Haematol 22: 277–279
Beall AC Jr, Holman MR, Moirris GC, DeBakey ME (1963) Mannitol-induced osmotic diuresis during vascular surgery. Arch Surg 86: 34–42
Bennett C (1979) The syndrome of malignant or accelerated hypertension. Cardiovasc Med 4: 1141–1161
Bennett WM, Wood CA, Kohlhepp SJ, Kohnen PW, Houghton DC, Gilbert DN (1987) Experimental gentamicin nephrotoxicity can be prevented by polyaspartic acid. Am Soc Nephrology p 206A
Berman LM, Smith LL, Chisholm GD, Weston RE (1964) Mannitol and renal function in cardiovascular surgery. Arch Surg 88: 239–243
Bird JE, Peterson OW, Blantz RC (1987) Early glomerular hemodynamic changes after ischemia and reflow: effect of antioxidant therapy. Am Soc Nephrology, p 206A
Boyce NW, Holdsworth SR (1986) Hydroxyl radical mediation of immune renal injury by desferrioxamine. Kidney Int 30: 813
Bradley VE, Shier MR, Lucas CE, Rosenberg IK (1974) Renal response to furosemide in critically ill patients. Surg Forum 25: 23–24
Brenner BM, Meyer TW, Hostetter TH (1982) Dietary protein intake and the progressive nature of kidney disease: The role of hemodynamically mediated glomerular injury in the pathogenesis of progressive glomerular sclerosis in aging, renal ablation, and intrinsic renal disease. N Engl J Med 307: 652–659
Brenner BM, Hostetter TH, Hebert SC (1987) Disturbances of renal function. In: Braunwald E, Isselbacher KJ, Petersdorf RG, Wilson JD, Martin JB, Fauci AS (eds) Harrison's principles of internal medicine. McGraw-Hill, New York
Brezis M, Rosen S, Epstein FH (1986) Acute renal failure. In: Brenner BM, Rector FC Jr (eds) The kidney, 3rd edn. WB Saunders, Philadelphia, pp 735–799
Brivet F, Roulot D, Poitrine A, Dormont J (1985) Reversible acute renal failure during enalapril treatment in a patient with chronic glomerulonephritis without renal artery stenosis. Lancet I: 1512
Brown CB, Cameron JS, Ogg CS, Bewick M, Stoff RB (1973) Established acute renal failure following surgical operations. In: Proceedings Acute Renal Failure Conference, DHEW Publication No. (NIH)74-608, Superintendent of Documents, US Government Printing Office Washington, p 187
Brown CB, Ogg CS, Cameron JS, Bewick M (1974) High-dose furosemide in acute reversible intrinsic renal failure. Scott Med J 19: 35–39
Brown CB, Ogg CS, Cameron JS (1981) High dose furosemide in acute renal failure: a controlled trial. Clin Nephrol 15: 90–96
Bullock WE, Luke RG, Nuttall CE, Bhathena D (1976) Can mannitol reduce amphoteracin B nephrotoxicity?: Double blind study and description of a new vascular lesion in kidneys. Antimicrob Agents Chemother 10: 555–563
Bullock WE, Umen AJ, Finkelstein M, Keane WF (1985) The assessment of risk factors in 462 patients with acute renal failure. Am J Kidney Dis 5: 97–103
Bunke M, Wilder L (1987) Effect of varapamil on glomerular prostaglandin production and glomerular filtration rate during cyclosporine administration. Am Soc Nephrology, p 208A
Burke TJ, Schrier RW (1983) Ischemic acute renal failure – pathogenetic steps leading to acute tubular necrosis. Circ Shock 11: 255–259
Burke TJ, Arnold PE, Gordon JA, Bulger RE, Dobyan DC, Schrier RW (1984) Protective effect of intrarenal calcium membrane blockers before or after renal ischemia. Functional, morphological, and mitochondrial studies. J Clin Invest 74: 1830–1841
Cantarovich F, Fernandez JC, Locatelli A, PerezLoredo J (1971) Furosemide in high doses in the treatment of acute renal failure. Postgrad Med J (Suppl) 47: 13–17
Cantarovich F, Galli C, Benedetti L et al. (1973) High-dose furosemide in established acute renal failure. Br Med J iv: 449–450
Capasso G, Anastasio P, Giordano D, Albarano L, DeSoto NG (1987a) Beneficial effects of atrial natriuretic factor on cisplatin-induced acute renal failure in the rat. Am J Nephrol 7: 228–234
Capasso G, Rosati C, Giordano DR, DeSanto NG (1987b) The protective effect of atrial natriuretic factor on cyclosporin nephrotoxicity. Am Soc Nephrology, p 209A

Chandra M, Agarwal SS, Mitra MK, Tandon NN, Gupta NN (1975) Some observations in the management of acute renal failure by massive intravenous frusemide therapy. J Assoc Physicians India 23: 415–422

Chapman PJ, Pascoe MD, van Zyl-Smit R (1986) Successful use of captopril in the treatment of "scleroderma renal crisis". Clin Nephrol 26: 106·108

Conger JD, Robinette JB, Guggenheim SJ (1981) Effect of acetylcholine on the early phase of reversible norepinephrine-induced acute renal failure. Kidney Int 19: 399–409

Coulie P, DePlaen JF, van Ypersele de Strikou C (1983) Captopril-induced acute reversible renal failure. Nephron 35: 108–111

Cronin RE, Newman JA (1985) Protective effect of thyroxine but not parathyroidectomy on gentamicin nephrotoxicity. Am J Physiol 248(3 Pt 2): F332–F339

Cronin RE, Brown DM, Simonsen R (1986) Protection by thyroxine in nephrotoxic acute renal failure. Am J Physiol 251(3 Pt 2): F408–F416

Cronin RE, Inman L, Spindler M (1987) Effect of thyroid hormone (T_4) on rate proximal tubular lysosomal volume after gentamicin. Am Soc Nephrology, p 209A

David JA, Abarzua M, Rajan T, Weinberg JM (1987) Glycine protects proximal tubules from injury by a variety of metabolic inhibitors. Am Soc Nephrology, p 210A

Davis RF, Lappas AG, Kirklin JK, Buckley MJ, Lowenstein E (1982) Acute oliguria after cardiopulmonary bypass: renal improvement with low dose dopamine infusion. Crit Care Med 10: 852–856

Dawson JL (1965) Postoperative renal function in obstructive jaundice: Effect of mannitol diuresis. Br Med J i: 82–86

Didlake R, Kirchner KA, Lewin J, Bower JD, Markov A (1985) Protection from ischemic renal injury by fructose-1-1,diphosphate infusion in the rat. Circ Shock 16: 205–212

Duggan KA, Macdonald GJ, Charlesworth JA, Pussell BA (1985) Verapamil prevents post-transplant oliguric renal failure. Clin Nehphrol 24: 289–291

Eisinger DR, Suranyi MG, Bracs P, Farnsworth A, Sheil AG (1985) Effects of verapamil in the prevention of warm ischaemia induced acute renal failure in dogs. Aust NZ J Surg 55: 391–396

Eknoyan G, Siegel MB (1971) Recovery from anuria due to malignant hypertension. JAMA 215: 1122–1125

Eknoyan G, Dobvan DC, Senekjian HO, Bulger RE (1983) Protective effect of oral clonidine in the prophylaxis and therapy of mercuric chloride-induced acute renal failure in the rat. J Lab Clin Med 102: 699–703

Eliahou HE (1964) Mannitol therapy in oliguria of acute onset. Br Med J i: 807–809

Eliahou HE, Bata A (1965) The diagnosis of acute renal failure. Nephron 2: 287–295

Eliahou HE, Iaina A, Solomon S, Gavendo S (1977) Alleviation of anoxic experimental acute renal failure in rats by beta-adrenergic blockade. Nephron 19: 158–166

Epstein M, Schneider NS, Befeler B (1975) Effect of intrarenal furosemide on renal function and intrarenal hemodynamics in acute renal failure. Am J Med 58: 510–516

Epstein FH, Brezis M, Silva P, Rosen S (1987) Physiological and clinical implications of medullary hypoxia. Artif Organs 11: 463–467

Etheredge EE, Levitan H, Nakamura K, Glenn WL (1965) Effect of mannitol on renal function during open-heart surgery. Ann Surg 161: 53–62

Farrow PR, Wilkinson R (1979) Reversible renal failure during treatment with captopril. Br Med J i: 1680

Feingold R, Weizman H, Winston J, Safirstein R (1987) Dietary protein intake affects the renal response to cyclosporine in uninephrectomized rats. Am Soc Nephrology, p 210A

Fink M (1982) Are diuretics useful in the treatment or prevention of acute renal failure? South Med J 75: 329–334

Fotino S, Sporn P (1983) Nonoliguric acute renal failure after captopril therapy. Arch Intern Med 143: 1252–1253

Fries D, Pozet N, Dubois N, Traeger J (1971) The use of large doses of furosemide in acute renal failure. Postgrad Med J 47: 18–20

Funck-Brentano C, Chatellier G, Alexandre JM (1986) Reversible renal failure after combined treatment with enalapril and frusemide in patient with congestive heart failure. Br Heart J 55: 596–598

Gaal K, Siklos J (1982) Effect of beta-receptor antagonists on $HgCl_2$-induced acute renal failure in rats. Renal Physiol 5: 245–255

Garnick MB, Mayer RJ, Abelson HT (1988) Acute renal failure associated with cancer treatment. In: Brenner BM, Lazarus JM (eds) Acute renal failure, 2nd edn. Churchill Livingstone, New York, pp 621–657

Garthoff B, Hirth C, Federmann A, Kazda S, Stasch JP (1987) Renal effects of 1.4-dihydropyridines in animal models of hypertension and renal failure. J Cardiovasc Pharmacol 9: Suppl 1: S8–S13

Gerstner G, Grunberger W (1980) Dopamine treatment for prevention of renal failure in patients with severe eclampsia. Clin Exp Obstet Gynecol 7: 219–222

Glenn WWL, Stansel HC, Hume M, Nakamura K (1964) Clinical experience with prolonged cardiopulmonary bypass. Circulation (suppl. 1) 29: 54–58

Goldfarb D, Iaina A, Serban I, Davendo S, Kapuler S, Elihous HE (1983) Beneficial effect of verapamil in ischemic acute renal failure in the rat. Proc Soc Exp Biol Med 172: 389–392

Gonzales-Vitale JC, Hayes DM, Cvitkovic E et al. (1977) The renal pathology in clinical trials of cis-platinum (II) diamminedichloride. Cancer 39: 1362–1371

Graziani G, Cantaluppi A, Casati S et al. (1984) Dopamine and frusemide in oliguric acute renal failure. Nephron 37: 39–42

Hayes DM, Cvitkovic E, Golbey RB et al. (1977) High dose cis-platinum diamminedichloride amelioration of renal toxicity by mannitol diuresis. Cancer 39: 1372–1381

Heidbreder E, Schafferhans K, Schramm D, Gotz R, Heidland A (1986) Toxic renal failure in the rat: Beneficial effects of atrial natriuretic factor. Klin Wochenschr 64:Suppl 6: 78–82

Henderson IS, Beattie TJ, Kennedy AC (1980) Dopamine hydrochloride in oliguric states. Lancet II: 827–828

Hou SH, Bushinsky DA, Wish JB, Cohen JJ, Harrington JT (1983) Hospital-acquired renal insufficiency: A prospective study. Am J Med 74: 243–244

Hricik DE (1985) Captopril-induced renal insufficiency and the role of sodium balance. Ann Intern Med 103: 222–223

Hricik DE, Browning PJ, Kopelman R, Goorno WE, Madia NE, Dzau VJ (1983) Captopril-induced functional renal insufficiency in patients with bilateral renal-artery stenoses or renal-artery stenosis in a solitary kidney. N Engl J Med 308: 373–376

Hull RW, Hasbargen JA (1985) No clinical evidence for protective effects of calcium-channel blockers against acute renal failure. N Engl J Med 313: 1477–1478

Iaina A, Solomon S, Eliahou HE (1975) Reduction in severity of acute renal failure in rats by beta-adrenergic blockade. Lancet II: 157–159

Iaina I, Serban I, Gavendo S, Kapuler SS, Elihous HE (1980) Alleviation of ischaemic acute renal failure by beta blockers: specific tubular receptor blockade or membrane stabilising effect? Proc Eur Dial Transplant Assoc Eur Ren Assoc 17: 686–689

Iaina A, Herzog D, Cohen D et al. (1986) Calcium entry-blockade with verapamil in cyclosporine A plus ischemia induced acute renal failure in rats. Clin Nephrol 25:Suppl 1, S168–S170

Isenberg GA, Hasday K, Oh J et al. (1981) Prevention of ischemic acute tubular necrosis with tris buffer or prostacyclin infusion. Mt Sinai J Med 48: 142–145

Ishigami M, Maeda T, Yabuki S, Stowe NT (1985) The effects of d-propranolol and captopril on post-ischaemic acute renal failure in rats. Proc Eur Dial Transplant Assoc Eur Ren Assoc 21: 843–848

James DW, Cleland LG, Robinson CW, Leoneilo PP (1982) Reversible renal failure associated with a beta-adrenergic receptor blocking drug and non-steroidal anti-inflammatory drugs. Med J Aust 1: 232–235

Janada A (1976) Dopamine therapy for acute postoperative renal failure. Prakt Anaesth 11: 33–38

Kahn DR, Cerny JC, Lee RWS, Sloan H (1965) The effect of dextran and mannitol on renal function during open-heart surgery. Surgery 57: 676–679

Kaufman RP Jr, Anner H, Kobzik L et al. (1987) Vasodilator prostaglandins (PG) prevent renal damage after ischemia. Ann Surg 205: 195–198

Kjellstrand CM (1972) Ethacrynic acid in acute tubular necrosis. Indications and effect on the natural course. Nephron 9: 337–348

Klein LA (1978) Propanolol protection in acute renal failure. Invest Urol 15: 401

Kleinknecht D, Ganeval D, Gonzalez-Duque LA, Fermanian J (1976) Furosemide in acute oliguric renal failure: A controlled trial. Nephron 17: 51–58

Ladeforged J (1977) Increase in renal blood flow in acute renal failure following intra-arterial infusion of acetylcholine. Scand J Clin Lab Invest 37: 709–716

Lee HA, Sharpstone P, Ames AC (1967) Parenteral nutrition in renal failure. Postgrad Med J 43: 81–91

Lee SM, Hillman BJ, Clark RL, Michael UF (1985) The effects of diltiazem and captopril on glycerol-induced acute renal failure in the rat. Functional, pathologic, and microangiographic studies. Invest Radiol 20:961–970

Levinsky NG, Bernard DB (1988) Mannitol and loop diuretics in acute renal failure. In: Brenner BM, Lazarus JM (eds) Acute renal failure, 2nd edn. Churchill Livingstone, New York, pp 841–856

Lewis RM, Rice JH, Patton MK et al. (1984) Renal ischemic injury in the dog: characterization and effect of various pharmacologic agents. J Lab Clin Med 104: 470–479

Lin JJ, Churchill PC, Bidani AK (1986) Effect of theophylline on the initiation phase of postischemic acute renal failure in rats. J Lab Clin Med 108: 150–154

Lin JJ, Churchill PC, Bidani AK (1988) Theophylline in rats during maintenance phase of postischemic acute renal failure. Kidney Int 33: 24–28

Lindner A (1983) Synergism of dopamine and furosemide in diuretic-resistant, oliguric acute renal failure. Nephron 33: 121–126

Lindner A, Cutler RE, Goodman G (1979) Synergism of dopamine plus furosemide in preventing acute renal failure in the dog. Kidney Int 16: 158–166

Loutzenhiser R, Epstein M, Horton C (1985) Reversal by the calcium antagonist nisoldipine of norepinephrine induced reduction of GFR: evidence for preferential antagonism of preglomerular vasoconstrictor. J Pharmacol Exp Ther 232: 382–387

Lucas CE, Zito JG, Carter KM, Cortez A, Stebner FC (1977) Questionable value of furosemide in preventing renal failure. Surgery 82: 314–320

Luderer JR, Schoolwerth AC, Sinicrope RA, Ballard JO, Lookingbill DP, Hayes AH (1981) Acute renal failure, hemolytic anemia and skin rash associated with captopril therapy. Am J Med 71: 493–495

Luft FC, Bloch R, Szwed JJ, Grim CM, Crim CE (1978) Minoxidil treatment of malignant hypertension. JAMA 240: 1985–1987

Luft FC, Aronoff GR, Evan AP, Connors BA, Weinberger MH, Kleit SA (1982) The renin-angiotensin system in aminoglycoside-induced acute renal failure. J Pharmacol Exp Ther 220: 433–439

Luke RG, Kennedy AC (1967) Prevention and early management of acute renal failure. Postgrad Med J 43: 280–289

Luke RG, Linton AL, Briggs JD, Kennedy AC (1965) Mannitol therapy in acute renal failure. Lancet I: 980–982

Luke RG, Briggs JD, Allison MEM, Kennedy AC (1970) Factors determining response to mannitol in acute renal failure. Am J Med Sci 259: 168–174

Magnusson MO, Rybka SJ, Stowe NT, Straffon RA (1983) Enhancement of recovery in postischemic acute renal failure with captopril. Kidney Int 24: S324–S326

Malis CD, Cheung JY, Leaf A, Bonventi JV (1983) Effects of verapamil in models of ischemic acute renal failure in the rat. Am J Physiol 245: F735–F742

Malis CD, Racusen LC, Solez K, Welton A (1984) Nephrotoxicity of lysine and of a single dose of aminoglycoside in lysine-treated rats. J Lab Clin Med 103: 660–676

Mandal AK, Lightfoot BO, Treat RE (1983) Mechanisms of protection in acute renal failure. Circ Shock 11: 245–253

Mann HJ, Fuhs DW, Hemstrom CA (1986) Acute renal failure. Drug Intell Clin Pharm 20: 421–438

Markov AK (1986) Hemodynamics and metabolic effects of fructose 1-6 diphosphate in ischemia and shock – experimental and clinical observations. Ann Intern Med 15: 1470–1477

Markov AK, Oglethorpe NC, Blake TM, Lehan PH, Hellems HK (1980) Hemodynamic, electrocardiographic and metabolic effects of fructose diphosphate on acute myocardial ischemia. Am Heart J 100: 639–646

Maschio G, Oldrizzi L, Tessitore N et al. (1982) Effects of dietary protein and phosphorus restriction on the progression of early renal failure. Kidney Int 22: 371–376

Mattern WD, Sommers SC, Kassirer JP (1972) Oliguric acute renal failure in malignant hypertension. Am J Med 52: 187–197

Mauk RA, Patak RV, Fadem SZ, Lifschmitz MD, Stein JH (1977) Studies on the effect of prostaglandin E administration in a nephrotoxic and a vasoconstrictor model of acute renal failure. Kidney Int 12: 122–130

McMurray SD, Luft FC, Maxwell DR, Hamberger RJ, Futty D, Szwed JJ, Lavelle KJ, Kleit SA (1978) Prevailing patterns and predictor variables in patients with acute tubular necrosis. Arch Intern Med 138: 950–955

Menasche P, Grousset C, Gauduel Y, Mouas C, Piwnica A (1987) Prevention of hydroxyl radical formation: a critical concept for improving cardioplegia. Protective effects of deferoxamine. Circulation 76: V180–185

Mills S, Shapiro J, Shanley P, Johnson G, Chan L (1987) The effect of L-thyroxine (T_4) on renal function and medullary thick ascending limb (TAL) morphology in the isolated kidney. Am Soc Nephrology, p 215A

Milsom SR, Nicholls MG (1986) Successful treatment of scleroderma renal crisis with enalapril. Postgrad Med J 62: 1059–1060

Minuth AN, Terrell JB Jr, Suki WN (1976) Acute renal failure: a study of the course and prognosis of 104 patients and of the role of furosemide. Am J Med Sci 271: 317–324

Mitch WE, Wilmore DW (1988) Nutritional consideration in the treatment of acute renal failure. In: Brenner BM, Lazarus JM (eds) Acute renal failure, 2nd edn. Churchill Livingstone, New York, pp 743–766

Moskowitz PS, Korobkin M, Rambo ON (1975) Diuresis and improved renal hemodynamics produced by prostaglandin E_1 in the dog with norepinephrine-induced acute renal failure. Invest Radiol 10: 284–299

Mourad G, Mimran A, Mion CM (1985) Recovery of renal function in patients with accelerated malignant nephrosclerosis on maintenance dialysis with management of blood pressure by captopril. Nephron 41: 166–169

Mroczek WJ, Davidov M, Gavrilovich L, Finnerty FA Jr (1969) The value of aggressive therapy in the hypertensive patient with azotemia. Circulation 40: 893–904

Muth RG (1973) Furosemide in acute renal failure. In: Proceedings Acute Renal Failure Conference, DHEW Publication No. (NIH)74-608, Superintendent of Documents, US Government Printing Office Washington, p 245

Nakamoto M, Shapiro JI, Shanley PF, Chan L, Schrier RW (1987) In vitro and in vivo protective effect of atriopeptin III on ischemic acute renal failure. J Clin Invest 80: 698–705

Neumayer HH, Wagner K, Groll J et al. (1985) Beneficial effects of long-term prostaglandin E_2 infusion on the course of postischemic acute renal failure. Long-term studies in chronically instrumented conscious dogs. Renal Physiol 8: 159–168

Neumayer HH, Seher-Thos U, Blossei M, Wagner K (1987) Effect of human atrial natriuretic factor (ANF) on postischemic acute failure in conscious dogs. Am Soc Nephrology, p 216A

Nguyen VD, Messana JM, Cieslinski DA, Humes HD (1987) Effect of glutathione depletion on hypoxia-induced injury to rabbit renal proximal tubule segments. Am Soc Nephrology, p 216A

Nuutinen LS, Kairaluoma M, Tuononen S, Larmi TKI (1978) The effect of furosemide on renal function in open heart surgery. J Cardiovasc Surg 19: 471–479

Oguagha C, Porush JG, Chou SY et al. (1981) Prevention of acute renal failure following infusion intravenous pyelography in patients with chronic renal insufficiency by furosemide. In: Proceedings of the Eighth International Congress on Nephrology, p 290

Oken DE, Sprinkler FM, Kirschbaum BB, Landwehr DM (1980) Amino acid therapy in the treatment of experimental acute renal failure in the rat. Kidney Int 17: 14–23

Olivero JJ, Lozano-Mendez J, Ghafary EM, Knoyan E, Suki WN (1975) Mitigation of amphoteracin B nephrotoxicity by mannitol. Br Med J i: 550–551

Orndorff MH, Hathaway S, Solomon S, Iaina D, Elihous HE (1978) B-blocking agents in acute renal failure. Proc West Pharmacol Soc 21: 209–213

Paller MS (1987) Protective effect of deferoxamine in glycerol-induced acute renal failure in the rat. Am Soc Nephrology, p 216A

Papadimitriou M, Alexopoulos E, Vargemezis V, Sakellariou G, Kosmidou I, Metasas P (1983) The effect of preventive administration of verapamil on acute ischaemic renal failure in dogs. Proc Eur Dial Transplant Assoc 20: 650–655

Papanicolaou N, Hatziantoniou C, Dontas A et al. (1987) Is thromboxane a potent antinatriuretic factor and is it involved in the development of acute renal failure? Nephron 45: 277–282

Patak RV, Fadem SZ, Lifschitz MD, Stein JH (1979) Study of factors which modify the development of norepinephrine-induced acute renal failure in the dog. Kidney Int 15: 227–237

Pichler M, Kleinberger G, Kotzaurek R, Pall H, Seeless S (1976) Clinical results with dopamine in acute renal failure. Wien Klin Wochenschr 88: 72–74

Pitman SW, Miller D, Weichaelbaum R et al. (1977) Weekly high dose methotraxate with leukovor in rescue as initial adjuvant therapy in advanced squamous cell carcinoma of the head and neck. In: Salmon SE, Jones JE (eds) Adjuvant therapy and cancer. North Holland Publishing Co, Amsterdam, p 467

Polson RJ, Park GR, Lindop MJ, Farman JV, Calne RY, Williams R (1987) The prevention of renal impairment in patients undergoing orthotopic liver grafting by infusion of low dose dopamine. Anaesthesia 42: 15–19

Pourrat JP, Douste-Blazy P (1984) Renal side effect of nifedipine. Clin Cardiol 7: 29–30

Powers SR, Boba A, Hostnik W, Stein A (1964) Prevention of postoperative acute renal failure with mannitol in 100 cases. Surgery 55: 15–23

Puschett JB (1985) Non-dialytic therapy of acute renal failure: a review. Int J Artif Organs 8: 249–256

Puschett JB (1987) Do calcium channel blockers protect against renal ischemia? Am J Nephrol 7(Suppl 1): 49–56

Rasmussen HH, Ibels LS (1982) Acute renal failure. Multivariate analysis of causes and risk factors. Am J Med 73: 211–218

Rasmussen S, Brahm M, Nielsen MD, Geise J, Larsen S, Brun C (1983) Postpartum renal failure and malignant hypertension treated with captopril. Scand J Urol Nephrol 17: 209–212

Ray JF, Winemiller RH, Parker JP, Myers WO, Wenzel FJ, Sautter RD (1974) Postoperative renal failure in the 1970's. A continuing challenge. Arch Surg 108: 576–583

Reams GP, Bauer JH (1986) Effect of enalapril in subjects with hypertension associated with moderate to severe renal dysfunction. Arch Intern Med 146: 2145–2148

Rigden SP, Dillon MJ, Kind PR, DeLeval M, Stark J, Barratt TM (1984) The beneficial effect of mannitol on post-operative renal function in children undergoing cardiopulmonary bypass surgery. Clin Nephrol 21: 148–151

Rose H, Philipson T, Puschett JB (1987) Effects of nitrendipine in a rat model of ischemic acute renal failure. J Cardiovasc Pharmacol 9(Suppl 1): 57–59

Rosman JB, TerWee PM, Meijer S, Sluiter WJ, Piers-Becht TP, Sluiter WJ, Donker AJ (1984) Prospective randomized trial of early dietary protein restriction in chronic renal failure. Lancet II: 1291–1296

Scanu P, Harault de Ligny B, Ryckelynck JP (1987) Reversible acute renal insufficiency with combination of enalapril and diuretics in a patient with single renal artery stenosis. Nephron 45: 321–322

Schafferhans K, Heidbreder E, Grimm D, Heidland A (1986a) Human atrial natriuretic factor prevents against norepinephrine-induced acute renal failure in the rat. Klin Wochenschr 64:Suppl 6: 73–77

Schafferhans K, Heidbreder E, Grimm D, Heidland A (1986b) Norepinephrine-induced acute renal failure: beneficial effects of atrial natriuretic factor. Nephron 44: 240–244

Schafferhans K, Heidbreder E, Schmatz R, Herdland A (1987) Atrial natriuretic peptide protects against gentamicin induced acute renal failure in the rat. Am Soc Nephrology, p 219A

Scheer RL (1965) The effect of hypertonic mannitol on oliguric patients. Am J Med Sci 250: 483–491

Schrier RW, Arnold PE, Burke T (1984) The calcium ion and calcium channel blockers in ischemic acute renal failure (ARF). Trans Am Soc Artif Intern Organs 30: 702–703

Schrier RW, Arnold PE, Van Putten VJ et al. (1987) Cellular calcium in ischemic acute renal failure: Role of calcium entry blockers. Kidney Int 32: 313–321

Schubiger G, Flury G, Nussberger J (1988) Enalapril for pregnancy-induced hypertension: Acute renal failure in a neonate. Ann Intern Med 108: 215–216

Schulte-Wissermann H, Straub E, Funke PJ (1977) Influence of L-thyroxine upon enzymatic activity in the renal tubular epithelium of the rat under normal conditions and in mercury-induced lesions. I. Histochemical studies of alkaline phosphatase, acid phosphatase, adenosine-tri-phosphatase and leucine-aminopeptidase. Virchows Arch [Cell Pathol] 23: 163–173

Scriabine A, Anderson CL, Janis RA et al. (1984) Some recent pharmacological findings with nitrendipine. J Cardiovasc Pharmacol 6(Suppl 7): S937–S943

Sevitt LH, Evans DJ, Wrong OM (1971) Acute oliguric renal failure due to accelerated (malignant) hypertension. Q J Med (New Series) 40: 127–144

Shallcross H, Padley SPG, Glynn MJ, Gibbs DD (1986) Fatal renal and hepatic toxicity after treatment with diltiazem. Br Med J 295: 1236–1237

Shapiro JI, Cheung JY, Itabashi A, Chan L, Schrier RW (1985) The effect of verapamil on renal function after warm and cold ischemia in the isolated perfused rat kidney. Transplantation 40: 596–600

Shaw SG, Weidmann P, Hodler J, Zimmerman A, Paternostro A (1987) Atrial natriuretic peptide protects against acute ischemic renal failure in the rat. J Clin Invest 80: 1232–1237

Shusterman N, Strom BL, Murray TG, Morrison G, West SL, Mailsin G (1987) Risk factors and outcome of hospital-acquired acute renal failure. Am J Med 83: 65–71

Siegel NJ, Gaudio KM (1988) Amino acids and adenine nucleotides in acute renal failure. In: Brenner BM, Lazarus JM (eds) Acute renal failure. Churchill Livingstone, New York, p 857

Siegel NJ, Gaudio KM, Katz LA et al. (1984) Beneficial effect of thyroxin on recovery from toxic acute renal failure. Kidney Int 25: 906–911

Simon NM, Graham MB, Kyser FA, Gashti EN (1979) Resolution of renal failure with malignant hypertension in scleroderma. Am J Med 67: 533–539

Smith LL, Berman LB, Chisholm GD (1963) Effect of mannitol on renal function during cardiovascular surgery. Surg Forum 14: 103–105

Snell A, Wallace M (1974) Beta-blockade in the presence of renal disease and hypertension. Br Med J ii: 672

Solez K (1984) Amino acids in acute renal failure, the controversy between the experimental and clinical data. In: Panel discussion, Acute renal failure revisited. Trans Am Soc Artif Intern Organs 30: 704–705
Solez K, Stout R, Bendush B et al. (1982) Adverse effect of amino acid solutions in aminoglycoside-induced acute renal failure in rabbits and rats. In: Eliahou H (ed) Acute renal failure. Libbey, London, pp 241–247
Sorensen LB, Paunicka K, Harris M (1983) Reversal of scleroderma renal crisis for more than two years in a patient treated with captopril. Arthritis Rheum 26: 797–800
Steinman TI, Silva P (1983) Acute renal failure, skin rash, and eosinophilia associated with captopril therapy. Am J Med 75: 154–157
Stoff JS, Clive DM (1986) Role of arachidonic acid metabolite in acute renal failure. In: Brenner BM, Lazarus JM (eds) Acute renal failure. Churchill Livingstone, New York, p 143
Stott RB, Ogg CS, Cameron JS, Bewick M (1972) Why the persistently high mortality in acute renal failure? Lancet II: 75–79
Stowe N, Emma J, Magnussen M et al. (1978) Protective effect of propranolol in the treatment of ischemically damaged canine kidneys prior to transplantation. Surgery 84: 265–270
Straub E (1976) Effects of L-thyroxine in acute renal failure. Res Exp Med (Berl) 168: 81–87
Swartz RD, Rubin JE, Leeming BW, Silva P (1978) Renal failure following major angiography. Am J Med 65: 31–37
Talley RC, Forland M, Beller B (1970) Reversal of acute renal failure with a combination of intravenous dopamine and diuretics. Clin Res 18: 518
Ter Wee PM, Rosman JB, Van der Geest S (1984) Acute renal failure due to diltiazem. Lancet II: 1337–1338
Tiller DJ, Mudge GH (1980) Pharmacologic agents used in the management of acute renal failure. Kidney Int 18: 700–711
Untura A (1979) Incidence and prophylaxis of acute post-operative renal failure in obstructive jaundice. Rev Med Chir Soc Med Nat Iasi 83: 249–252
Valdes ME, Landau SE, Shah DM et al. (1979) Increased glomerular filtration rate following mannitol administration in man. J Surg Res 26: 473–477
Valido A, López-Novoa JM, Hernando L (1977) Papaverine effect on postischemic acute renal failure in rats. Biomedicine 27: 278–280
Vincenti F, Goldberg LI (1978) Combined use of dopamine and prostaglandin A_1 in patients with acute renal failure and hepatorenal syndrome. Prostaglandins 15: 463–472
Wagner K, Schultze G, Molzahn M, Neumayer HH (1986) The influence of long-term infusion of the calcium antagonist diltiazem on postischemic acute renal failure in conscious dogs. Klin Wochenschr 64: 135–140
Wagner K, Albrecht S, Neumayer HH (1987) Prevention of posttransplant acute tubular necrosis by the calcium antagonist diltiazem: a prospective randomized study. Am J Nephrol 7: 287–291
Wait RB, White G, Davis JH (1983) Beneficial effects of verapamil on postischemic renal failure. Surgery 94: 276–282
Walker PD, Shah SV (1987) Potential role of hydroxyl radical in glycerol-induced acute renal failure. Am Soc Nephrology, p 221A
Warren DJ, Swainson CP, Wright N (1974) Deterioration in renal function after beta-blockade in patients with chronic renal failure and hypertension. Br Med J ii: 193–194
Wasner C, Cooke CR, Fries JF (1978) Successful medical treatment of scleroderma renal crisis. N Engl J Med 299: 873–875
Watson AJ, Stout RL, Adkinson NF, Solez K, Whelton A (1986) Selective inhibition of thromboxane synthesis in glycerol-induced acute renal failure. Am J Kidney Dis 8: 26–30
Webb WR (1985) Metabolic effects of fructose diphosphate in hypoxic and ischemic states. J Thorac Cardiovasc Surg 88: 863–866
Weub R, Clark WF, Lindsay RM, Jones EO, Turnbull DI, Linton AL (1978) Protective effect of prostaglandin (PGE_2) in glycerol-induced renal failure in rats. Clin Sci Mol Med 55: 505–507
Wheeler DC, Feehally J, Walls J (1986) High risk acute renal failure. Q J Med (New Series) 61: 977–984
Woods JW, Blythe WB (1967) Management of malignant hypertension complicated by renal insufficiency. N Engl J Med 277: 57–61
Woods JW, Blythe WB, Huffines WD (1974) Malignant hypertension and renal insufficiency. N Engl J Med 291: 10–14
Yasmineh DJ, Schirger JA, Edwards BS, Schwab TR, Heublein DW, Burnett JC Jr (1987) Atrial natriuretic factor prevents acute renal dysfunction induced by hypotensive hemorrhage in the dog. Am Soc Nephrology, p 222A

Yeboah ED, Petrie A, Pead JL (1972) Acute renal failure and open heart surgery. Br Med J i: 415–418
Yeh TJ, Brackney EL, Hall DP, Ellison RG (1964) Renal complications of open-heart surgery. Predisposing factors, prevention and management. J Thorac Cardiovasc Surg 47: 79–97
Zager RA, Venkatachalam MA (1983) Potentiation of ischemic renal injury by amino acid infusion. Kidney Int 24: 620–625
Zawada ET Jr, Clements PJ, Furst DA, Bloomer HA, Paulus HE, Maxwell MH (1981) Clinical course of patients with scleroderma renal crisis treated with captopril. Nephron 27: 74–78

Discussion

Dr Bion opened the discussion by making a comment concerning the use of dopamine to improve spanchnic blood flow. He emphasized that whilst no one investigator had demonstrated conclusively an increase in renal blood flow associated with the administration of dopamine in critically ill patients, it seemed that this drug might also increase blood flow to the gut. This might be very important in maintaining the integrity of the gut and in the amelioration of multiple organ failure. It might also have a role in preventing the development of stress ulceration and this would account for the apparent decrease in bleeding from the gastrointestinal tract in patients requiring intensive care. Dr Lazarus was questioned closely about the data available in humans, that renal blood flow actually increased when low dose dopamine was prescribed. Dr Bihari thought that so called "low dose dopamine" might also affect systemic haemodynamics, produce an increase in cardiac output, and also change the renal perfusion pressure. All these things had to be taken into account in the assessment of the renal protective effects of dopamine. Dr Myers made the distinction between the prescription of dopamine as a prophylactic agent in patients with an intact circulation but with nephrotoxic acute renal failure, in contrast with other cases in whom acute circulatory failure was present. In the latter, he thought it was most unlikely that dopamine could overcome the effects of other vasoconstrictors that were released in response to the failing circulation.

Dr Neild returned the discussion to the problem of volume loading. He wondered whether the administration of mannitol or just volume loading alone was sufficient in many patients to prevent the development of acute renal failure. Dr Myers thought that the effects of mannitol in lowering renovascular resistance and causing a high rate of proximal tubule fluid flow, would disperse the brush border and other accumulating debris and relieve obstruction, whilst increasing peritubular blood flow. Similarly, a large volume load might also achieve the same effects. All participants believed that mannitol and volume loading were acting in the same way.

Dr Epstein made a comment about thyroxine. He mentioned that in animal studies of acute renal failure in which renal dysfunction was produced by clamping the renal artery for 45 minutes, thyroxine had a rational place in so far as it induces an increase in the pump enzyme, sodium, potassium-ATPase, in proximal tubules. Thus, these cells which usually swell up and exhibit the signs of necrosis might be more likely to reduce their swelling through the increased activity of the membrane pump. Dr Epstein emphasized that for thyroxine to be useful in the prevention and treatment of acute renal failure in humans it would be necessary to give a sufficient amount of the hormone to make the patient hyperthyroid. Moreover, thyroxine does not appear to act in the distal tubule or the thick ascending limb of the loop of Henle – two sections of the nephron most likely to be damaged in ischaemic acute renal failure. He thought it was unlikely that this compound would be of much use in the management of patients.

Chapter 25

Appropriate Renal Support in the Management of Acute Renal and Respiratory Failure: Does Early Aggressive Treatment Improve the Outcome?

K. Simpson, M. Travers and M. Allison

Introduction

Before dialysis was available acute renal failure carried a mortality of around 91% (Bywaters and Beall 1941). With the introduction of renal replacement therapy, the mortality for patients with acute renal failure fell to 50% and for those with acute renal and respiratory failure, it fell to around 70% (Kennedy et al. 1973). Despite enormous advances in intensive care, no further significant reduction in mortality has been noted.

Kleinknecht et al. (1972) suggested that early and frequent dialysis improved the prognosis for patients with acute renal failure, presumably by relieving the uraemic state. In 1982 Kramer et al. described spontaneous arterio-venous haemofiltration, a technique which has proved to be extremely useful in the treatment of critically ill patients. The use of biocompatible membranes with high hydraulic permeability reduced many of the untoward reactions induced by contact between blood and the membrane surface. It also permitted high volume filtration at pressures available from an arterial blood supply: an ability which might at first sight remove the need for expensive monitoring equipment. Unfortunately the clearances available are limited by the practical problems of reinfusing enormous quantities of replacement fluid and we remain unconvinced that a spontaneous, unmonitored extra-corporeal circuit is as safe as we can make it (Simpson et al. 1988).

There is also some evidence that early attention to nutrition and the provision of energy can help to decrease mortality (Abel et al. 1973; Blumenkrantz et al. 1978; Mault et al. 1983). The composition of the diet best suited to patients with acute renal failure is still the subject of intense debate (Solez 1984).

Shoemaker and his group have shown that all critically ill patients can benefit from resuscitation with colloid, which reduces extravascular oedema and the associated abnormal diffusion path for oxygen from capillaries to mitochondria.

These fluids also raise cardiac output and in the well-oxygenated patient, oxygen delivery (Hauser et al. 1980). Despite, or perhaps because of, the improved immediate survival that these treatment methods have produced, we are now more than ever aware of the central role of infection and the uncontrolled acute inflammatory response. These reactions can damage organs remote from the primary focus of infection and may ultimately lead to the demise of critically ill patients (Cerra 1987).

We are conducting a study in which patients with acute multi-organ failure (at least renal and respiratory failure) are randomly allocated to receive either CUPID (continuous ultrafiltration and continuous bicarbonate haemodialysis) or conventional haemodialysis therapy. It is our thesis that a determined attempt to remove "toxins" – whether they are the classical uraemic toxins or the mediators of the acute inflammatory response – may be rewarded by a more benign clinical course and by improved mortality.

Methods

After obtaining consent from the immediate relatives, ventilator-dependent patients with acute multi-organ failure who have been referred to our intensive care unit are randomly allocated to receive one of the two treatments.

Conventional renal replacement therapy consists of sufficient dialysis with a cuprophane membrane, daily or on alternate days, to keep the morning serum urea concentration at 30 mmol l^{-1}. Ultrafiltration is performed during each session to allow the administration of blood, plasma protein solution, drugs and nutrition.

The second group of patients are treated according to our new regimen, which combines continuous, volumetrically controlled machine-driven ultrafiltration with continuous bicarbonate haemodialysis across a polysulphone membrane (CUPID) (Simpson et al. 1987). During the first 48 hours of CUPID therapy, the acute disequilibrium syndrome is prevented by initially limiting the average creatinine clearance to 20 ml min^{-1}. This is slowly increased by increasing the dialysate flow rate (Qd). Blood flow rate (Qb) is kept at 150–200 ml min^{-1}. Eventually sufficient clearance (100–140 ml min^{-1}) is achieved to return the peripheral blood urea and creatinine concentrations to our laboratory's reference range (Table 25.1).

All anticoagulants are given into the arterial side of the dialyser. CUPID patients receive a continuous infusion of heparin at a dose sufficient to keep the whole blood clotting time at 30 min (500–1500 U h^{-1}) and prostacyclin (Flolan Wellcome) at 15 ng kg^{-1} min^{-1}. Changes in prostacyclin dose are made at a rate of 1 ng kg^{-1} min^{-1} every hour. Patients on the conventional arm of the trial receive a bolus injection of 2000–3000 units of heparin at the beginning of dialysis and extra doses of 500–1000 units are given if the clotting time falls below 30 min.

Vascular access is, if possible, via a Scribner shunt but both single and double lumen central venous catheters have been used successfully.

Table 25.1. Comparison of the two methods

	Conventional	CUPID
Dialysis membrane	1.1 m² Cuprophane	0.65 m² Polysulphone
Dialysate composition	Reverse osmosis pre-treated tapwater. Bicarbonate buffered (PGS22, Fresenius)	
Dialysate potassium	Adjusted daily as necessary	4 mmol l^{-1}
Dialysate temperature	37 °C	37 °C
Machine	Fresenius A2008C/D	
Blood flow rate	150–200 ml min^{-1}	
Average dialysate flow rate	500 ml min^{-1}	0, increasing to 500 ml min^{-1} over the first 48 h of treatment
Ultrafiltration rate	100–500 ml h^{-1}	
Fluid replacement	2500 ml parenteral nutrition daily	8500–10500 ml parenteral nutrition daily
Anticoagulant	Heparin	Heparin + prostacyclin
Nutrition	18 gN (144 cal gN^{-1}, per 70 kg patient)	

Patients in both groups receive parenteral nutrition containing 18 g of nitrogen per day with 144 calories gN^{-1}, of which a third are derived from lipid. Trace metals, fat- and water-soluble vitamins are given daily (Neo range, Kabivitrum).

Patients in both groups receive the H$_2$-receptor antagonist ranitidine (Zantac, Glaxo Laboratories) 50 mg i.v. three times a day.

As well as the "routine biochemistry" and the clinical outcome the following are measured:

Beta 2-microglobulin	– Radioimmunoassay
C3a, C5a	– Radioimmunoassay
Granulocyte elastase	– Immunoenzymatic
Lymphocyte mitogenesis	– [^{3}H]thymidine uptake following stimulation with PWM, ConA, PhA

Statistical analysis is performed with Student's unpaired t test.

Results

The mean 8 am serum urea was significantly reduced in the CUPID group (Fig. 25.1). The peaks and troughs that are normally seen with conventional dialysis therapy are "smoothed out" by this graph. For patients on CUPID, these fluctuations really are removed and there is a smooth reduction of nitrogenous waste levels and serum electrolytes are returned to reference values. For patients on conventional therapy, each dialysis session is of course associated with a peak and trough.

Serum beta-2 microglobulin (B2MG, MW 11 800) concentration was significantly reduced ($p<0.05$) in CUPID patients on day 5 (17.6 mg l^{-1} ± 9.2 SD, $n=9$) whereas conventionally treated patients have a mean B2MG concentration of

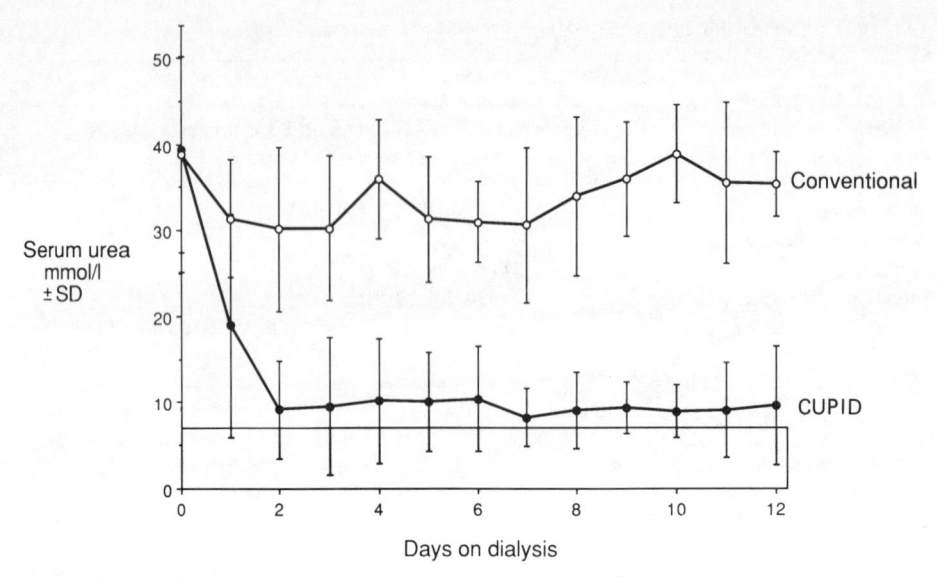

Fig. 25.1. The 8 am serum urea concentrations during the first 12 days of treatment with CUPID or conventional dialysis.

32.4 mg l^{-1} (± 8.9 SD, $n=7$). These figures may not all be due to improved clearance because exposure of blood to cuprophane membranes is known to stimulate the release of B2MG from lymphocytes (Vincent et al. 1978).

The total white blood count rose dramatically in CUPID patients to an average of $30 \times 10^9 l^{-1}$ at the end of five days' treatment. The incidence of infection in this group was not increased and their polymorphonuclear leucocytes were less "activated" as assessed by the lower serum concentration of granulocyte elastase. At the end of the first three hours of treatment the mean plasma elastase concentration in CUPID patients was 250 µg ml^{-1} while in the conventionally treated group it was 540 µg ml^{-1}.

Acute exposure to the artificial membrane caused a rise in C3a and C5a in both patient groups and although it was more marked in the conventionally treated group, this difference does not reach statistical significance. For C3a the peak response was seen at 15 min (CUPID, 4145 ng ml^{-1} ± 3258 (SD), $n=10$; conventional, 6516 ng ml^{-1} ± 2854 (SD), $n=9$). At day 5 C3a in CUPID patients had a mean value of 1166 ng ml^{-1} (± 628 (SD), $n=9$), and in the conventional group mean C3a was 2200 ng ml^{-1} (± 1722 (SD), $n=4$). Table 25.2 illustrates C5a levels. The peak in the conventional group occurred at 15 minutes (62 ng ml^{-1}) whereas in the CUPID group peak levels were lower and occurred at 1 hour. Thereafter C5a concentrations decreased in both groups.

Blood for mitogenesis studies was drawn before treatment, at 15 minutes, 1 hour, 3 hours and then at day 3 and day 7. Lymphocytes were prepared from this blood on a sucrose density grading and the mitogen response to pokeweed, concanavalin A and phytohaemagglutinin was assessed by the uptake of tritiated thymidine. Preliminary results show that when compared to healthy controls the response in both groups of patients with renal failure was depressed to the same extent and did not differ from that of other ITU patients (Fig. 25.2). The dialysis regime did not appear to influence the mitogen responses.

^{3}H THYMIDINE UPTAKE CPM x 10^3

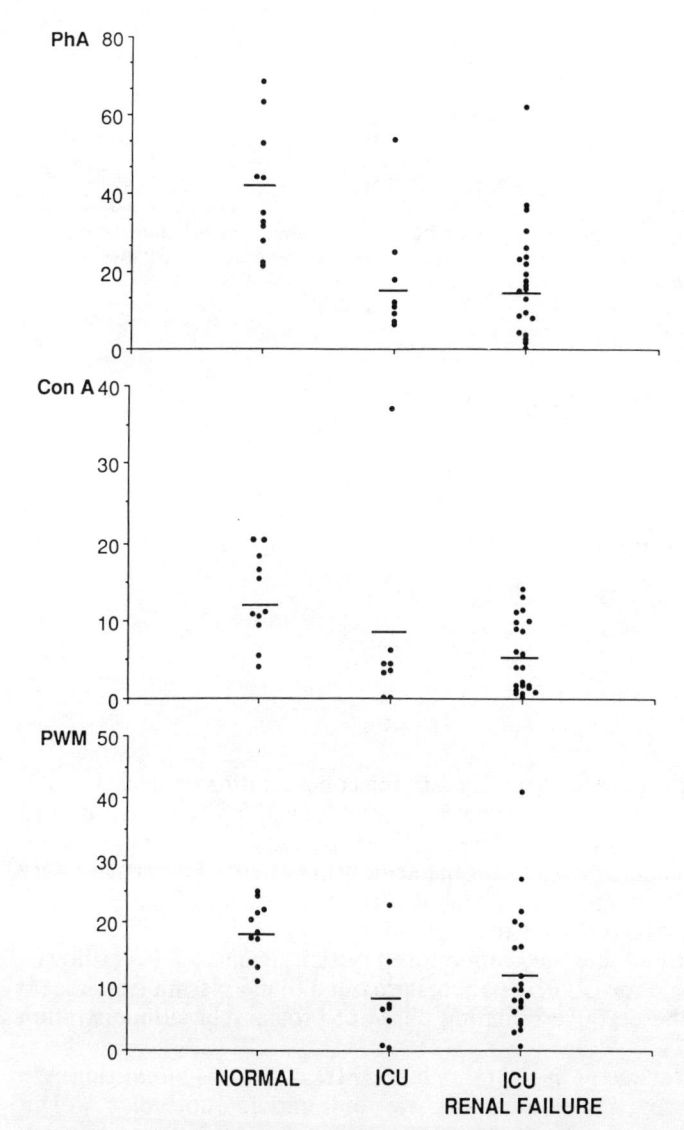

Fig. 25.2. Tritiated thymidine uptake of lymphocytes from normal control subjects, general intensive care unit patients with respiratory failure but normal renal function and intensive care unit patients with renal and respiratory failure, following stimulation with phytohaemagglutinin (*PhA*), concanavalin A (*Con A*) or pokeweed (*PWM*).

Table 25.2. Mean arterial blood C5a concentration (ng ml^{-1})

	Pre	15 min	60 min	180 min	Day 5	Day 14
CUPID	16	21	35	16	8	12
SD	6	21	34	16	5	11
n	10	10	10	3	8	6
Conventional	37	62	24	17	7[a]	12[a]
SD	45	38	11	10	3	5
n	10	10	10	7	6	2
p	NS	<0.025	NS	NS	NS	NS

[a] Samples from patients in the conventional group for days 5 and 14 were drawn before dialysis and therefore do not represent the response to acute exposure to dialysis on that day. Patients in the CUPID group were continuously exposed to the membrane.

Mortality

Sixty one patients have now entered the trial.

Group	Survived	Died	Mean age	Mortality
CUPID	13	17	47	57%
Conventional	7	24	52	77%

The decrease in mortality is interesting and encouraging but not statistically significant.

Discussion

CUPID can render the serum urea and creatinine concentrations normal even in the most catabolic patient. Virtually unlimited quantities of fluid can be removed in a controlled fashion and parenteral feeding and other fluids can be prescribed freely. The dialysis machine provides for the acutely ill patient, the normal safety features that would be regarded as essential for the treatment of patients with chronic renal failure. We feel that these standards should not be discarded in favour of an apparently simple but unmonitored system. Remarkable cardiovascular stability is the rule for CUPID patients provided that a plasma expander is given slowly during the early vasodilating phase of prostacyclin administration (Simpson et al. 1987).

The suggested improvement in mortality in CUPID patients is tantalizing. We have shown an improved clearance of low and middle molecular weight substances, the deleterious effects of which are suspected but not proved. Contact activation is reduced as assessed by complement fraction generation and granulocyte elastase production. This is probably useful in acutely ill patients although it must be said that these features have not been shown to correlate well with adverse symptoms or long-term survival in patients with chronic renal failure on haemodialysis.

The mitogenesis studies are the most direct way of examining the ability of B and T cells to divide. We found that lymphocytes from patients in both of our treatment groups had an impaired mitogenic response and that their behaviour was the same as those of other ventilator-dependent ITU patients without overt renal failure. We were unable to identify any consistent improvement during CUPID treatment. We hope that the polymorph function studies currently under way will throw some light on the importance of the marked leucocytosis that is seen in CUPID patients and that this will provide information which will be of use in the management of all patients with acute renal failure. This clinical study is still in progress and as far as we are aware, it remains the only randomized prospective trial of renal replacement therapy in critically ill patients.

References

Abel R, Beck CH, Abbott WM, Ryan JA, Barnett GO, Fischer JE (1973) Improved survival from acute renal failure after treatment with intravenous essential L-amino acids and glucose. N Engl J Med 288: 695–699
Blumenkrantz MJ, Kopple JD, Koffler A, Kamdar AK, Healy MD, Einstein EI, Massry SG (1978) Total parenteral nutrition in the management of acute renal failure. Am J Clin Nutr 31: 1831
Bywaters ELG, Beall D (1941) Crush injuries with impairment of renal function. Br Med J i: 427–432
Cerra FB (1987) The hypermetabolism organ failure complex. World J Surg 11: 173–181
Cerra FB, Siegel JH, Border J, Coleman B (1979) Correlations between metabolic and cardiopulmonary measurement in patients after trauma, general surgery and sepsis. J Trauma 19: 621–628
Hauser CJ, Shoemaker WC, Turpin I, Goldburg SJ (1980) Oxygen transport responses to colloids and crystalloids in critically ill surgical patients. Surgery 150: 811–816
Kennedy AC, Burton JA, Luke RG, Briggs JD, Lindsay RM, Allison MEM, Edward N, Dargie HJ (1973) Factors affecting the prognosis and acute renal failure: a survey of 251 cases. Q J Med 42: 73–86
Kleinknecht D, Jungers P, Chanard J, Barbanel C, Ganeval D (1972) Uraemic and non uraemic complications in acute renal failure: evaluation of early and frequent dialysis on prognosis. Kidney Int 1: 190–196
Kramer P, Bohler A, Kehr HJ, Grone J, Schrader D, Matthaei D, Scheler R (1982) Intensive care potential of continuous arterio-venous haemofiltration. Trans Am Soc Artif Intern Organs 28: 28–32
Mault JR, Barlett RH, Dechert RE, Clark SF, Swartz RD (1983) Starvation: a major contribution to mortality in acute renal failure. Trans Am Soc Artif Intern Organs 29: 390–395
Simpson HKL, Allison MEM, Telfer ABM (1987) Improving the prognosis in acute renal and respiratory failure. Renal Failure 10: 45–54
Simpson HKL, Allison MEM, Telfer ABM (1988) Continuous haemodialysis (letter). Br Med J 297: 616–617
Solez K (1984) Amino acids in acute renal failure, the controversy between the experimental and clinical data. Trans Am Soc Artif Intern Organs 30: 704–705
Vincent C, Revillard JP, Galland M, Traeger J (1978) Serum beta$_2$ microglobulin in haemodialysed patients. Nephron 21: 260–268

Discussion

Dr Simpson was asked whether he had stratified his patients using the APACHE II system. He replied that this had been done and that the APACHE II scores were the same for both groups of patients with mean values around 18 and 19 points respectively. He went on to emphasize that the patients on conventional therapy were much more likely to develop haemodynamic instability. Dr Bihari asked about the prostacyclin infusion and whether this caused any side effects. Dr Simpson explained that prostacyclin was introduced at 1 ng kg^{-1} min^{-1} and then increased slowly over 15 h to 15 ng kg^{-1} min^{-1}, whilst heparin was added as necessary to keep the whole blood clotting time at 30 min. Dr Simpson explained that on this dose of prostacyclin the blood pressure tended to rise. This was rather unusual, since prostacyclin is a known vasodilator and, if anything, tends to lower the blood pressure. Dr Epstein asked Dr Simpson whether all his patients were in both respiratory and renal failure. Dr Epstein also asked whether there was any difference in the incidence of bleeding in the two groups. Dr Simpson replied that indeed all patients were in combined respiratory and renal failure and there was no difference in the incidence of bleeding in the two groups. However, the CUPID treatment had to be terminated in two patients for a short period because of bleeding. One of them occurred following a perioperative liver biopsy, whereas the other episode resulted following surgery in a patient when small vessels started to bleed and the patient had to go back to theatre. Dr Epstein went on to ask whether the final figures of percentage mortality were analysed on an intention to treat basis. Dr Simpson replied that this had been the basis for his analysis and he paid tribute to the nursing staff of his unit who had worked so hard to create these improvements in survival. All participants agreed that the complexity of the renal replacement technique added greatly to the work of the nurses and in some cases it was necessary to have 1½ or 2 nurses per patient which greatly increased the cost of care. Dr Bihari asked whether the quoted survival rates were the ICU survival or hospital discharge survival rates. Moreover he questioned the use of the Scribner shunt as a primary form of vascular access in so far as once such a shunt has been inserted it needs to stay there and is difficult to change if the patient should develop a fever or appear to become septicaemic. The advantage of a double lumen catheter in the subclavian/jugular/fermoral vein was that it could be easily changed quickly with no need for further surgery. Dr Bihari's third point was the cost of the CUPID technique compared with the technique of haemodialysis of continuous arteriovenous haemodiafiltration. It was obvious to all participants that episodic haemodialysis was one of the cheapest techniques to use, but all agreed that one used it at the patient's peril. Dr Simpson reiterated the gut feeling of many nephrologists that Scribner shunts seem to become infected very much less frequently than central lines. Whether this is related to their position or to the flow through the shunt remains unknown. In general, these shunts are left intact unless there is obvious infection of the incision sites.

The discussion then centred on the use of prostacyclin in addition to heparin to anticoagulate the extracorporeal circuit used in the technique of CUPID. Several discussants voiced their concern that prostacyclin was not being used in the conventional treatment group. There was concern that prostacyclin might have some other effects such as an improvement in tissue perfusion, a reduction in the activation of platelets and white cells, together with its cytoprotective qualities. Dr Smithies asked how the anticoagulation had been assessed. Dr Simpson had difficulty answering some of these points. Most of the conventional tests of clotting are not useful for assessing the anticoagulation of extracorporeal circuits and whilst he recognized that prostacyclin had many other effects other than just acting as an antiplatelet agent, one just had to accept this as a possible defect in the trial design.

Chapter 26

The Role of Spontaneous and Pumped Haemofiltration

J. C. Mason

Although haemodialysis (HD) remains the mainstay of management in acute renal failure (ARF) (Broyer et al. 1983), the rapid and widespread espousal of continuous arteriovenous haemofiltration (CAVH) initially described by Kramer et al. (1977), perhaps resulted from its fusion of two ideas which had long been attractive to nephrologists. The first of these was continuity of therapy, with its aspiration towards the maintenance of a steady state in the internal environment and avoidance of the oscillations inherent in intermittent therapy. Peritoneal dialysis (PD) of course has this quality but in the contemporary spectrum of cases of ARF, particularly those attracting the interest of the intensive care specialist, it is commonly precluded by prior surgical attentions to the abdomen or technical problems – infections, leakage and notably failure to achieve fluid removal. Continuous HD was considered almost 30 years ago (Scribner et al. 1960) but only recently has technical advance made this a realistic possibility (Geronemus and Schneider 1984).

The second idea was that haemofiltration might preclude the haemodynamic disturbances, hypotension and dysrhythmias, frequently experienced in HD, and by avoiding further ischaemic insults to the kidney create conditions favourable for renal recovery. Although ultrafiltration had been used from the early days of dialysis (Leonards et al. 1951) to achieve fluid removal, it was the development during the 1960s of polysulphone membranes of high hydraulic conductivity that enabled Henderson et al. (1967) to demonstrate that pressure-driven convective exchange could provide an alternative method for renal replacement therapy. The interest in haemofiltration was enhanced by the observation (Bergstrom et al. 1976) that hypotension, associated with fluid removal during dialysis of the overloaded patient, was ameliorated if the periods of ultrafiltration and dialysis were organized sequentially. Further reports (Quellhorst et al. 1983; Baldamus et al. 1978) have confirmed the benefits of haemofiltration as maintenance therapy for patients with end-stage disease, in terms of patient well-being, avoidance of symptomatic hypotension and control of hypertension. Shaldon et al. (1983) have debated the physiological mechanisms underlying this improvement. Economic considerations, however, have prevented the adoption of haemofiltration on any substantial scale.

If the benefits of continuity and circulatory stability remained insufficiently attractive, proponents of CAVH could additionally point to its simplicity. The original circuit, devoid of blood pumps and dependent only on arterial blood pressure, did not require sophisticated monitors or specialist attendants but merely attention to simple burettes for the measurement of filtration and substitution flows. The potential to remove care of those with ARF away from the dialysis unit has certainly played a part in the commercial promotion of CAVH but whether it can reliably offer complete replacement therapy merits further consideration.

Performance of CAVH

Rigorous descriptions of solute and water transport during haemofiltration are available (Colton et al. 1975). The following approximations illustrate general principles:

$$J_s = J_v\, C_f = J_v\, C_w\, S \tag{1}$$

where

$$S = C_f/C_w \tag{2}$$

J_s is the rate of solute flow per unit time and unit membrane area, J_v is the rate of volume flow of water per unit time and unit membrane area, C_f and C_w are the concentrations of solute in ultrafiltrate and plasma water respectively and S is the sieving coefficient determined by the relative size of the solute molecule and membrane pores. The volume flow J_v is determined by the hydraulic conductivity of the membrane (L_p), membrane area A and the net hydrostatic (ΔP) and osmotic ($\Delta \pi$) pressure gradients across the membrane.

$$J_v = L_p\, A\, (\Delta P - \Delta \pi) \tag{3}$$

Equation (3) implies a linear relation between volume flow rate and applied pressure but in practice this is not found. The increment in flow rate is progressively less as P increases. The convective flow causes accumulation of protein and other large molecules at the membrane surface ("concentration polarization") which exerts an osmotic pressure greater than that predicted from the bulk phase concentration. This effect is amplified by the non-ideal relation between colloid osmotic pressure and protein concentration. However, the protein concentration gradient at the surface of the membrane will tend to be dissipated by diffusion and also by shear forces caused by the axial flow of blood. This suggests that the filtration rate will be related to the rate of blood flow through the haemofilter and we, like others (Olbricht et al. 1985), have found this to be the case. Vascular access using femoral catheters generally provides blood flows and filtration rates superior to that achieved with shunts (Olbricht et al. 1985). Both of these flows are inversely related to plasma protein concentration and haematocrit (Eisenhauer 1985), although these are determined by other clinical considerations.

Although there is great individual variation, by using Amicon D20 membranes with standard circuits, femoral arterial and venous catheters (Vygon 3 mm i.d.), we found a mean systemic blood pressure of 77 mmHg, and in the extracorporeal circuit average pressures were: arterial line 57 mmHg, venous line 27 mmHg and so within the filter a pressure of about 42 mmHg. The bed was elevated so that the filtrate collecting point was one metre below the heart, applying approximately 70 mmHg negative pressure to the filtrate. The net transmembrane hydrostatic gradient was therefore approx. 110 mmHg, almost two-thirds being provided by the negative pressure resulting from the low collecting point. Colloid osmotic pressure in these patients who are usually hypoalbuminaemic, is unlikely to exceed 15 mmHg, and the filtration fraction is usually less than 0.25. Under these circumstances it is unlikely that filtration equilibrium is reached proximal to the venous end of the filter, as has been suggested by others (Bosch 1986).

During spontaneous haemofiltration the blood flow through the device varies considerably but is usually in the range 50–140 ml min^{-1}, most commonly 80–100 ml min^{-1}. Similarly the filtration rates are highly variable but we found an average of 624 ml h^{-1}, similar to the values of others (Frisch et al. 1986). The time involved in filter changes reduces this by approx. 10% so that the average daily filtration rate was 13.1 l, equivalent to a GFR of 9.1 ml min^{-1}. The average replacement by substitution fluid was 9.9 l, the balance consisting of nutritional fluids, blood products and drugs.

Metabolic control varies with the filtration rate. The average values at the start and finish of treatment respectively were for plasma creatinine 560 and 375 µmol l^{-1}, and for urea 38.5 and 34.4 mmol l^{-1}. It is not uncommon to fail to reduce blood urea below 50 mmol l^{-1}. The progressive reduction in creatinine presumably reflects muscle wasting despite nutritional support.

Finally the life expectancy of the haemofilter during CAVH is also unpredictable. In our series of 87 filters in 31 patients, the average was 51 hours but the distribution is skewed with a few exceeding one week. All who have practised this technique will recognize the substantial proportion of patients in whom flows are poor and loss of the filter occurs within a few hours.

Metabolic Control in CAVH

Even the prescription of dialysis in stable patients on maintenance HD therapy is not entirely straightforward and it required a survey of the magnitude of the National Cooperative Dialysis Study (Lowrie and Laird 1983) to provide general recommendations and to quantify the morbidity consequent on insufficient treatment. Although there is evidence pointing to the benefits of early and frequent treatment in ARF (Kleinknecht et al. 1972), no information of equivalent precision is available among this highly heterogeneous group of patients. The uncertainties are still greater with haemofiltration. Although the selectivity of the membranes differ with the possible advantage of greater removal of molecules of intermediate size, the base of experience in chronic maintenance therapy is comparatively small. There has, however, been a move towards larger exchange volumes when intermittent haemofiltration is used in the maintenance therapy for patients with end-stage disease. Baldamus (1985) has suggested that small molecule clearance should approach that of HD i.e. approx. 3×30 l week^{-1}. Given the hiiih catabolic rates characteristic of ARF, it is reasonable to anticipate that daily exchange volumes in excesss of 20 l will be reliably required.

Evidence that there is widespread anxiety concerning the adequacy of metabolic control during spontaneous CAVH is provided by the proliferration of variations on the theme (Table 26.1). The transmembrane pressure gradient has been increased by the application of suction to the filtrate compartment (Kaplan et al. 1983), although this approach is limited by the non-linearity of the pressure/flow relationship outlined above. Moreover, this produces a high filtration fraction whose adverse rheological consequences may predispose to early filter failure. Introduction of the substitution fluid upstream of the filter (predilution) requires a higher filtration rate and more substitution fluid to achieve the same clearance (Colton et al. 1975). However, axial flow through the filter is increased and the haematocrit and plasma protein concentration are reduced with a possible benefit to overall performance (Kaplan 1985). Filter geometry has also been modified in an attempt to improve flow and prolong filter life. The possible advantages of short filters (Ronco et al. 1986), and relatively high membrane areas have been discussed (Henderson et al. 1986). Filters with increased fibre internal radii (280 µm in comparison with the more usual 200 µm) are available but no single design has yet established itself as pre-eminent.

Table 26.1. Modifications of spontaneous CAVH to provide increased solute clearance

1. CAVH
   Predilution
   Ultrafiltrate suction
   Modification of filter geometry
2. Pumped CAVH/CVVH
   Simple roller pump
   Dialysis pump module with safety monitors
   Gravimetric filtrate monitor/automated substitution
3. CAVHD (combined diffusional exchange)
   Slow continuous ultrafiltration/intermittent HD
   Continuous HD
     "Manual" dialysis
     Pumped dialysis
     "CUPID"

CAVH has been widely used as an adjunct to intermittent HD (Paganini and Nakamoto 1980; Dodd et al. 1983). Slow rates of filtration (5 l day^{-1}) suffice to correct any pre-existing volume overload and to compensate intravenous therapy, while metabolic control is achieved by conventional HD, perhaps at the reduced frequency of every second or third day. Combination with continuous haemodialysis (CAVHD) has also been advocated, with levels of sophistication ranging from simple elution of the filtrate compartment with dialysis fluid, regulated "manually" (Geronemus and Schneider 1984) to the use of automatic volumetrically controlled dialysis machines ("CUPID") (Simpson et al. 1987).

The alternative approach to improved metabolic control in haemofiltration is to increase blood flow and filtration rate by incorporation of a blood pump into the extracorporeal circuit. The use of an isolated peristaltic pump is mentioned only to condemn it. There seems little point in reliving the difficulties of the early days of HD in the cause of "simplicity" and conventional arterial, venous and air monitors should be mandatory. This can be achieved with a conventional dialysis pump module. Alternatively, a fully automated machine, with gravimetric substitution, of the type used in intermittent haemofiltration may be cycled continuously for many days. The attributes of spontaneous CAVH and its pumped variant are summarized in Table 26.2. The essential difference is that to provide satisfactory metabolic control CAVH must consistently operate towards its maximum potential. However, the addition of a pump introduces ample spare capacity, and it can operate towards the lower end of its range with low circuit pressures.

Table 26.2. A comparison of spontaneous and pumped CAVH

	Spont. CAVH	Pumped CAVH/CVVH
1. Access	Arterial	Venous or arterial
2. Monitors	? No	Yes
3. Blood flow ml min^{-1}	50–100	120–180
4. Filtrate l day^{-1}	5–20	20–40
5. Filter life	Variable	Usually >2 days
6. Clearance supplementation	Common	No – single modality
7. Dialysis staff	No	No

Regulation of Volume Flows

The assessment of fluid status is far from easy in this group of patients with ARF, commonly in the context of multi-system failure. Clinical indices such as tissue turgor and peripheral perfusion may have to be interpreted in the light of hypoproteinaemia and possible venous or lymphatic obstruction to the peripheries following trauma. Circulatory measurements such as CVP or pulmonary wedge pressure are important guides in optimizing cardiac function but only indirectly reflect extracellular volume. They may remain "normal" in the face of significant dehydration which may delay renal recovery. Body weight is the gold standard in assessing day-to-day variation in fluid status but its measurement may prove impractical in the face of orthopaedic traction or special pressure distributing beds. Fluid balance charts remain a mainstay but they are inherently arithmetically inaccurate and cannot take account of unmeasured secretions such as losses into the gut.

The additional imposition of regulating and charting the large volume flows intrinsic to CAVH presents a significant burden to nursing staff. CAVHD offers no solution to this problem since the measurements must be just as accurate whether the flows are purely filtrational or include a component of dialysate. Widespread practice involves the hourly measurement and delivery of flows with equipment varying from simple calibrated vessels to volumetric pumps (I-Vac, IMED), ultrasonic "urinometers" (Vitalmetrics) and gravimetric scales (Sartorius). Kramer et al. (1979) implicitly recognized this difficulty in an early paper which includes the description of a weight-driven device for automatic delivery of substitution fluid appropriate to the filtration rate. This was technically unsatisfactory but automatic substitution has been achieved with an ingenious and simple mechanical device based on the constancy of the combined mass of filtrate and substitution fluid (Schurek et al. 1985). The gravimetric, microprocessor-controlled systems used for pumped intermittent haemofiltration (e.g. Sartorius, Gambro) are complex and expensive, as are the coupled volumetric pumps available in certain HD machines capable of controlling high filtration flows. Arithmetic charting of such data and its adjustment to all other fluid exchanges with the patient is still required.

Computer Monitoring of Continuous Haemofiltration

Difficulties in the management of the high flows necessary when CAVH was used as sole replacement therapy prompted us to develop an automatic monitoring system, sufficiently comprehensive to incorporate the whole of the patient's fluid balance. This coincided with a generally new approach to instrumentation on the ICU (Cowell 1983) using microcomputers as core units to serve multiple purposes such as multi-channel pressure monitoring, temperature recording, cardiac output studies, respiratory gas spectrometry and intracardiac electrocardiography. The integral analogue to digital converter of the BBC microcomputer made it a particularly suitable instrument for this application. The haemofiltration system has been described in detail elsewhere (Mason et al. 1985) and is illustrated in Fig. 26.1. Changes in weight following changes of volume of the haemofiltrate or replacement solution cause variations in the analogue outputs of the two force gauges. The computer converts the signals into digital form and automatically provides a continuous display on a VDU of the prevailing flow rates and volumes transferred (Fig. 26.1, HF in and HF out). All other fluid inputs and

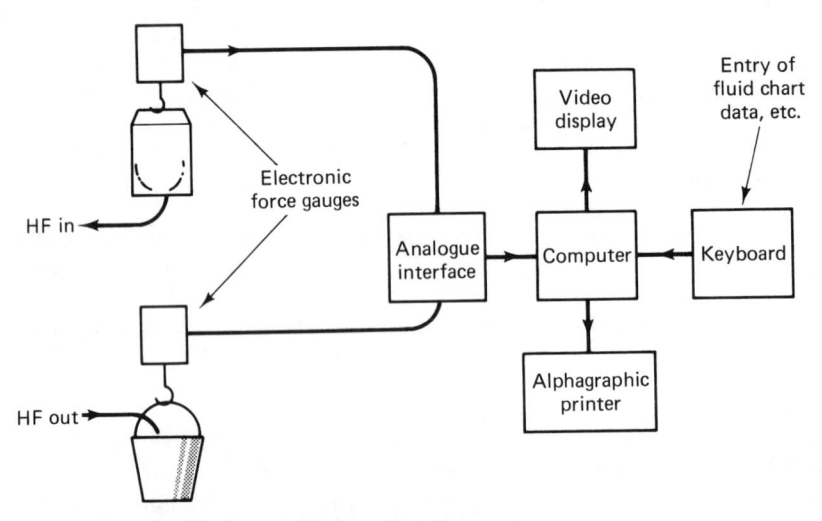

Fig. 26.1. Schematic diagram of haemofiltration monitor.

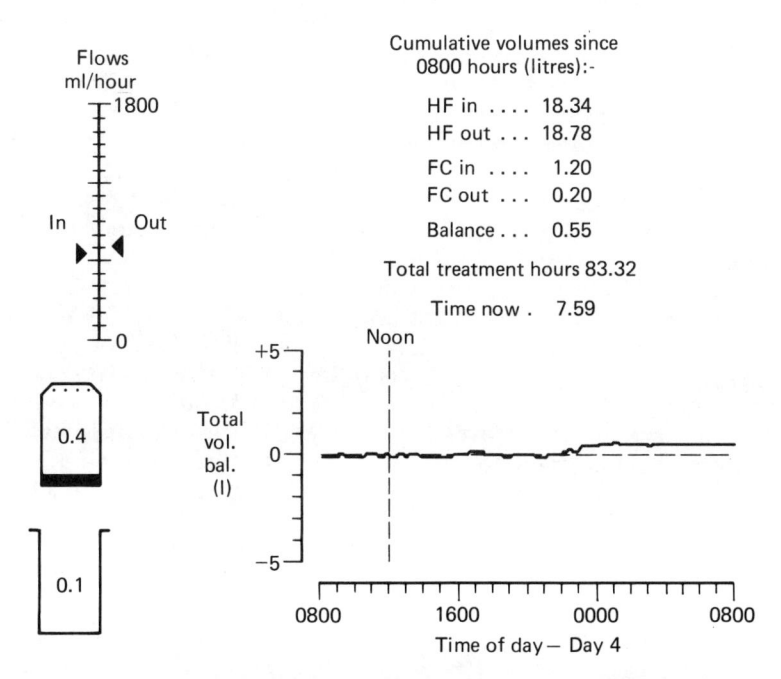

The Role of Spontaneous and Pumped Haemofiltration

Fig. 26.2. VDU screen display on completion of one day's treatment. See text for explanation.

outputs are entered, approximately hourly, through the computer keyboard by the nurse. The net fluid balance is calculated and displayed continuously, both numerically and graphically (Fig. 26.2). All fluid chart entries (FC in and FC out) are timed and printed while a second line of print provides the cumulative quantities of each item up to that time. At the end of each day the completed screen display is transferred to print, the fluid registers are re-zeroed and the graphical display cleared, permitting immediate resumption of monitoring for the next day. This process does not require any intervention by the operator. "Friendly" sub-routines guide the nurse through procedures such as emptying the filtrate container, replacing the substitution fluid bag or making "fluid chart" entries. All arithmetic and manual charting are entirely eliminated. The system is ideally suited to cope with the greater flows offered by pumped haemofiltration which have been routinely achieved by incorporation of a dialysis pump module (Gambro AK10 or Hospal Monitral).

Conclusions

The advances offered by continuous haemofiltration in terms of continuity of therapy, haemodynamic stability and volume control, are beyond dispute. Yet despite this and allied progress in cardiovascular, respiratory and nutritional management, the mortality in ARF remains high (Cameron 1986). In a prospective study the mortality of the group treated by CAVH exceeded 80% (Wing et al. 1985). Sepsis and the number of organ systems affected remain important determinants of survival (Cameron 1986). Any analysis of the contribution of a particular renal replacement technique to survival will require careful stratification of the patients according to disease severity.

The simplicity of CAVH has been overemphasized in the literature. The purpose of relatively sophisticated adjuncts such as the computer monitor described above is to reduce workload and improve accuracy. It has been readily assimilated by nurses without prior dialysis experience, in several centres.

Spontaneous CAVH will certainly not provide adequate exchange rates for satisfactory metabolic control in a significant proportion of patients. Centres lacking access to more-advanced techniques should consider this before embarking upon therapy. In those cases with poor blood flows in the extracorporeal circuit and early, repetitive filter loss, only the use of a blood pump, whether for dialysis or filtration, is likely to prove satisfactory. No clear therapeutic advantage has yet been demonstrated for any of the variety of methods and it is likely that units will continue to choose that most convenient for their individual circumstances.

References

Baldamus CA (1985) Problems in hemofiltration. Contrib Nephrol 44: 212–222
Baldamus CA, Schoeppe W, Koch KM (1978) Comparison of hemodialysis and post dilutional hemofiltration on an unselected dialysis population. Proc Eur Dial Transplant Assoc Eur Ren Assoc 15: 228–234
Bergstrom J, Asaba H, Furst P, Oules R (1976) Dialysis, ultrafiltration and blood pressure. Proc Eur Dial Transplant Assoc Eur Ren Assoc 13: 293–300
Bosch JP (1986) Continuous arteriovenous hemofiltration. In: LaGreca G, Fabris A, Ronco C (eds) International Symposium on CAVH, Vicenza 1986. Wichtig Editore, Milan, pp 9–35
Broyer M, Brunner FP, Brynger H et al. (1983) Combined report on regular dialysis and transplantation in Europe, XIII 1982 Acute (reversible) renal failure. Proc Eur Dial Transplant Assoc Eur Ren Assoc 20: 64–66
Cameron JS (1986) Acute renal failure – the continuing challenge. Q J Med 59: 337–343
Colton CK, Henderson LW, Ford CA, Lysaght MJ (1975) Kinetics of hemodiafiltration. I. In vitro transport characteristics of a hollow-fibre blood ultrafilter. J Lab Clin Med 85: 355–371
Cowell TK (1983) The BBC model B microcomputer in clinical instrumentation. J Med Eng Technol 7: 79–82
Dodd NJ, O'Donovan RM, Bennett-Jones DN et al. (1983) Arteriovenous haemofiltration: a recent advance in the management of renal failure. Br Med J 287: 1008–1010
Eisenhauer T (1985) Development and actual performance of continuous arteriovenous hemofiltration (CAVH). In: Sieberth HG, Mann H (eds) Continuous arteriovenous hemofiltration (CAVH). International conference on CAVH, Aachen 1984. Karger, Basel, pp 1–13
Frisch J, Kindler J, Schmitter H et al. (1986) Performance of CAVH in ARF therapy In: LaGreca G, Fabris A, Ronco C (eds) International Symposium on CAVH, Vicenza 1986. Wichtig Editore, Milan, pp 283–288
Geronemus R, Schneider N (1984) Continuous arteriovenous hemodialysis: A new modality for treatment of acute renal failure. Trans Am Soc Artif Intern Organs 30: 610–613
Henderson LW, Besarab A, Michaels A et al. (1967) Blood purification by ultrafiltration and fluid replacement (diafiltration). Trans Am Soc Artif Intern Organs 13: 216–222
Henderson LW, Leypoldt JK, Frigon RP (1986) The impact of membrane area on solute clearance in continuous hemofiltration. In: LaGreca G, Fabris A, Ronco C (eds) International Symposium on CAVH, Vicenza 1986. Wichtig Editore, Milan, pp 37–47

Kaplan AA (1985) Predilution vs postdilution for continuous arteriovenous hemofiltration. Trans Am Soc Artif Intern Organs 31: 28–31
Kaplan AA, Longnecker RE, Folkert VW (1983) Suction-assisted continuous arteriovenous hemofiltration. Trans Am Soc Artif Intern Organs 29: 408–413
Kleinknecht D, Jungers P, Chanard J et al. (1972) Uraemic and non-uraemic complications in acute renal failure: Evaluation of early and frequent dialysis on prognosis. Kidney Int 1: 190–196
Kramer P, Wigger W, Rieger J et al. (1977) Arteriovenous haemofiltration: A new and simple method for the treatment of overhydrated patients resistant to diuretics. Klin Wochenschr 55: 1121–1122
Kramer P, Seegers R, DeVivie D et al. (1979) Therapeutic potential of hemofiltration. Clin Nephrol 11: 145–149
Leonards JR, Skeggs LT, Kahn JR (1951) Fed Proc 10: 214
Lowrie EG, Laird NM (eds) (1983) The national cooperative dialysis study. Kidney Int 23: Suppl 13 S1–S122
Mason JC, Cowell TK, Hilton PJ, Wing AJ (1985) Continuous arteriovenous haemofiltration (CAVH) as complete replacement therapy in acute renal failure: management of fluid balance assisted by computer monitoring. In: Sieberth HG, Mann H (eds) Continuous arteriovenous hemofiltration (CAVH). International Conference on CAVH, Aachen 1984. Karger, Basel, pp 37–44
Olbricht CJ, Schurek HJ, Stolte H, Koch KM (1985) The influence of vascular access modes on the efficiency of CAVH. In: Sieberth HG, Mann H (eds) Continuous arteriovenous hemofiltration (CAVH). International conference on CAVH, Aachen 1984. Karger, Basel, pp 14–24
Paganini EP, Nakamoto S (1980) Continuous slow ultrafiltration in oliguric acute renal failure. Trans Am Soc Artif Intern Organs 21: 201–203
Quellhorst E, Scheuneman B, Hildebrand U (1983) Long term results of regular hemofiltration. Blood Purific 1: 70–79
Ronco C, Bosch JP, Lew S, Fecondini L et al. (1986) Technical and clinical evaluation of a new hemofilter for CAVH: theoretical concepts and practical application of a different blood flow geometry. In: LaGreca G, Fabris A, Ronco C (eds) International Symposium on CAVH, Vicenza 1986. Wichtig Editore, Milan, pp 55–61
Schurek HJ, Biela JD, Bergmann KH (1985) Further improvement of a mechanical device for automatic fluid balance in CAVH. In: Sieberth HG, Mann H (eds) Continuous arteriovenous hemofiltration (CAVH). International conference on CAVH, Aachen 1984. Karger, Basel, pp 67–75
Scribner BH, Caner JEZ, Buri R, Quinton W (1960) The technique of continuous dialysis. Trans Am Soc Artif Intern Organs 6: 88–103
Shaldon S, Baldamus CA, Koch KM, Lysaght MJ (1983) Of sodium, symptomatology and syllogism. Blood Purific 1: 16–24
Simpson HKL, Allison MEM, Telfer ABM (1987) Improving the prognosis in acute renal and respiratory failure. Renal Failure 10: 45–54
Wing AJ, Broyer M, Brunner FP et al. (1985) Combined report on regular dialysis and transplantation in Europe, XV 1984 Acute (reversible) renal failure. Proc Eur Dial Transplant Assoc Eur Ren Assoc 22: 48–51

Discussion

The discussion opened with a consideration of the advent of continuous arteriovenous haemodiafiltration (CAVHD). The mania for this technique has swept the United Kingdom and a number of intensive care physicians seem to be using this form of renal replacement therapy to support patients in small district general hospitals, so that these cases are not referred to regional renal units until late on in their disease. Dr Smithies and Dr Bihari expressed concern that this technique did not achieve the control of uraemia that was required in patients with multiple organ failure in whom the aim was to reduce the serum creatinine to less than 200 µmol l^{-1} with a blood urea of less than 15 mmol l^{-1}. Dr Smithies thought that CAVHD might have the advantage of using smaller volumes to achieve an exchange that improved clearance of small molecules. Dr Mason did not think this was the case. He pointed out that to achieve a certain clearance of urea it was necessary either to increase the haemofiltration volume or to add a diffusional element in the form of pumped dialysate through the dialysate compartments of the filter. In either case there had to be accurate measurements of the volumes either filtrated from the patient or infused into the filter. He also went on to emphasize that middle molecular clearance appeared to be greater using a filtration system rather than a diffusional system. This might be important in clearing the various mediators which could contribute to the development of multiple organ failure. Dr Simpson pointed out that if one had infinitely slow dialysis and the dialysate fluid was completely equilibrated with the plasma water, then the clearance with dialysis would be the same as the clearance using filtration of molecules that can be dialysed across a membrane. However, for any system that was not infinitely slow, there would not be complete equilibration between the dialysate fluid and blood so that the clearance of a particular molecular species would be less using dialysis compared with haemofiltration per litre of fluid filtered or infused. Dr Simpson emphasized that the physics of dialysis and filtration across these very high flux membranes was complex. Dr Bihari reported that it had been quite difficult to introduce CAVHD into the Royal North Shore Hospital in Sydney, since there was an excellent haemodialysis service already in action. However, in that institution four patients had recently been treated in the intensive care unit with acute respiratory failure and polyuric acute renal failure and who had become anuric during the course of the illness. Oligoanuria had coincided with the first two episodes of haemodialysis and as usual haemodialysis in these critically ill patients had been associated with mild hypotension and the institution of increased inotropic support. Since that time, CAVHD had been instituted with great success, and the pump system of high volume venous–venous haemofiltration was also in use. This had put some pressure on the nurses in the intensive care unit to learn the technique and to supervise a blood pump functioning continuously in the ITU. This did not seem to be a problem after the first two or three patients. Dr Lazarus commented that the urine output often fell in patients started on haemodialysis. It was not necessary to lower the blood pressure to make the urine flow rate disappear to nothing. In his hands he said CAVHD also made the urine flow rate reduce. He thought that CAVHD was a rapidly evolving procedure in the States at the present time. Dr Linton replied that its introduction was being limited somewhat in Canada. He knew of two trials in which it was being examined and he thought that until it had been shown to be of proven benefit over and above haemodialysis it should continue to be used only in the context of a controlled clinical trial.

Dr Schrier took up the problem of middle molecules. He told the workshop that these molecules had been originally described in the early 1960s when two patients with a uraemic neuropathy improved on peritoneal dialysis. He was highly sceptical concerning the toxicity or existence of middle molecules and warned against the development of techniques which emphasized their clearance. Dr Mason replied that he had not invoked middle molecular clearance as an important component of the haemofiltration system. Nevertheless in the absence of a positive identification of the toxins involved in the uraemic process, clearance of molecular weight substances from 0 to 20 000 daltons should be the basis for renal support.

Dr Parsons pursued this problem of clearance of middle molecules. He was particularly concerned about the clearance of the various mediators, particularly cytokines – interleukin-1 and tumour necrosis factor – in patients developing multiple organ failure. He wondered whether a patient should be treated by a period of plasmapheresis, 50 ml kg^{-1} plasma exchange over 4 hours followed by 20 h of haemofiltration. Dr Bihari referred to the data of Gottlieb et al. who had measured various different mediators – endorphins, eicosanoids etc. – in the haemofiltrate of a number of patients with acute respiratory and other organ failure. They demonstrated that haemofiltration could improve lung function and also effectively clear a variety of mediators.

Dr Neild asked about the practicalities of parenteral nutrition in patients receiving continuous arteriovenous or venous–venous haemofiltration. Dr Mason thought that about 5% of the sugar and the amino acids were lost directly into the filtrate. Naturally, this percentage is related to the actual volume filtered. At about 25 litres of filtrate a day, a loss of 5% of the calories and nitrogen administered, can be expected.

Chapter 27

Renal Replacement Therapy in the ICU: Approaches in Switzerland

P. M. Suter, R. Malacrida, M Levy and H. Favre

Introduction

Different techniques for efficient kidney replacement therapy are used in the intensive care unit (ICU). During the last 10 years, a progressive shift from classical haemodialysis towards the use of continuous arterio-venous haemofiltration has been observed for the treatment of acute renal failure in the critically ill (Bartlett et al. 1986; Kramer 1985; Stevens et al. 1988; Teschan et al. 1980). This method has the advantage of making possible a more efficient control of the water and metabolic balances even in patients with unstable haemodynamic parameters who can be poorly managed by conventional haemodialysis techniques (Keskaviah and Shapiro 1982; Mault et al. 1987). However, this very simple method has some limitations in patients with insufficient blood flow to generate adequate ultrafiltration to compensate for uraemia. To overcome this problem, a vacuum pump has been attached to the filtrate port (Kaplan et al. 1983; Milant et al. 1985), or the addition of a blood pump to the system has been used and proved to be efficient (Favre et al. 1987; Höfliger et al. 1984). These additions have altered the original concept of simplicity of a technique which was conceived to avoid the use of any mechanical support (Kramer et al. 1977, 1982).

Survey of 52 Medical, Surgical or Multidisciplinary ICUs
(Malacrida et al. 1988)

To assess the most frequent indications for extracorporeal renal replacement therapy in the intensive care units in Switzerland, a questionnaire was sent to the

64 units recognized for the official 2-year training for ICU nurses; 52 questionnaires were returned completed, corresponding to a return rate of 81%. Table 27.1 shows the preferred kidney replacement therapies for the years 1982 and 1985. The shift towards continuous haemofiltration is evident.

Table 27.1. Preferred kidney replacement techniques in the ICU in Switzerland for 1982 and 1985, and for different underlying conditions

	1982	1985	Aetiology of acute renal failure		
			Post-traumatic	Postoperative	Cardiogenic shock
Haemodialysis (%)	83.3	38	40	40	14
Continuous haemofiltration (%)	2.7	45	45	53	57
Peritoneal dialysis (%)	14	17	15	7	29

From Malacrida et al. (1988).

Kidney Replacement Therapy in a Surgical ICU

In our surgical ICU, 45 patients were treated in 1986 and 1987 with continuous veno-venous haemofiltration (CVVH). Patients' data and underlying diagnosis are summarized in Table 27.2. The mean age ± SD was 55 ± 7 years. About one-third were patients who sustained multiple trauma, involving the central nervous system and chest, abdomen and skeletal injury in most cases. Another third of the patients presented with acute kidney failure after cardiac or major vascular surgery in high-risk cases. In the group presenting after abdominal surgery, acute pancreatitis or peritonitis were the underlying diagnoses in 10 of the 12 patients.

Table 27.2. Patient data, diagnosis and treatment

No. of patients	Diagnosis	Infection present	Mean systolic and diastolic BP	Vasopressive drugs	Mechanical ventilation
14	Polytrauma	12	110 ± 2 / 80 ± 3	14	14
14	Cardiac or vascular surgery	8	90 ± 4 / 60 ± 5	13	12
12	Abdominal surgery	12	90 ± 5 / 60 ± 5	12	12
5	Other	2	100 ± 3 / 60 ± 4	5	4
45	Total	34 (76%)		44 (98%)	42 (93%)

The mean duration of CVVH was 9 ± 2 days (range 1–23 days). All patients had parenteral nutrition on day 1 of CVVH; in 12 of these enteral nutrition was started during CVVH. As can be seen from Table 27.2, all patients had a number of other organ failures, mostly cardiocirculatory (98% of all patients) and respiratory (93%) insufficiency. The mean number of organ failures for the whole group was 3.7. The ICU mortality rate was 66%, the hospital mortality 70%.

Technique of CVVH

Venous access was obtained by cannulation of the femoral, internal jugular or subclavian vein with a double lumen catheter (VasCath^R Gambro) using the Seldinger technique. Three different haemofilters were used: FH 66 (Gambro), Diafilter D 30 (Amicon) and Hospal SCU CAVH. Before use, all the filters were rinsed with 1 litre of saline solution containing 5000 IU heparin and flushed with another litre of isotonic saline solution. The haemofilters were connected to the double lumen catheter using conventional haemodialysis lines. The blood flow was maintained at a constant rate of 100–150 ml min^{-1} by a blood circulating pump to obtain a pressure in the haemofilter of about 70 mmHg.

This resulted in the removal of 800–1300 ml of ultrafiltrate per hour. The haemodynamic condition remained stable on vasoactive drugs. A negative fluid balance could be achieved in all patients, but in some cases only after 2–3 days of CVVH.

Monitoring and safety features of the system included a venous pressure sensor, an air detector and an automatic clamp on the venous line using the corresponding AK5 module (Gambro). Anticoagulation of the extracorporeal circuit was initiated by the intravenous administration of 1000–2000 IU heparin as a bolus injection followed by a constant infusion of heparin at a rate of 250–750 IU h^{-1}. The substitution fluid was given in the post-dilution mode using a standard solution containing (in mmol l^{-1}): Na 142, K 0, lactate 44.5, Mg 1.5, Ca 1.25, Cl 100. If the patient presented with a metabolic acidosis at the beginning of the procedure (arterial pH < 7.3) substitution was achieved with a 1/2 v/v 1.3% bicarbonate solution/standard solution. As the output of ultrafiltrate remained constant throughout the procedure, fluid balance was adjusted according to the condition of the patient by adapting hourly the rate of intake, i.e. substitution fluid plus the amount of fluid required for parenteral alimentation and vehicle of drugs. Efficiency of the metabolic control was assessed by measurement of serum urea and creatinine. Effect of haemofiltration on the pulmonary function was evaluated by the ratio arterial pO_2/F_IO_2 in the patients who were on mechanical ventilation. Finally blood parameters including haematocrit, leucocytes and platelets were controlled regularly.

Antibiotics were prescribed according to a dosage adapted for a GFR of 20 ml min^{-1} since creatinine clearance averaged 18 ml min^{-1}. This estimation was proven to be correct by measurements of the blood levels of the most commonly used antibiotics.

CVVH was associated with a decrease in plasma urea and creatinine levels to plateau values of 25–45 mmol l$^-$ and 220–320 μmol l^{-1} respectively. The ratios

pO_2/F_IO_2 were 255 ± 122 at initiation of the procedure versus 222 ± 81 at day 3. No significant changes were observed in haematocrit, leucocytes and platelets during the first 3 days of CVVH.

Conclusions

The treatment of acute renal failure in the ICU with CVVH has made the management of patients with multiple organ failure much easier. The ability to remove large amounts of fluid allows normalization of the extracellular volume and adequate parenteral nutrition (Lauer et al. 1983; Mault et al. 1984). The pump-driven CVVH permits a constant flow through the filter despite haemodynamic instability and a decrease of clotting in the circuit. Our experience has shown that ICU-trained nurses can be rapidly instructed in CVVH and take responsibility without the help of specialized personnel.

The advantages of CVVH (Table 27.3) have made its introduction as the preferred technique of kidney replacement therapy in most ICUs of our country a reality.

Table 27.3. Advantages and disadvantages of different kidney replacement therapies cited by ICU physicians

Advantages	Disadvantages
Classical haemodialysis	
Good + fast elimination of urea, creatinine, K	Requires specific personnel
Treatment periods limited to 3–5 hours per day	Fluid balance more difficult to achieve
Continuous arteriovenous haemofiltration	
Simple technical equipment, no pump necessary	Filtration rate depends on arterial pressure + cardiac output
Can be handled by ICU nurses	Danger of air embolism
Good elimination of water	Slow clearance of urea, creatinine, K, etc.
Continuous venovenous haemofiltration	
Good monitoring of line permeability	Costly equipment with specific "gags"
Filtration rate easy to regulate	
Can be handled by ICU nurses	
Good elimination of water	Slow clearance of urea, creatinine, K, etc.

References

Bartlett RH, Mault JR, Dechert RE, Palmer J, Swartz RD, Port FK (1986) Continuous arteriovenous hemofiltration: improved survival in surgical acute renal failure? Surgery 2: 400–408

Favre H, Levy M, Klohn M, Suter PM (1987) Continuous veno-venous hemofiltration. In: Paganini E, Geronemus R (eds) Proceedings of Third International Symposium on Acute Continuous Renal Replacement Therapy. Kidney Foundation, pp 87–93

Höfliger N, Keusch G, Biswanger U (1984) Spontaneous arteriovenous hemofiltration in the treatment of acute renal failure. Kidney Int 25: 988

Kaplan AA, Longnecker RE, Folkert VW (1983) Suction assisted continuous arteriovenous hemofiltration. Trans Am Soc Artif Intern Organs 29: 408–413

Keskaviah P, Shapiro FL (1982) A critical examination of dialysis-induced hypotension. Am J Kidney Dis 2: 290

Kramer P (1985) Arteriovenous hemofiltration. A kidney replacement therapy for the intensive care unit. Springer-Verlag, Berlin Heidelberg New York

Kramer P, Wigger W, Rieger D, Matthaei D, Scheler F (1977) Arteriovenous hemofiltration: A new and simple method for treatment of overhydrated patients resistant to diuretics. Klin Wochenschr 55: 1121–1122

Kramer P, Bohler J, Kehr A, Grone HJ, Schrader J, Matthaei D, Scheler F (1982) Intensive care potential of continuous arteriovenous hemofiltration. Trans Am Soc Artif Intern Organs 28: 28–32

Lauer A, Saccaggi A, Ronco C, Belledonne M, Glabman S, Bosch J (1983) Continuous arteriovenous hemofiltration in the critically ill patient. Ann Intern Med 99: 455–460

Malacrida R, Fritz ME, Genoni M, Spira JC, Suter PM (1988) Verfahren der künstlichen Niere auf der Intensivstation. Med Klinik 83: 832–835

Mault JR, Kresowik RF, Dechert RE, Arnoldi DK, Swartz RD, Bartlett RH (1984) Continuous arteriovenous hemofiltration: The answer to starvation in acute renal failure? Trans Am Soc Artif Intern Organs 30: 203–206

Mault JR, Dechert RE, Lees P, Schwartz RD, Port FK, Bartlett RH (1987) Continuous arteriovenous filtration: An effective treatment for surgical acute renal failure. Surgery 101: 478–484

Milant T, Toupance O, Lavaud S, Melin JP, Seys GA, Chanard J (1985) Hémofiltration artérioveineuse continue dans l'insuffisance rénale aiguë. Intérêt de la régulation du débit d'ultrafiltration. Néphrologie 6: 239

Stevens PE, Davies SP, Brown EA, Riley B, Gower PE, Kox W (1988) Continuous arteriovenous haemodialysis in critically ill patients. Lancet I: 150–152

Teschan PE, Ahmad S, Hull AR, Nolph KD, Shapiro FL (1980) Daily dialysis–applications and problems. Trans Am Soc Artif Intern Organs 26: 600

Discussion

Dr Lazarus wondered how one could get an air embolus with an arteriovenous passive non-pumped system. Professor Suter explained that this could occur in patients who developed a markedly negative intrapleural pressure during respiration. If the venous return cannula is situated in the subclavian vein, then the negative pleural pressure during inspiration can be responsible for sucking air into the system. This problem was less important when the femoral vein was used as a form of access. Professor Suter was asked about the average nurse:patient ratio in Swiss intensive care units. Dr Bion wondered whether line disconnection and air embolism could be avoided if appropriate ratios were maintained. Apparently, on the early shift in the morning, there is an average of one nurse per patient, in a Swiss ICU. However, in the afternoon this ratio falls and on the night shift there is one nurse for every two patients. However, patients with three-organ failure or more, on average have 0.8 nurses per patient over a period of 24 hours. Dr Bion asked Professor Suter whether he thought that the complication rate of haemofiltration and dialysis was related to the intensity of nursing care. Professor Suter, and all participants, agreed that this was certainly the case. Nevertheless, complications can occur even in the presence of exceptional nurses and can be extremely hazardous, especially when no monitoring is in place. Professor Suter and Dr Bihari both emphasized that this was much more likely with spontaneous arteriovenous systems which lacked an alarm system for monitoring blood flow and preventing the introduction of air.

Dr Myers was curious to get a sense of how widespread the use of haemofiltration (CAVH) was in the management of patients with acute renal failure. He emphasized that the Stanford Unit had been through this phase and had abandoned the technique. He had modelled the technique carefully and thought that most of the resistance on the venous side was exerted by the cannula and the choice of the cannula was critical. The Stanford group had returned to an older technique that was essentially the same as that described by Dr Simpson – daily sequential filtration followed by haemodialysis during which no fluid was removed. Dr Myers was astonished at the rarity of unmanageable hypotension using this technique. He emphasized that the Stanford group were not inhibited in giving vasopressor drugs such as noradrenaline since there was now clear evidence in animal models that there is no autoregulatory capacity in the failed ATN kidney. Flow in the failed ATN kidney appears to be entirely pressure dependent as demonstrated by Congar et al. from Dr Schrier's institution. He wondered whether other centres had abandoned CAVH. Dr Bihari was pleased to hear his own prejudices confirmed by the words of Professor Suter in Switzerland and Dr Myers in the United States. He described how the Middlesex Hospital Intensive Care Unit had moved from haemodialysis to CAVH and then on to a pumped veno-venous haemofiltration system during the period 1983 to 1986. In general Dr Bihari thought that most intensivists felt that a pump was essential. It allows one to perform renal support in all patients independently of their arterial blood pressure with the ability to produce clearances that allows an extremely tight control of the uraemic state. Dr Lazarus disagreed, and thought that CAVHD in which the dialysate was run in at 15 ml min^{-1} was clearly as effective as haemodialysis. He was concerned about giving a blood pump into the charge of the average nurse in an American ICU. It was not clear that they could cope with such a device and he thought that the installation of an unmanned pump operating at 100–150 ml min^{-1} was a dangerous activity. This was the minority view and Dr Simpson spoke for the majority. He said that the important point from the safety angle was that if one had a pump, then you had to monitor pump flow with a bubble trap in the circuit. Providing there were adequate alarms to detect air, then a blood pump was a very safe device to have in an intensive care setting. An unpumped circuit will work, but occasionally it makes fluid balance impossible and clearances are often far from adequate. At this stage the discussion was terminated.

Chapter 28

Anticoagulation and Extracorporeal Circuits: The Role of Prostacyclin

M. J. Weston

That the application of advanced technology in the intensive care unit is in the patient's best interests is too often taken for granted by those unfamiliar with its use and unwary of possible harmful effects of such technology. For example, the pioneers of haemodialysis recall how the technique was nearly abandoned because it often caused hypotension. This was shown to be due to hypovolaemia from unrecognized ultrafiltration and once understood, haemodialysis gradually became an accepted technique for the treatment of acute renal failure and later for chronic renal failure, although more subtle unwanted effects such as complement activation with pulmonary dysfunction and the effects of acetate in the dialysate on the heart have continued to emerge from time to time.

Hypotension was again to prove to be a problem in the development of charcoal haemoperfusion for the treatment of acute liver failure (Weston et al. 1977b). During investigation of this phenomenon platelet aggregates were found in the blood returning to the patient from the charcoal column and the role of heparin as the routine choice of anticoagulant for the extracorporeal circulation of blood was called into question.

The very existence of the platelet was still in doubt a hundred years ago and thought by some to be an artefact on the blood film. The vast sums of money now spent by the pharmaceutical industry to develop drugs to try to inhibit these "artefacts" testifies to the importance of platelets in the pathogenesis of atheroma, a major cause of death and disease today. If platelets can cause trouble on the native endothelium how much more likely are they to react when blood is pumped over the foreign surfaces of extracorporeal circuits?

Early attempts at haemodialysis were hampered by clotting and although hirudin obtained from the pressing of leaches paved the way for anticoagulation it was not until the discovery of heparin that haemodialysis began to make progress. It has taken several decades though to recognize the heterogeneous nature of heparin and the different biological properties of its various fragments (Salzman 1986). Low-molecular-weight fragments have less inhibitory activity for thrombin but more against activated factor X. Together with less platelet activating characteristics this has suggested to some that low-molecular-weight heparin could provide anticoagulation (factor Xa inhibition) without the risk of bleeding (less thrombin inhibition). Whether low-molecular-weight heparin will prove to be a cost-effective improvement on unfractionated heparin remains to be proven but the importance of protecting platelets during extracorporeal circulation is beginning to be recognized and is discussed below.

The first indication that commercially prepared unfractionated heparin might not provide comprehensive anticoagulation was that, used in higher dosage, it did not prevent the formation of platelet aggregates which could be detected by screen filtration pressure techniques in aliquots of blood leaving charcoal columns being used to treat patients with liver failure (Fig. 28.1). The appearance of these platelet aggregates coincided with sudden and severe hypotension (Fig. 28.2). Indeed, in experimental haemoperfusion circuits, platelet aggregation seemed to result in sudden shortening of thrombin clotting times (used to monitor the biological activity of heparin) implying the release of heparin neutralizing material (Weston et al. 1977a).

Perhaps platelets, in the process of aggregation, released their contents, some of which may have depressed the blood pressure and others neutralized heparin. Vasodepressant material in platelets has never been identified although it is known that if rat blood is allowed to clot the supernatant serum can depress blood pressure. In contrast with liver failure haemoperfusion on activated charcoal for exogenous poisoning and as an adjunct in the treatment of chronic renal failure by haemodialysis does not seem to lower blood pressure catastrophically (J. F. Winchester, personal communication 1978) and this raises a number of intriguing questions. For example, does the complex derangement of clotting and platelet function in hepatic necrosis render the patient more difficult to anticoagulate for extracorporeal circulation? Do the platelets of these patients absorb biologically active amines, peptides, amino acids, fatty acids or any of the other numerous compounds thought to accumulate in plasma and brain only to release them again with depressant effects on blood pressure when prompted to aggregate by the charcoal column?

Some but not all of these questions have been answered indirectly by the use during extracorporeal circulation of prostacyclin, the most potent inhibitor of platelet aggregation known to man.

Prostacyclin, now also called epoprostenol, is a very short-acting product of arachidonic acid metabolism. It is synthesized in endothelium, mesothelium and the kidney and in the latter organ in particular it has important vasodilatory properties. Its discovery and synthesis by the team at Wellcome in the United Kingdom led by John Vane has opened up the possibility of palliation of many disease processes mediated by vascular occlusion. Its use during extracorporeal circulation was suggested by Vane who had been approached to help identify the curious relationship between hypotension and the formation of platelet aggregates during charcoal haemoperfusion. This relationship seems to have been confirmed since use of prostacyclin during extracorporeal circulations of different types stops the formation of platelet aggregates and stabilizes blood pressure (Fig. 28.3) so long as insufficient of this potent vasodilator reaches the systemic circulation (Weston 1983). Moreover, the anticoagulant effect of heparin is potentiated by prostacyclin permitting in haemodialysis for chronic renal failure a reduction of heparin dosage of approximately 50% (Fig. 28.4) (Rylance et al. 1984). Platelet protection and heparin sparing with prostacyclin combine to

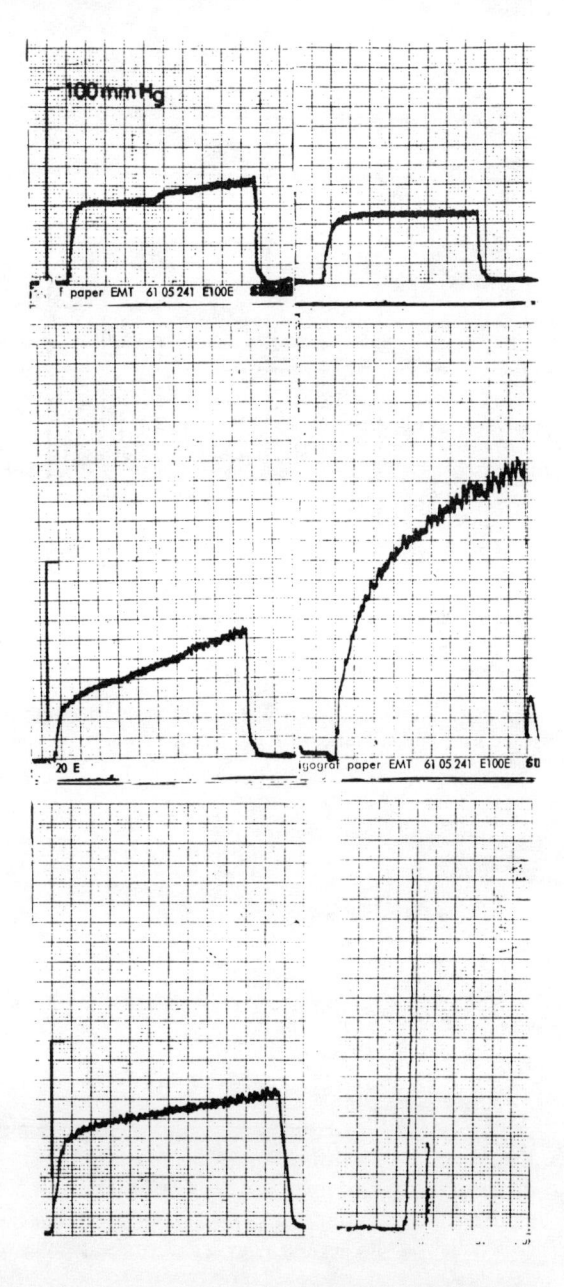

Fig. 28.1. Screen filtration pressure curves from aliquots of blood entering charcoal column (*on left*) and leaving the column (*on right*) at 10 minutes (*top*), 15 minutes (*middle*) and 20 minutes (*bottom*) after the start of haemoperfusion.

reduce blood loss after cardiopulmonary bypass and to make haemodialysis safer in patients with acute renal failure who may be at risk of bleeding for several different reasons, not least of which is the surgery that they might so often be in need of (Keogh et al. 1984).

The most dramatic demonstration of heparin sparing was shown during charcoal haemoperfusion in healthy dogs (Woods et al. 1980, Fig. 28.5). Although it was not possible to haemoperfuse these animals for long with

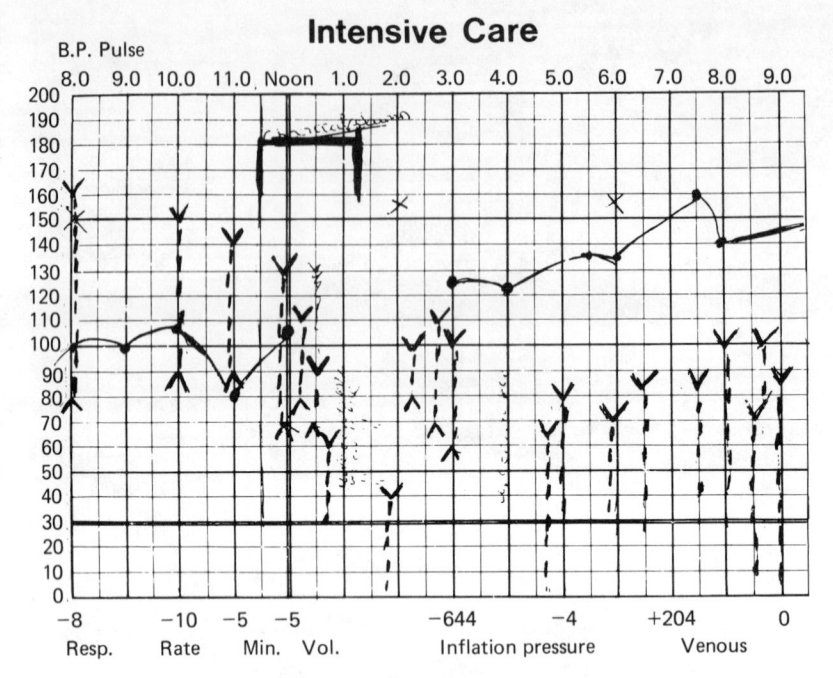

Fig. 28.2. Part of an Intensive Care Chart showing the decrease in blood pressure in a patient with acute liver failure being treated by charcoal haemoperfusion.

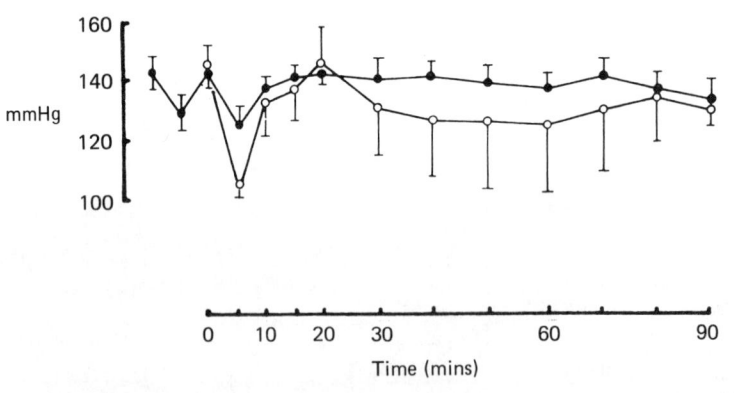

Fig. 28.3. Mean systolic blood pressures during haemodialysis experiments in healthy dogs. *Open circles*, dialysis with heparin alone. *Filled circles*, dialysis with heparin and prostacyclin.

prostacyclin alone because clotting occurred this was not the case with haemodialysis in this species (Woods et al. 1978). An infusion of prostacyclin into the dialyser inlet line enabled dialysis to proceed without clotting in the circuit and raised the possibility that patients with renal failure, at risk of bleeding or already doing so, could be dialysed without heparin (see below). Interestingly, prostacyclin does not abolish the extraction of platelets that occurs early during dialysis due to adhesion to the cuprophane membranes but it abolishes the later decrease

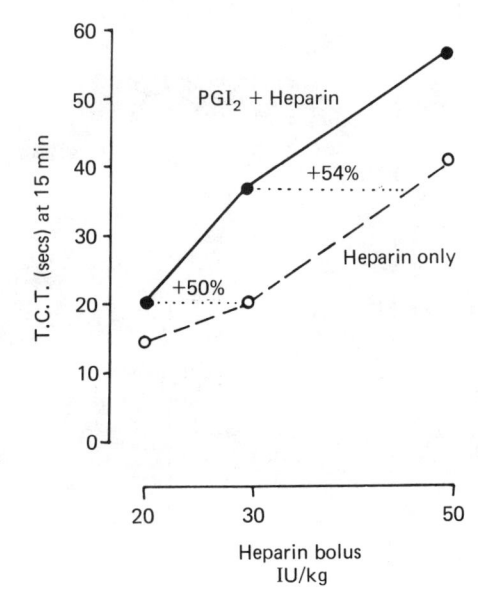

Fig. 28.4. Thrombin clotting times (TCT) in patients with chronic renal failure dialysed with various boluses of heparin showing that infusion of prostacyclin (PGI$_2$) requires approximately 50% less heparin to produce an equivalent prolongation of the thrombin clotting time.

in platelets that results from formation of aggregates (Fig. 28.6). The screen filtration pressure technique to detect platelet aggregates is not applicable to patients with renal failure, probably because of the low haematocrit of such patients, but use of prostacyclin during human haemodialysis for chronic renal failure can be shown to protect platelets in other ways (Turney et al. 1980). First, the thrombocytopenia that occurs, although much more modest than in healthy animals, is minimized, rises in plasma beta thromboglobulin, a platelet-specific protein, are reduced and the effect of heparin is enhanced (implying inhibition of release of an antiheparin substance known as platelet factor 4). Platelets also contain Factor VIII although the endothelium is probably the richest source of this coagulation substrate. Widening of the ratio between antigenically determined Factor VIII and its coagulant activity is an indicator of disseminated intravascular coagulation and may be found in many patients with acute renal failure in whom sepsis is the cause. On the other hand a widened ratio of the Factor VIII moieties is often found in patients with chronic uraemia suggesting a state of low-grade consumptive coagulopathy and this ratio is widened further by haemodialysis which raises the plasma concentrations of the antigenic moiety. Use of prostacyclin in this group of patients during dialysis prevents this rise in antigenic Factor VIII but it is not clear whether this is an effect on the platelet or endothelium or both (Turney et al. 1981).

How can these experimentally demonstrated effects of prostacyclin be put to use for the benefit of the patient in the intensive therapy unit? Caution is required before extrapolating the results of experiments in healthy animals to patients who have different diseases requiring different forms of extracorporeal support. Apart from species differences in the haemostatic mechanisms the diseases themselves affect platelets and coagulation in different ways. Although a bleeding diathesis may be seen in uraemia and liver failure this is the result of very different mechanisms. In the former an acquired platelet defect affecting Factor VIII-mediated platelet adhesion to endothelium predominates but in liver

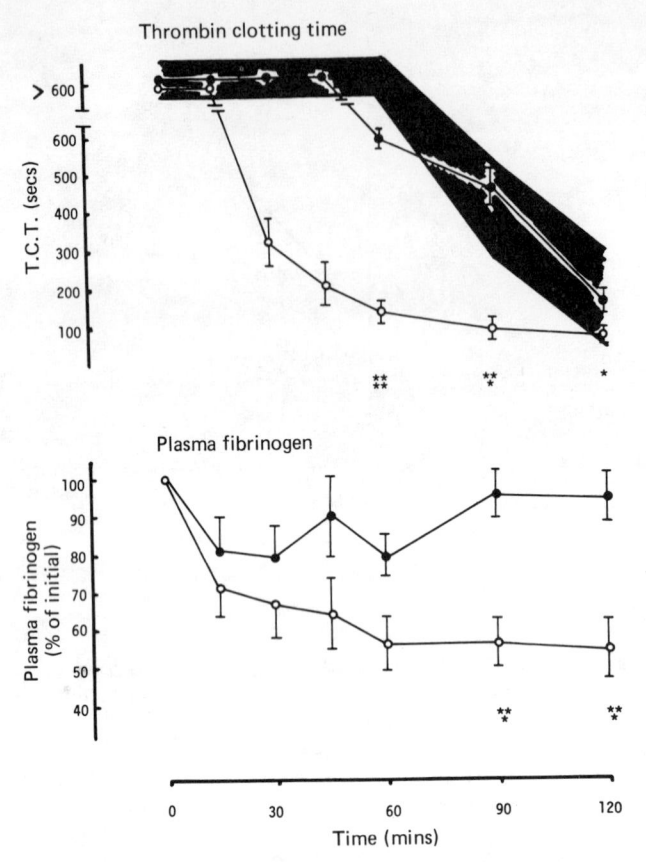

Fig. 28.5. *Upper panel*: thombin clotting times after injection of a bolus of heparin in healthy dogs (*shaded area*); after the same dose of heparin followed by charcoal haemoperfusion (*open circles*); and after the same treatment plus infusion of prostacyclin (*filled circles*). *Lower panel*: conservation of fibrinogen levels with prostacyclin (*filled circles*).

failure there is a failure to synthesize a wide range of clotting factors and possibly failure of the liver to release thrombopoietin needed for the maturation of healthy platelets. Consumption of clotting factors and platelets may make variable contributions to both kidney and liver failure. Lastly, the stimulus to the haemostatic mechanisms by cuprophane dialysis membranes is probably less than that from a column of activated charcoal. Despite these reservations clinical experience has been gained in both liver failure and kidney failure employing prostacyclin during extracorporeal perfusion. First, there seems little doubt that if charcoal haemoperfusion for acute liver failure is helpful (Gimson et al. 1980) then the use of prostacyclin to prevent platelet aggregation and its consequences during haemoperfusion has a place until column design or improvements in heparin production and administration can be shown to overcome the problem (Weston 1978). Second, at Dulwich Hospital a combination of low doses of heparin and prostacyclin infusion has been used in over a hundred haemodialyses in patients who were bleeding or at risk of doing so without aggravating the problem in any instance. The regime used is as follows:

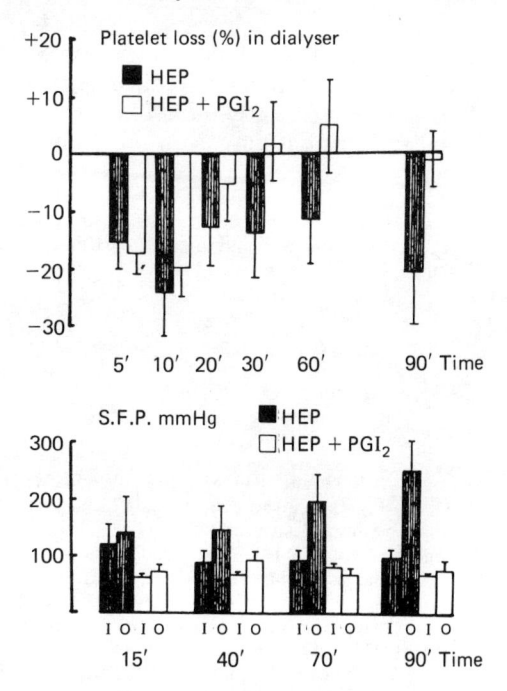

Fig. 28.6. Haemodialysis in healthy dogs with heparin (HEP) or heparin plus prostacyclin (PGI$_2$). *Upper panel*: platelet extraction by dialyser. *Lower panel*: screen filtration pressure (SFP). *I*, dialyser inlet line, *O*, dialyser outlet line.

1. Add 0.5 mg prostacyclin to 50 ml glycine buffer in syringe pump.
2. Infuse intravenously for 30 minutes at
   1.5 ml h^{-1} for body weight < 60 kg
   2.0 ml h^{-1} for body weight 60–80 kg
   2.5 ml h^{-1} for body weight > 80 kg.
3. Measure baseline Hemochron (activated clotting time).
4. Start haemodialysis with 30 unit kg^{-1} bolus of heparin.
5. Resite prostacyclin infusion to dialyser inlet line.
6. Infuse further boluses of heparin every 30 minutes to keep Hemochron time 15%–20% above baseline value.

If the dialysis has to be interrupted for any reason turn off the prostacyclin infusion to avoid a hypotensive bolus when restarting the dialysis and infuse more heparin to avoid clotting in the static circuit.

Although there are reports that haemodialysis can be carried out without any anticoagulation at all, blood flow rates have to be high and the circuit may have to be irrigated with saline at intervals during the dialysis. It would appear that such techniques have no particular advantage and it is difficult to imagine that they preserve coagulation factors and platelets and thus could conceivably aggravate any bleeding the patient may have.

Comparison of anticoagulation regimes for haemodialysis in acute renal failure is not really amenable to evaluation in controlled clinical trials because of the large number of variables, but further clinical experience is needed to evaluate the place of prostacyclin in extracorporeal circulation. The evidence so far is that prostacyclin is a potent in vivo inhibitor of platelet reactivity. Its use during extracorporeal circulation conserves platelets and may prevent other derangements of coagulation and reduce heparin requirements, so minimizing the risk of bleeding. Its use early on in illnesses characterized by platelet consumption and renal impairment may even pre-empt the need for dialysis, but that is another story!

Acknowledgements. This short review draws on the work of many colleagues at Dulwich Hospital and King's College Hospital and in particular I must thank H. F. Woods, J. H. Turney, N. Dodd, P. B. Rylance, G. Ash, M. Fewell, M. P. Gordge and the nurses on the Renal Unit at Dulwich Hospital.

References

Gimson AES, Hughes RD, Mellon PJ, Woods HF, Langley PG, Canalese J, Williams R, Weston MJ (1980) Prostacyclin to prevent platelet activation during charcoal haemoperfusion in fulminant hepatic failure. Lancet I: 173–175

Keogh AM, Rylance PB, Weston MJ, Parsons V (1984) Prostacyclin (epoprostenol) haemodialysis in patients at risk of haemorrhage. Proc Eur Dial Transplant Nurses Assoc 13: 51–54

Rylance PB, Gordge MP, Ireland H, Lane DA, Weston MJ (1984) Haemodialysis with prostacyclin (epoprostenol) alone. Proc Eur Dial Transplant Assoc Eur Ren Assoc 21: 281–286

Salzman EW (1986) Low-molecular-weight heparin. Is small beautiful? N Engl J Med 315: 957–959

Turney JH, Williams LC, Fewell MR, Parsons V, Weston MJ (1980) Platelet protection and heparin sparing with prostacyclin during regular dialysis therapy. Lancet II: 219–222

Turney JH, Woods HF, Fewell MR, Weston MJ (1981) Factor VIII complex in uraemia and effects of haemodialysis. Br Med J 282: 1653–1656

Weston MJ (1978) Platelet function in fulminant hepatic failure and effects of charcoal haemoperfusion. MD Thesis, Cambridge University

Weston MJ (1983) Prostacyclin and extracorporeal circulation. Br Med Bull 39: 285–288

Weston MJ, Hanid MA, Rubin MH, Langley PG, Mellon PJ, Williams R (1977a) Biocompatibility of coated and uncoated charcoal during haemoperfusion in healthy dogs. Eur J Clin Invest 7: 401–406

Weston MJ, Langley PG, Rubin MH, Hanid MA, Mellon PJ, Williams R (1977b) Platelet function in fulminant hepatic failure and effect of charcoal haemoperfusion. Gut 18: 897–902

Woods HF, Ash G, Weston MJ, Bunting S, Moncada S, Vane JR (1978) Prostacyclin can replace heparin in haemodialysis in dogs. Lancet II: 1075–1077

Woods HF, Weston MJ, Bunting S, Moncada S, Vane JR (1980) Prostacyclin eliminates the thrombocytopenia associated with charcoal haemoperfusion and heparin and fibrin consumption. Int J Artif Organs 3: 127–132

Discussion

The first question that arose in the discussion of the use of prostacyclin was its cost. Dr Weston emphasized it was expensive, but then good intensive care was also expensive. He agreed with Dr Bihari that it was all very well spending enormous amounts of money looking after these patients with multiple organ failure – nurses' salaries, unit overheads, expenditure on other consumables – but then quibbling over the cost of a single drug, which might actually improve the outcome of the patient. Dr Bihari asked several rhetorical questions; What was the cost of catastrophic bleeding in a patient requiring acute haemodialysis or arteriovenous haemofiltration in the intensive care unit, and did the administration of prostacyclin reduce the time spent on renal support? Similarly, by preserving the patency of the circuit did prostacyclin reduce the number of filters required in treatment and did it reduce the nursing time required for priming the extracorporeal circuits in those that clot up? Of course, no one was (or is able) to put a figure on all this; all that was concluded was that the drug itself is expensive and it makes dialysis and haemofiltration a more expensive procedure.

Dr Bion asked whether it might be more appropriate to infuse the prostacyclin directly into the patient, rather than infusing the drug into the arterial limb of the extracorporeal circuit. Dr Weston agreed that it might be appropriate to pre-treat the patient for half an hour with prostacyclin before starting the extracorporeal circulation of blood. The regimen used widely in the United Kingdom consists of pre-treating the patient for 30 minutes with 5 ng kg^{-1} min^{-1} and providing the blood pressure does not fall, increasing the dose by 1 ng kg^{-1} min^{-1} every 10–15 minutes once the extracorporeal circulation was in place. A maximum of 10–20 ng kg^{-1} min^{-1} is the usual dose tolerated with few side effects. Several participants had observed increases in blood pressure associated with the administration of prostacyclin in some patients as myocardial function had improved. Dr Smithies emphasized the importance of maintaining adequate cardiac filling pressures during the infusion of prostacyclin as there was no doubt that the vasodilatation could produce relative hypovolaemia. Dr Weston referred to his other experiences of using prostacyclin in the management of patients with cerebral malaria, the haemolytic uraemic syndrome and other consumptive coagulopathies. He thought that if there was no response in the latter case to the administration of fresh plasma, plasma exchange and heparin, then it might be worthwhile infusing prostacyclin. Certainly, the paediatricians had had great success in treating meningococcal septicaemia with prostacyclin infusions. Dr Bihari pointed out that whilst there was an enormous amount of clinical experience with the use of prostacyclin in patients requiring intensive care, there were very few controlled clinical trials available to assess its efficacy. The data remain incredibly anecdotal, but in general many clinicians have been impressed by the drug in certain conditions.

Chapter 29

Nutritional Support in Acute Renal Failure in the Critically Ill

R. A. Little, I. T. Campbell, C. J. Green, R. Kishen and S. Waldek

In the assessment of nutritional requirements and the efficacy of support, it is important to identify precisely those groups of critically ill patients to be considered.

This short review will, of necessity, be limited to those patients in acute renal failure (ARF) who are being treated in an Intensive Therapy Unit (ITU). They can, therefore, be compared to the hypercatabolic ARF or Group 3 patients described by Lee (1980). Such cases have a rapid daily increase in blood urea concentration (> 12 mmol l^{-1}) and are often already suffering from severe multiple injuries and/or the septic complications of surgery. Thus in such patients the development of ARF is one of the features of multiple organ failure which is still associated with an unacceptably high morbidity and mortality rate (Bihari 1987). Their nutritional management, often parenteral, should already be a matter of concern as it has been suggested that attention to such matters markedly improves the prognosis of patients with major intra-abdominal sepsis (Irving et al. 1985). The development of ARF ought not be taken as a sign that such nutritional support should be stopped, indeed as succinctly stated previously, "the metabolic/nutritional care of acute renal failure patients is of paramount importance in the total body concept whilst that of dialysis is of secondary importance. Thus if a patient's nutritional/metabolic requirements are of a certain magnitude then these should not be curtailed to reduce the frequency of dialysis but, on the contrary, dialysis be undertaken as frequently as is necessary to accommodate a patient's requirements" (Lee 1980).

A consideration of the metabolic disturbances characteristic of trauma and sepsis will be followed by discussion of those features of ARF and its treatment (haemodialysis or haemofiltration) which might modify these responses before the nutritional management of ARF is considered.

Metabolic Responses to Injury and Sepsis

We are concerned with the "flow" phase pattern of response (Cuthbertson 1942) which is characterized by an increase in metabolic rate, the extent of which is directly related to the severity of injury and sepsis (Wilmore 1977). Multiple long-bone fractures increase metabolic rate by some 10%–20%, rises of 30%–40% are seen in severe sepsis but the largest rises (100% increase) are seen after major burns (Davies 1982) and after severe head injuries (Clifton et al. 1986). The real increases may be larger than these, since the flow phase is superimposed on a declining background level of resting energy expenditure due to reductions in food intake and physical activity. It is important to realize, however, that even in severe sepsis measured metabolic rates in excess of 2500 kcal day^{-1} are uncommon (Stoner et al. 1983). The increase in metabolic rate may be limited by restrictions imposed by the cardiovascular and respiratory systems. It is a prime function of intensive therapy to ensure that oxygen delivery is maintained by appropriate respiratory and cardiovascular support as it has been clearly demonstrated that increases in oxygen consumption are associated with improvements in survival in septic shock (Shoemaker 1986). There are some critically ill patients who have a persistent low oxygen uptake in spite of a high oxygen delivery and in these it has been suggested that there is a microcirculatory defect which might be amenable to pharmacological manipulation (Bihari 1987).

The pathogenesis of the hypermetabolism is unclear and there may be a number of factors involved, the relative contributions of which may depend on the underlying conditions (Stoner 1987; Little 1988). There is good evidence that after burns there is enhanced sympatho-adrenal activity secondary to a central resetting of metabolic activity (Wilmore 1977). There may also be a need to provide the latent heat of evaporation of water from the surface of a burned wound or a laparostomy. The wound itself – the "extra" organ – will contribute to the increased glucose–lactate cycling, an energy-consuming process and will also increase metabolic rate in other ways (Wilmore 1986). It has a high oxygen consumption and a hyperaemic circulation which is not under nervous control and will, therefore, require an increase in cardiac output, incurring extra energy expenditure by the heart. Other factors which may be involved include substrate cycling (Wolfe et al. 1987), the generation of O_2-free radicals and, of course, the Q_{10} effect of the raised body temperature.

The hypermetabolism is accompanied by changes in the control of substrate metabolism. Insulin resistance is the hallmark of glucose metabolism in the "flow" phase and reflects abnormalities in both liver and muscle. Studies in thermally and non-thermally injured patients have shown a decreased glucose disposal in the face of supra-physiological plasma concentrations of insulin and at least a part of the insulin resistance is in skeletal muscle (Black et al. 1982; Brooks et al. 1984; Little et al. 1987). Similar observations have been made in septic surgical patients (Gump et al. 1974; White et al. 1987). The mechanism of this insulin resistance is not known, although it seems to be a post-receptor defect (Black et al. 1982; Henderson 1988). Immobility may contribute (e.g. Dolkas and Greenleaf 1977) as may the counter-regulatory hormones glucagon, cortisol, growth hormone and the catecholamines. For example, the infusion in normal subjects, of adrenaline, glucagon and cortisol, with or without noradrenaline, resulted in peripheral insulin resistance and increases in nitrogen excretion and metabolic rate (e.g. Bessey et al. 1984). The changes produced were, however, quantitatively rather modest and other factors may also be involved e.g. one of the interleukins and/or tumour necrosis factor. A role for interleukin-1 is attractive in that its release from activated macrophages provides a link between the local and general responses to injury and sepsis; unfortunately initial studies have not been very encouraging (Watters et al. 1986).

During the "flow" phase the rate of fat oxidation is higher than expected from the plasma non-esterified fatty acid (NEFA) concentration (Birkhahn et al. 1980; Frayn et al. 1984). The turnover of NEFA is also increased although there is no obvious relationship between NEFA turnover and oxidation (Nordenström et al. 1983). Normally fat oxidation is suppressed by the administration of large quantities of exogenous glucose owing to the release of insulin. Hypermetabolic septic and burns patients as well as those after major surgery behave abnormally in that this suppression is not complete even when plasma insulin concentrations are controlled (Nordenström et al. 1983; Stoner et al. 1983; White et al. 1987). The reasons for this preferential oxidation of fat are not clear although it has been suggested that further stimulation of sympathetic activity by the administered glucose overrides the effects of insulin (Nordenström et al. 1981).

The metabolism of free fatty acids is facilitated by carnitine which is involved in the transport of long chain fatty acids into the mitochondria. Carnitine is normally derived from the diet or is synthesized from the two amino acids lysine and methionine. In the absence of any dietary intake this means that carnitine has to be synthesized from the breakdown of endogenous protein. Urinary carnitine losses are increased in trauma (Cederblad et al. 1983), burns (Cederblad et al. 1981) and infection (Tanphaichitr and Lerdvuthisopon 1981). The amount of carnitine lost after injury seems to bear a positive correlation with urinary nitrogen and 3-methyl histidine excretion. (Cederblad et al. 1983). There is also some evidence that it is reduced by branched chain amino acid administration. (Cederblad et al. 1983).

There are also changes in the balance between whole body protein synthesis and breakdown during the "flow" phase (reviewed by Rennie 1985). Patients undergoing elective surgery showed a negative nitrogen balance arising mainly from a decreased rate of protein synthesis with a normal or even decreased rate of breakdown. More severely injured patients show increased protein breakdown with, in some cases, an increased rate of protein synthesis. It has been suggested that the changes observed represent an interaction between the degree of injury and nutritional state; increasing severities of injury cause increasing rates of both synthesis and breakdown, whereas undernutrition tends to depress synthesis (Clague et al. 1983). A major site of the net protein loss during the hypercatabolic "flow" phase is skeletal muscle with a marked efflux of amino acids occurring from all skeletal muscle beds, not just those directly damaged. Liver is the other tissue in which protein turnover is of particular interest at this time. There is an increase in the synthesis of the acute phase reactants while the synthesis of other proteins, such as albumin, decreases (Fleck et al. 1985).

Metabolic Changes Associated with ARF

Acute renal failure in intensive care arises most frequently as a complication of other conditions – trauma, sepsis etc. – and these in themselves may promote increased levels of energy expenditure and abnormalities in protein, fat and carbohydrate metabolism. There are few data on the energy requirements of acutely ill patients in renal failure. Measurements of energy balance in acute illness also suffer from the methodological problems of measuring energy expenditure. Oxygen consumption (energy expenditure) is frequently measured over a limited period and 24 hour energy expenditure extrapolated from the results. The validity of doing so, however, is questionable.

The alternative of measuring oxygen consumption continuously is impracticable in the "free-living" individual but it is possible in the ventilated patient. In one study 24 hour energy expenditure measurements have been made in ventilated patients in acute renal failure (Green et al. in press). They were studied for between 3 and 25 days and showed a median level of energy expenditure of 124% (range 90%–148%) of basal energy expenditure predicted by the Harris Benedict equation (based on height, weight, sex and age). This compared with 116% (range 95%–129%) in a comparable group of intensive care patients not in renal failure. The contribution of protein metabolism (calculated from urinary nitrogen and urea production rates) to total energy expenditure was 22.3 (± 1.8)% in the renal failure patients and was significantly higher than the 16.4 (± 1.8)% seen in the patients whose kidneys continued to function. The implication is that although energy expenditure of intensive care patients in acute renal failure does not appear to be very much greater than non-renal failure patients in similar circumstances the range of values of individual levels of expenditure is wider and protein appears to make a proportionately greater contribution.

A number of metabolic disturbances with direct relevance to the discussion above have been associated with ARF although, as mentioned above, it is often difficult to disassociate the responses to ARF from those to the underlying critical illness following injury or sepsis. Glucose intolerance has been widely reported in ARF (e.g. Westervelt and Schreiner 1962; Briggs et al. 1967; Luke et al. 1968) and it seems that the disappearance rate of glucose is improved by dialysis (e.g. Alfrey et al. 1967). Early studies suggested that the disturbance in glucose metabolism in uraemia did not seem to be related to defective insulin production or release but rather to the presence of dialysable antagonists and/or increased insulin degradation (Briggs et al. 1967; Alfrey et al. 1967; Fröhlich et al. 1978). For example, the activity of the plasma insulinase system found in the liver may be potentiated in ARF by glutathione (Westervelt and Schreiner 1962) and cysteine and guanidine which are capable of degrading insulin are present in uraemic serum (Alfrey et al. 1967). The situation is, however, complicated by recent experiments in acutely uraemic dogs, following bilateral nephrectomy, which have shown a reduction in both the production and hepatic removal of insulin (Cianciaruso et al. 1987). It has been suggested that the insulin resistance in uraemia is mediated by a post-receptor defect (Smith and DeFronzo 1982) and therefore may be analogous to that seen in trauma and sepsis. The counter-regulatory hormones may also be involved; for example, an increase in tissue sensitivity to glucagon, which is normalized by dialysis, has been reported (Sherwin et al. 1976).

There is some, rather inconclusive, evidence that carnitine is lost in haemodialysis and this may well affect fatty acid metabolism. Bohmer et al. (1978) and Battistella et al. (1978) have described decreases in plasma and muscle carnitine concentrations during dialysis, recovering over the ensuing 1–2 days. Lacour et al. (1980) were able to improve lipid profiles in patients on chronic haemodialysis by supplementing their diet with carnitine. Serum triglycerides decreased and high-density lipoprotein cholesterol increased to normal levels. However, it has been shown recently that carnitine supplementation in uraemic patients on chronic haemodialysis with depleted plasma levels of free carnitine did not affect whole body fat oxidation (Lundholm et al. 1988).

The clearance of NEFA (and fat emulsions) is also reduced in ARF (Lee et al. 1968; Lee 1980; Losowsky and Kenward 1968; Cramp et al. 1975) and once again this defect is improved by dialysis. The mechanism of the impaired clearance is unclear although it is possible that the usual binding sites for NEFA on albumin are blocked by other compounds (Lee et al. 1968). One hypothesis was that the increase in NEFA after dialysis was due to the use of heparin which increases the activity of lipoprotein lipase (e.g. Becker et al. 1955) although this has been disputed (Lawson 1965).

Considerable attention has been paid to protein metabolism in ARF because of the changes in nitrogen excretion and frequent claims that it is a catabolic state in which the loss of muscle mass can be extreme. Once again it is difficult to dissect out the effects of ARF from the markedly catabolic states with which it is commonly associated. However enhanced protein degradation and release of amino acids from skeletal muscle have been reported in acutely uraemic rats. These animals also show an increased hepatic production of glucose and urea (Lacy 1969; Fröhlich et al. 1974). Insulin resistance (Smith and DeFronzo 1982; Mitch et al. 1987), metabolic acidosis (May et al. 1986), the release of proteinases into the circulation (Heidland et al. 1988) and changes in the metabolism of branched chain amino acids (Mitch and Clark 1984) may all play a role in the increased protein degradation associated with ARF.

Nutritional Management of ARF

In most of the patients in ARF treated in an ITU nutritional support will be given parenterally and the safety of this technique in such patients is well established (Lee et al. 1967). Any complications that may arise seem to be those attributable to the technique of parenteral nutrition rather than to ARF *per se*. There has been considerable discussion on the value of nutritional therapy in ARF and although there seems to be a consensus that the provision of calories is of benefit the relative merits of different amino acid mixtures are far from clear.

Early studies showed that patients in chronic renal failure could be put into positive nitrogen balance if they were given essential amino acids (Giordano 1963). These patients seem to be able to utilize their own urea nitrogen for protein synthesis, a process in which the intestinal flora play an important role (Fürst et al. 1978). Although these organisms may also adversely affect uraemic patients by enhancing catabolism through the release of toxins, this process can be prevented by the use of appropriate antibiotics (Mitch 1978). The situation in ARF is much more complex and it is extremely difficult, if not impossible, to achieve positive nitrogen balance (Giordano et al. 1978). However, it has been suggested that the intravenous administration of essential amino acids and hypertonic glucose might be useful adjuncts in the treatment of ARF (Wilmore and Dudrick, 1969; Dudrick et al. 1970). In a prospective double-blind study Abel et al. (1973) showed, in a group of patients with postoperative ARF, that the administration of glucose and amino acids, as compared with glucose alone, enhanced the recovery of renal function although the overall survival rate was not improved. It should, perhaps, be emphasized that septic and/or trauma patients were excluded from this study. These encouraging results were supported by a larger study showing decreased mortality and morbidity in ARF patients receiving a fibrin hydrolysate as part of their parenteral nutrition (Baek et al. 1975). An experimental basis for these clinical observations is provided by studies using a model of acute tubular necrosis in the rat which showed that treatment with amino acids enhanced renal regeneration (Toback 1977).

The promise engendered by these studies has not been fully realized although it stimulated the development of a range of mixtures of amino acids – the "renal failure solutions". A randomized prospective study failed to show a difference in negative nitrogen balance, rate of recovery of renal function or survival in two groups of ARF patients infused either with dextrose and amino acids or dextrose alone (Leonard et al. 1975). It can always be argued that insufficient calories or amino acids have been given but studies using equal amounts of essential and non-essential amino acids (a total of 42 g day^{-1}) and hypertonic glucose failed to show an improvement in nitrogen balance or survival when compared to intravenous therapy with just 21 g day^{-1} of essential amino acids and glucose (Blumenkrantz et al. 1978; Kopple and Feinstein 1983). In a comprehensive review, Toback (1980) concluded that amino acid treatment has not been shown to improve survival in those patients who are the most severely ill. However, the use of branched-chain amino acids and especially their keto-analogues, in limiting protein degradation (e.g. Blackburn et al. 1978; Sapir et al. 1983) may repay further study. A note of caution to the uncritical use of amino acids must be sounded, there is evidence for nephrotoxicity in rats when mixtures of non-essential amino acids are infused in clinically relevant doses. They cause an abrupt decrease in glomerular filtration rate and may sensitize the kidney to ischaemic or toxic injury (Zager 1987).

No matter what nutrition regimen is used it must be remembered that dialysis itself can modify the availability of calories and amino acids. Haemodialysis removes not only "uraemic toxins" but also glucose and amino acids together with the hormones which may be involved in their utilization. For example 1–3 g of amino acids can be lost every hour and indeed the loss can be such that in patients on a protein-free diet repeated dialysis can lead to a deterioration in nutritional state (Young and Parsons 1966). The losses incurred during dialysis will depend on the efficiency of the equipment used and the composition of the dialysis solution. Manipulation of the concentration gradients between this solution and blood can prevent or even reverse the loss of glucose and amino acids from the blood (Di Palo et al. 1978). The addition of acetate to the dialysis solution can also contribute calories to the patient although in those with severe metabolic acidosis this gain should be forgone in favour of the use of bicarbonate.

Much of the concern about fluid overload in ARF can be overcome by the use of continuous arterio venous haemofiltration (CAVH). This technique has been shown to be effective in the treatment of the critically ill anuric patient with cardiovascular instability (Lauer et al. 1983), as well as those with diuretic resistant and terminal cardiac failure (Morgan et al. 1985), massive fluid overload (Silverstein et al. 1974) and multiple organ failure (Clarke 1985). Our own experience is that this form of therapy works very well, especially in septic patients with renal and multiple organ failure. Even in hypercatabolic patients haemodialysis can often be avoided particularly with continuous "high-flux" haemofiltration. We have achieved high fluid exchange rates of 30–35 l day^{-1} without undue cardiovascular disturbance with a net fluid loss of 2–5 l day^{-1}. In critically ill unstable patients this is often more than adequate to provide space for total parenteral nutrition (TPN) which can be continued without any restraint imposed by the need for fluid restriction. The TPN is infused on the venous side of the haemofilter without any apparent adverse effects.

Summary

In conclusion it seems that the development of ARF in the severely catabolic patient on the ITU should not greatly modify their nutritional management. The calorie requirements can be met by mixtures of carbohydrate and fat. The latter is often very useful as the preferential oxidation of fat is a feature of critical illness and fears that fat emulsions may adversely affect the filters used in haemodialysis have not been substantiated (Lee et al. 1967).

References

Abel RM, Beck CH, Abbott WM, Ryan JA, Barnet GO, Fischer JE (1973) Improved survival from acute renal failure after treatment with intravenous essential L-amino acids and glucose. N Engl J Med 288: 695–699

Alfrey AC, Sussman KE, Holmes JH (1967) Changes in glucose and insulin metabolism induced by dialysis in patients with chronic uremia. Metabolism 16: 733–740

Baek SE, Makabali GG, Bryan-Brown CW, Kusek J, Shoemaker WC (1975) The influence of parenteral nutrition on the course of acute renal failure. Surg Gynecol Obstet 141: 405–408

Battistella PA, Angelini C, Vergani L, Bertoli M, Lorenzi S (1978) Carnitine deficiency induced during haemodialysis. Lancet I: 939

Becker GH, Rall TW, Grossman MI (1955) Effect of heparin on the distribution of intravenously administered C^{14} labelled soya bean oil emulsions in rats. J Lab Clin Med 45: 786–791

Bessey PQ, Watters JM, Aoki TT, Wilmore DW (1984) Combined hormonal infusion simulates the metabolic response to injury. Ann Surg 196: 420–435

Bihari DJ (1987) Mismatch of the oxygen supply and demand in septic shock. In: Vincent JL, Thijs LG (eds) Septic shock – a European view. Springer-Verlag, Berlin Heidelberg New York, pp 148–160 (Update in intensive care and emergency medicine, vol 4)

Birkhahn RH, Long CL, Fitkin DL, Geiger JW, Blakemore WS (1980) Effects of major skeletal trauma on whole body protein turnover in man measured by L-[1, ^{14}C]-leucine. Surgery 88: 294–300

Black PR, Brooks DC, Bessey PQ, Wolfe RR, Wilmore DW (1982) Mechanisms of insulin resistance following injury. Ann Surg 196: 420–435

Blackburn GL, Etter G, MacKenzie T (1978) Criteria for choosing amino acid therapy in acute renal failure. Am J Clin Nutr 31: 1841–1853

Blumenkrantz MJ, Kopple JD, Koffler et al. (1978) Total parenteral nutrition in the management of acute renal failure. Am J Clin Nutr 31: 1831–1840

Bohmer T, Bergrem H, Eiklind K (1978) Carnitine deficiency induced during intermittent haemodialysis for renal failure. Lancet I: 126–128

Briggs JD, Buchanan KD, Luke RG, McKiddie MT (1967) Role of insulin in glucose intolerance in uraemia. Lancet I: 462–464

Brooks DC, Bessey PQ, Black PR, Aoki TT, Wilmore DW (1984) Post-traumatic insulin resistance in uninjured forearm tissue. J Surg Res 37: 100–107

Cederblad G, Larsson J, Nordstrom H et al. (1981) Urinary excretion of carnitine in burned patients. Burns 8: 102–109

Cederblad G, Schildt B, Larsson J, Liljedahj S-O (1983) Urinary excretion of carnitine in multiple injured patients on different regimes of parenteral nutrition. Metabolism 32: 383–389

Cianciaruso B, Saccià L, Terracciano V et al. (1987) Insulin metabolism in acute renal failure. Kidney Int 32: S109–S112

Clague MB, Keir MJ, Wright DD, Johnston IDA (1983) The effects of nutrition and trauma on whole-body protein metabolism in man. Clin Sci 65: 165–175

Clarke GM (1985) Multiple system organ failure. Clin Anaesthesiol 3: 1027–1053

Clifton GI, Robertson CS, Choi SC (1986) Assessment of nutritional requirements of head-injured patients. J Neurosurg 64: 895–901

Cramp DG, Moorhead JF, Wills MR (1975) Disorders of blood-lipids in renal disease. Lancet I: 672–673

Cuthbertson DP (1942) Post-shock metabolic response. Lancet I: 433–437

Davies JWL (1982) Physiological responses to burning injury. Academic Press, New York

DiPalo FQ, Buccianti G, Valenti GF, Miradoli R, Polli EE (1978) Nutritive hemodialysis in renal failure. Dial Transplant 7: 457–462

Dolkas CB, Greenleaf JE (1977) Insulin and glucose responses during bed rest with isotonic and isometric exercise. J Appl Physiol 43: 1033–1038

Dudrick SJ, Steiger E, Long JM (1970) Renal failure in surgical patients. Treatment with intravenous essential amino acids and hypertonic glucose. Surgery 68: 180–186

Fleck A, Colley CM, Myers MA (1985) Liver export proteins and trauma. Br Med Bull 41 (3): 265–273

Frayn KN, Little RA, Stoner HB, Galasko CSB (1984) Metabolic control in non-septic patients with musculo-skeletal injuries. Injury 16: 73–79

Fröhlich JJ, Schölmerich J, Hoppe-Seyler G et al. (1974) The effect of acute uraemia on gluconeogenesis in isolated perfused rat livers. Eur J Clin Invest 4: 453–458

Fröhlich J, Schollmeyer P, Gerok W (1978) Carbohydrate metabolism in renal failure. Am J Clin Nutr 31: 1541–1546

Fürst P, Ahlberg M, Alvestrand A, Bergström J (1978) Principles of essential amino acid therapy in uremia. Am J Clin Nutr 31: 1744–1755

Giordano C (1963) Use of exogenous and endogenous urea for protein synthesis in normal and uremic subjects. J Lab Clin Med 62: 231–246

Giordano C, De Santo NG, Senatore R (1978) Effects of catabolic stress in acute and chronic renal failure. Am J Clin Nutr 31: 1561–1571

Green CJ, McLelland P, Gilbertson AA, Wilkes RG, Bone JM, Campbell IT (in press) Energy balance in acute illness. Br J Nutr

Gump FE, Long C, Killian P, Kinney JM (1974) Studies of glucose intolerance in septic injured patients. J Trauma 14: 378–388

Heidland A, Schaefer RM, Heidbreder E, Hörl WH (1988) Catabolic factors in renal failure: therapeutic approaches. Nephrol Dial Transplant 3: 8–16

Henderson A (1988) Euglycaemic clamping in injured patients. MD Thesis, University of Manchester

Irving MH, White RH, Tresadern J (1985) Three years experience with an intestinal failure unit. Ann R Coll Surg Engl 67: 2–5

Kopple JD, Feinstein EI (1983) Nutritional therapy for patients with acute renal failure. In: Johnston IDA (ed) Advances in clinical nutrition. MTP Press, pp 113–122

Lacour B, Guilio SDi, Chanard J et al. (1980) Carnitine improves lipid anomalies in haemodialysis patients. Lancet II: 763–765

Lacy WW (1969) Effect of acute uremia on amino acid uptake and urea production by perfused rat liver. Am J Physiol 216: 1300–1305
Lauer A, Saccagi A, Ronco C et al. (1983) Continuous arteriovenous haemofiltration in the critically ill patient. Ann Intern Med 99: 455–460
Lawson LJ (1965) Parenteral nutrition in surgery. Br J Surg 52: 795–800
Lee HA (1980) The management of acute renal failure. In: Chapman A (ed) Acute renal failure. Churchill Livingstone, Edinburgh, pp 104–124 (Clinics in critical care medicine)
Lee HA, Sharpstone P, Ames AC (1967) Parenteral nutrition in renal failure. Postgrad Med J 43: 81–91
Lee HA, Hill LF, Ginks WR, Pohl JEF (1968) Some aspects of parenteral nutrition in the treatment of renal failure. In: Berlyne GM (ed) Nutrition in renal disease. Livingstone, Edinburgh, pp 216–227
Leonard CD, Luke RG, Siegel RR (1975) Parenteral essential amino acids in acute renal failure. Urology 6: 154–157
Little RA (1988) Metabolic rate and thermoregulation after injury. In: Ledingham IMcA (ed) Recent advances in critical care medicine, vol 3. Churchill Livingstone, Edinburgh, pp 159–173
Little RA, Henderson A, Frayn KN, Galasko CSB, White RH (1987) The disposal of intravenous glucose studied using glucose and insulin clamp techniques in sepsis and trauma in man. Acta Anaesth Belg 38: 275–279
Losowsky MS, Kenward DH (1968) Lipid metabolism in acute and chronic renal failure. J Lab Clin Med 71: 736–743
Luke RG, Briggs JD, McKiddie MT, Kennedy AC (1968) Studies in carbohydrate metabolism in renal failure. In: Berlyne GM (ed) Nutrition in renal disease. Livingstone, Edinburgh, pp 170–187
Lundholm K, Persson H, Wennberg A (1988) Whole body fat oxidation before and after carnitine supplementation in uremic patients on chronic haemodialysis. Clin Physiol 8: 417–426
May RC, Kelly RA, Mitch WE (1986) Metabolic acidosis stimulates protein degradation in rat muscle by a glucocorticoid-dependent mechanism. J Clin Invest 77: 614–621
Mitch WE (1978) Effects of intestinal flora on nitrogen metabolism in patients with chronic renal failure. Am J Clin Nut 31: 1594–1600
Mitch WE, Clark AS (1984) Specificity of the effect of leucine and its metabolites on protein degradation in skeletal muscle. Biochem J 222: 579–586
Mitch WE, May RC, Clark AS, Maroni BJ, Kelly RA (1987) Influence of insulin resistance and amino acid supply on muscle protein turnover in uremia. Kidney Int 32: S104–S108
Morgan SH, Mansell MA, Thompson FD (1985) Fluid removal by haemofiltration in diuretic resistant cardiac failure. Br Heart J 54: 218–219
Nordenström J, Jeevanandam M, Elwyn DH et al. (1981) Increasing glucose intake during total parenteral nutrition increases norepinephrine excretion in trauma and sepsis. Clin Physiol 1: 525–534
Nordenström J, Carpentier YA, Askanazi J et al. (1983) Free fatty acid mobilization and oxidation during total parenteral nutrition in trauma and infection. Ann Surg 198: 725–735
Rennie MJ (1985) Muscle protein turnover and the wasting due to injury and disease. Br Med Bull 41(3): 257–264
Sapir DG, Walser M, Moyer ED et al. (1983) Effects of α-ketoisocaproate and of leucine on nitrogen metabolism in postoperative patients. Lancet I: 1010–1014
Sherwin RS, Bastl C, Finkelstein FO et al. (1976) Influence of uremia and haemodialysis on the turnover and metabolic affects of glucagon. J Clin Invest 57: 722–731
Shoemaker WC (1986) Haemodynamic and oxygen transport patterns in septic shock: physiologic mechanisms and therapeutic implications. In: Sibbald WJ, Sprung CL (eds) Perspectives on sepsis and septic shock. Society of Critical Care Medicine, California, pp 203–234
Silverstein ME, Ford CA, Lysaght MJ, Henderson LW (1974) Treatment of severe fluid overload by ultrafiltration. N Engl J Med 291: 747–751
Smith D, DeFronzo RA (1982) Insulin resistance in uremia mediated by a post-binding defect. Kidney Int 22: 54–62
Stoner HB (1987) Interpretation of the metabolic effects of trauma and sepsis. J Clin Pathol 40: 1108–1117
Stoner HB, Little RA, Frayn KN, Elebute AE, Tresadern J, Gross E (1983) The effect of sepsis on the oxidation of carbohydrate and fat. Br J Surg 70: 32–35
Tanphaichitr V, Lerdvuthisopon N (1981) Urinary carnitine excretion in surgical patients on total parenteral nutrition. JPEN 5: 505–509
Toback FG (1977) Amino acid enhancement of renal regeneration after acute tubular necrosis. Kidney Int 12: 193–198

Toback FG (1980) Amino acid treatment of acute renal failure. In: Brenner BM, Stein JH (eds) Acute renal failure. Churchill Livingstone, Edinburgh, pp 202–228 (Contemporary issues in nephrology, vol 6)

Watters JM, Bessey PQ, Dinarello CA, Wolff SM, Wilmore DW (1986) Both inflammatory and endocrine mediators stimulate host responses to sepsis. Arch Surg 121: 179–189

Westervelt FB, Schreiner GE (1962) The carbohydrate intolerance of uraemic patients. Ann Intern Med 57: 266–276

White RH, Frayn KN, Little RA, Threlfall CJ, Stoner HB, Irving MH (1987) Hormonal and metabolic responses to glucose infusion in sepsis studied by the hyperglycaemic glucose clamp technique. JPEN 11: 345–353

Wilmore DW (1977) The metabolic management of the critically ill. Plenum Medical, New York

Wilmore DW (1986) The wound as an organ. In: Little RA, Frayn KN (eds) The scientific basis for the care of the critically ill. Manchester University Press, Manchester, pp 45–59

Wilmore DW, Dudrick SJ (1969) Treatment of acute renal failure with intravenous essential L-amino acids. Arch Surg 99: 669–673

Wolfe RR, Herndon DN, Jahoor F, Miyoshi H, Wolfe M (1987) Effect of severe burn injury on substrate cycling by glucose and fatty acids. N Engl J Med 317: 403–408

Young GA, Parsons FM (1966) Amino nitrogen loss during haemodialysis, its dietary significance and replacement. Clin Sci 31: 299–307

Zager RA (1987) Amino acid hyperalimentation in acute renal failure: a potential therapeutic paradox. Kidney Int 32: S72–S75

Discussion

Dr Myers opened the discussion by emphasizing the similarity between a patient in the intensive care unit with acute renal failure and an unfortunate human being who develops kwashiorkor; in both cases oedema with a low serum albumin is present, and there is activation of the renin–angiotensin system. Whilst he accepted that there was a real lack of good information on the use of nutritional support in acute renal failure, he could not accept that the right thing to do was to abandon the use of amino acid solutions. Profound protein malnutrition was unacceptable in patients supported in intensive care, and adequate nutrition forms an important part of their care. Dr Myers had made a very careful analysis of nitrogen balance in patients with acute renal failure, but in his studies, had not been able to achieve nitrogen balance in this population of patients. This was in spite of administering an apparently adequate mixture of amino acids and a reasonable, non-protein calorie load. He also deplored the development of further immunosuppression associated with malnutrition, and thought that nutritional support was one method of dealing with this problem that occurred in septic, uraemic patients. He agreed with Dr Little that one had to measure the metabolic rate in such cases and feed the patient the substrate that he appeared to be using.

Dr Little agreed that studies of the forearm were probably the most appropriate means of assessing utilization. Measurements of amino acid uptake by skeletal muscle in the forearm would be one method of monitoring. He agreed with Dr Myers that the toxicity argument of amino acids was a complete red herring. The only evidence of toxicity was Zager's study, and there were many other studies which had shown some benefit of amino acid infusions. Dr Linton interjected that the reason he had mentioned the meta-analysis of the various clinical studies of amino acids in patients with acute renal failure was to emphasize the fact that the evidence that amino acids are of benefit did not exist. Dr Linton thought that the discussants simply had to accept this finding and stop kidding themselves that they knew what they were doing was right. Of course, that was not to say that patients in intensive care should be starved; they should be fed as a part of the intensive care package in the face of the absence of knowledge that conclusively demonstrates this approach improves outcome.

Dr Arieff thought that it was inappropriate to use statistical analyses to write off nutritional support. An emphasis towards the metabolic processes by determining balance, metabolic rate and so forth was probably more appropriate. Dr Little was asked about anabolic hormones and whether they could be used in some patients who were wasting away in the intensive care unit. Dr Little did not know the answer to this, but pointed out that there was now some evidence that beta-receptor agonists might cause an increase in protein mass especially in skeletal muscle. These techniques of reducing muscle wasting were now under investigation.

Chapter 30

The Prevention of Severe Combined Acute Respiratory and Renal Failure in the Intensive Therapy Unit

D. J. Bihari

Introduction

Clinicians who work regularly in the Intensive Therapy Unit (ITU) recognize that survival from acute renal failure associated with critical illness depends upon many different factors. The epidemiological studies of Knaus and his colleagues (Knaus et al. 1985a; Knaus and Zimmerman 1985) have demonstrated that age, chronic health status, severity of illness and diagnosis are four important variables which affect outcome in general intensive care patients. More importantly perhaps, since it is impossible to influence these "patient-dependent" variables which are present on admission to a general ITU, has been the identification of other factors which may be manipulated to improve outcome (Knaus et al. 1986). These include the quality of nursing care, the presence or absence of a specialist director of intensive care, the success or otherwise of the various professional relationships existing in the ITU between medical, nursing and paramedical staff and, finally, the form of treatment. These patient-independent "unit" factors which may be described as the "process of care" reflect not only the smaller issues such as the use of colloid or crystalloid to resuscitate a patient from septic shock (Demling 1986), or the form of renal replacement therapy – haemofiltration or haemodialysis (Simmonds and Mansell 1986) – locally available, but also the global problems of administration, staffing, enthusiasm and the availability of resources. In this context, it has been particularly difficult to assess the various attempts to prevent or treat patients with severe combined acute respiratory and renal failure, so-called SCARRF (Wardle 1982; Cameron 1986; Bartlett et al. 1986; Simpson et al. 1987).

Although SCARRF is no more than a variant of multiple organ failure associated with severe sepsis and massive trauma (Cerra and Bihari 1989), its emergence as a clinical entity has been related primarily to the problems of defining the "multiple organ failure syndrome" in the ITU. In general, it has been difficult to obtain a working definition of "failure" (and/or "dysfunction") which lends itself to an assessment of each individual organ system function with the construction of a useful scoring system. A number have been proposed and although the most widely applied has been that of Knaus et al. (1985b), this too suffers from a number of limitations. One specific limitation of the system is the absence of criteria for the assessment of hepatic, gut, endocrine, skin, skeletal muscle and immune system function. By contrast, the requirement for renal replacement therapy in patients who are ventilator dependent immediately defines a population of patients with a substantially increased mortality rate compared with patients with acute renal or acute respiratory failure alone (Sweet et al. 1981; Cameron 1986; Wheeler et al. 1986). Nevertheless, it remains somewhat artificial to subdivide this group from the main body of patients in whom the primary problem is multiple organ failure associated with sepsis, particularly since the mechanisms of cell injury are limited in number and probably unrelated to the organ system involved.

The Pathogenesis of Multiple Organ Failure Associated with Sepsis and Trauma – the Prevailing Hypothesis

Most investigators now agree that cell damage and organ dysfunction in sepsis and massive trauma arise initially through two different but inter-related mechanisms (Cerra and Bihari 1989). First, the inappropriate and uncontrolled release of the various mediators of the acute inflammatory response may be directly cytotoxic (Movat et al. 1987; Beutler and Cerami 1987) whilst contributing to the second mechanism – the development of a maldistribution of blood flow (and hence the oxygen supply) within the microcirculations of actively respiring tissues (Bihari 1987a) (Tables 30.1 and 30.2). This second process, the consequence of inappropriate vasoconstriction, endothelial cell damage, microembolism, thrombosis and interstitial oedema leading directly to hypoxia-related cell dysfunction and death, has been brought to our attention through the description of "flow-dependent oxygen consumption" that often occurs in patients with severe sepsis and respiratory failure despite the presence of an apparently adequate oxygen supply (Cain 1984; Gutierrez and Pohil 1986; Schumacker and Cain 1987; Astiz et al. 1987; Bihari 1988a; Bryan-Brown 1988). Similarly, some patients with acute renal failure associated with sepsis also appear to suffer from this disturbance in the matching between oxygen demand and systemic oxygen transport. Measurements of blood flow and oxygen uptake, although difficult, are more easily obtained than those of the various different mediators. For this reason, confusion still surrounds the exact role of endotoxin itself together with the activation of the complement system, white cells (neutrophils, monocytes), fixed tissue macrophages, platelets, the coagulation and kinin cascade systems with the release of their various mediators in the pathogenesis of organ failure (Westaby 1986; Hyers et al. 1987).

A third mechanism of importance is the effects of reperfusion on ischaemic tissue (Tables 30.3 and 30.4). There is now considerable evidence to suggest that much of the cellular injury associated with ischaemia occurs on reperfusion with the re-establishment of an oxygen supply and a source of extracellular calcium

Table 30.1. Mechanisms of organ failure: potential mediators of cytotoxicity and the maldistribution of blood flow associated with severe sepsis and trauma

1. Endotoxin, other bacterial cell wall products (e.g. FLMP) and exotoxins
2. Active products of the complement system (C_{3a}, C_{5a})
3. Neutrophil activation and degranulation products
   Eicosanoids (PGs, LTs)
   PAF
   Proteases (cathepsins, elastase etc)
   Oxygen free radicals
4. Monocyte / macrophage release products
   Cytokines (especially IL-1 and TNF)
   Eicosanoids (PGs, LTs)
   PAF
   Proteases (cathepsins, elastase etc)
   Oxygen free radicals
   Growth factors
5. Platelet release products
   TXA_2
   Histamine
   5-HT
6. Endothelial cell peptides and other products
   IL-1
   PGI_2
   EDRF
   Endothelin
7. Products of coagulation and the kinin systems
8. Other vasoactive circulating hormones

Table 30.2. Mechanisms of organ failure: maldistribution of blood flow within the microcirculation of actively respiring tissues

Maldistribution of blood flow related to:
1. Direct effects of endotoxin on endothelial cells with mediator generation and release (e.g. IL-1, PGI_2, EDRF, endothelin) and endothelial cell swelling (leading to the "no-reflow" phenomenon)
2. Microembolic phenomena (related to white cells, platelets and local fibrin deposition)
3. Interstitial oedema and capillary compression
4. The activation of the various cascades systems (complement, coagulation, kinins), the cellular elements in blood (polymorphs, monocytes and platelets) and fixed tissue macrophages with the release of vasoactive compounds

Leads to "low/no perfusion injury" through simple hypoxia

This may occur in the presence of:
1. An apparently adequate cardiac output
2. Normal arterial and mixed venous oxygenation
   and in the absence of a lactic acidosis

(Farber 1982; Weinberg 1984; McCord 1985; Halliwell 1987; Brezis et al. 1988; McCoy et al. 1988; Paller and Sikora 1988) – the so-called "oxygen and calcium paradox". Since the severity of the reperfusion injury is most probably related to the length of the ischaemic period, and given that tissue survival ultimately depends on an adequate blood flow, reperfusion must, in principle, be brought about as soon as possible. Thus, the "no perfusion" injury is more deleterious in the long run than "reperfusion" but an understanding of the various damaging processes that go on during the reperfusion period might allow some further therapeutic intervention aimed at their inhibition (Gardner et al. 1983; Schrier et al. 1987; Machlin and Bendich 1987).

Table 30.3. Mechanisms of organ failure: reperfusion of previous ischaemic tissues

Development of a *reperfusion injury* related to:
1. Increased calcium delivery to ischaemic/hypoxic cells with uncontrolled rise in intracellular concentration
2. Oxygen free radical generation through the metabolism of xanthine and hypoxanthine by the oxidase form of the enzyme (formed by calcium-induced phosphorylation of xanthine dehydrogenase)
3. Increased delivery of cellular elements and other mediators in blood leading to an acute inflammatory response, further microembolism with mediator release, and direct cytotoxicity

Table 30.4. Mechanisms of organ failure: effects of an uncontrolled rise in the intracellular calcium concentration

Loss of calcium homeostasis and rise in intracellular calcium levels related to cellular energy failure:
1. Influx from extracellular space
2. Efflux from mitochondria and endoplasmic reticulum

Resulting in:
1. Activation of a number of cytosolic calcium-dependent proteases by phosphorylation

Leads to breakdown of cytoskeleton, conversion of xanthine dehydrogenase into the oxidase form
2. Activation of phospholipase A_2 with the subsequent release of PAF, eicosanoids and oxygen free radicals whilst amplifying the acute inflammatory response

The primary stimulus which precipitates activation of the cellular and contact systems with the release of mediators is unknown (Carrico et al. 1986; Goris et al. 1985). Bacterial cell wall products, in particular endotoxin, are the most likely candidates (Morrison and Ulevitch 1978; Wardle 1982; Brigham and Meyrick 1986) and in the absence of septicaemia or a known focus of infection, bacterial/endotoxin translocation through a leaky, ischaemic or oedematous gut mucosa may account for these phenomena – the so-called gut leak–liver prime hypothesis of multiple organ failure (Baker et al. 1988; Cerra et al. 1988). Why the lungs and the kidneys should be so susceptible to injury is unknown. Both organ systems receive a very high blood flow relative to their weight whilst being unrelated to their metabolic demand. This might contribute to their susceptibility in providing them with a very much greater toxic mediator "load" compared with other tissues. In the case of the lungs, this "dosing" effect might be even more important since this organ system is the first to receive the venous effluent from septic or traumatized tissue. Moreover, both organ systems are at substantial risk in the ITU from injury with an iatrogenic component (Table 30.5). High inspired oxygen concentrations and peak inspiratory pressures during mechanical ventilation markedly potentiate any acute lung injury (Kolobow et al. 1987; Gattinoni et

Table 30.5. Iatrogenic complications of critical illness contributing to the development of multiple organ failure

---

1. *Central venous/pulmonary arterial catheterization*
   Pneumothorax
   Arterial puncture with bleeding
   Infection
   Knotting of catheters
   Arrhythmias
   Pulmonary infarction associated with prolonged wedging
   Vascular perforation and pulmonary artery rupture
2. *Fluid therapy*
   Unrecognized hypovolaemia
   Overtransfusion with crystalloid and colloid
   Excessive reductions in oncotic pressure (crystalloids)
3. *Mechanical ventilation*
   Barotrauma related to high peak inspiratory pressures
   Haemodynamic disturbances
   Immunosuppression, hypotension and muscle wasting related to sedation and muscle relaxants
4. *Hyperalimentation*
   Hepatic steatosis from excessive calorie intake
   Hyperglycaemia
   Ventilatory embarrassment related to excessive carbon dioxide production
   Pulmonary dysfunction related to excessive lipid
5. *Administration of other toxic substances*
   Pulmonary toxicity related to high (>60%) inspired oxygen concentrations for prolonged periods
   Non-steroidal anti-inflammatory drugs
   Steroids
   Aminoglycosides
   (? H_2 antagonists)

---

al. 1988) whereas a raised mean airway pressure has profound effects on cardiac output, renal blood flow and function (Falke and Steinhoff 1985; Miller and Anderson 1987; Pingleton 1988). Nephrotoxicity from aminoglycosides on the one hand, and pulmonary dysfunction as a consequence of excessive fluid administration on the other, are two common problems that may contribute to disturbances in function although it is fair to say that in both cases, more patients get into trouble from being underdosed with both forms of treatment. Finally, given their substantial blood flow, neither organ system should be susceptible to a "low/no perfusion" ischaemic/hypoxic injury in sepsis. Yet, this is certainly not the case in the renal medulla according to Epstein's hypothesis (Epstein et al. 1982; Brezis et al. 1984). Any reduction in flow rate in the vasa recta would markedly exaggerate the proposed oxygen diffusional shunt from arteriole to venule, substantially reducing oxygen tension at the tip of the loops. A disturbance in the distribution of blood flow within the kidney, sludging of red cells in the medulla as suggested by Mason et al. (1984) together with a decrease in arterial oxygen content might well be enough to create such a condition. The lung too, paradoxically, could well be at risk from ischaemic/hypoxic injury; abnormal alveoli which are injured (infection/atelectasis) and receive little ventilation also receive a greatly reduced pulmonary arterial blood flow through the process of hypoxic pulmonary vasoconstriction (HPV). Whilst this reflex maintains the matching of perfusion with ventilation and prevents early severe arterial hypoxaemia in patients with an acute lung injury, it could produce critical reductions in "nutrient" blood flow to diseased alveoli (Bihari 1987b). This possible mechanism of injury is discussed more fully below.

Given this rather hazy understanding of the process of cell injury associated with severe sepsis and trauma together with the temporal difficulties in relating mediator release to tissue damage (Demling 1988), it is not surprising that the "magic bullet" approach to mediator inhibition has been unsuccessful in preventing or reversing the process. The majority of investigators have demonstrated a surprising degree of naïvety in supposing that a standard, randomized, controlled clinical trial of a single compound is likely to demonstrate a positive effect on survival in such a complex, unstandardized condition. Therefore, the less than critical introduction of individual forms of anti-inflammatory therapy (steroids or non-steroidal anti-inflammatory drugs (NSAIDs) or vasodilatory prostaglandins) in an attempt to reduce the severity of the tissue injury was almost bound to lead to disappointment. The same concern now surrounds the structure of the various clinical trials which have been proposed, and in some cases, initiated, to examine the protective effects of calcium channel antagonists, by themselves, in episodes of renal (and indeed cerebral) ischaemia.

The Possible Beneficial Effects of Prostacyclin (PGI_2) in Preventing Multiple Organ Failure Associated with Sepsis

For some time, the King's College and Middlesex Hospital groups have had an interest in PGI_2 as an anticoagulant of extracorporeal circuits – specifically charcoal haemoperfusion, as a form of artificial liver support (Gimson et al. 1982) and continuous high volume haemofiltration as a form of renal support (Wendon et al. 1989, in press). A natural extension of these studies has been the assessment of the many other actions of this prostaglandin in the critically ill, and in particular, its effect on tissue perfusion (Bihari et al. 1986; Bihari et al. 1987). Similar investigations have gone on in the US and Japan using the related prostaglandin compound, PGE_1 (Tokioka et al. 1985; Shoemaker and Appel 1986; Holcroft 1986). These two agents, of which PGI_2 is the more potent by five times, have a number of properties which make them attractive as agents which might reduce the tissue damage associated with sepsis (Table 30.6). Given the increased potency of prostacyclin, and the pulmonary degradation of PGE_1 which limits systemic circulating levels (and hence the incidence of undesirable side effects such as systemic hypotension), it may be that PGI_2 is the more logical therapeutic choice. The effects of sepsis are such that widespread tissue damage can occur throughout the organism so that some form of systemic protection is required. Nevertheless, given as a continuous infusion at a high enough dose in the presence of reduced pulmonary metabolism associated with severe adult respiratory distress syndrome (ARDS) (Gillis et al. 1986), PGE_1 can probably achieve the same results.

Table 30.6. Possible beneficial effects of prostacyclin (PGI_2) and prostaglandin E_1 and E_2 in the prevention of multiple organ failure associated with sepsis and the adult respiratory distress syndrome

1. *Improvements in microcirculatory blood flow with the prevention of tissue hypoxia*
   Vasodilatation (especially post-capillary venule)
   Inhibition of platelet activation and aggregation with a reduction in thromboxane A_2 release
   Increased red cell deformability

2. *Inhibition of polymorphonuclear leukocyte activation and adhesion to damaged vascular endothelium*

3. *Inhibition of monocyte–macrophage activation*

4. *Cytoprotection*

5. *Pulmonary vasodilatation with a reduction in pulmonary artery pressure and calculated resistance*

6. *Increased delivery of antimicrobial agents to septic foci*

Vasodilatation with Prostacyclin

The most important effect of these compounds is the profound vasodilatation of the microcirculation that occurs in a manner which is very different from other more conventional vasodilators such as nitroprusside. Using a laser doppler system for the measurement of red cell transit in the dermis of human volunteers, we have observed increases with PGI_2 in the size and frequency of the oscillations of blood flow associated with "vasomotion" within the microcirculation. In general (in common with the septic process itself), other vasodilators, especially alpha-blockers, tend to reduce or paralyse this vasomotion so that tissue perfusion changes with preferential capillary flow in short vessels (George and Tinker 1983). There is some evidence that PGI_2 has a more profound effect on the postcapillary venule (FitzGerald et al. 1981) so that as flow increases, capillary hydrostatic pressure tends to fall. This may be of some importance in the later stages of septic shock in which postcapillary resistance is thought to increase substantially compared with precapillary resistance leading to interstitial oedema (George and Tinker 1983). In general, the presumed PGI_2-induced increases in red cell transit time and red cell deformability, together with transcapillary refill (and fall in haemotocrit) related to the reduction in intracapillary pressure, all contribute to an improvement in whole blood fluidity and flow within the microcirculation. Moreover, PGI_2 produces substantial vasodilatation within the splanchnic bed, increasing blood flow to the often ischaemic gut and liver. This effect may be particularly important in maintaining gastrointestinal integrity and preventing translocation of endotoxin and bacteria. Our studies in patients with sepsis and acute respiratory failure have demonstrated that in some patients, prostacyclin (at 5 ng kg^{-1} min^{-1} will increase both the oxygen delivery to tissues and the extraction ratio (Bihari et al. 1987; Bihari 1988b). We have interpreted these observations to suggest that prostacyclin improves not only the oxygen supply but also its distribution within the microcirculation. This effect on tissue perfusion in patients with sepsis is now well documented but as yet, prostacyclin has not been compared in this patient group with other (cheaper) vasodilators. Anecdotal comparisons with nitroprusside in patients with heart failure, or following cardiopulmonary bypass (Bihari, unpublished data) and especially in children with shock (Mathews and Levine, personal communication) are consistent with our hypothesis that prostacyclin is much superior in improving "nutrient" blood flow and correcting any lactic acidosis.

Effects on Platelet and White Cell Function

Another important aspect of the function of these prostaglandin compounds in sepsis is thought to be their effects on white cell and platelet activation. Prostacyclin, which is not only the most potent inhibitor of platelet activation so far described but also produces the dispersal of formed platelet aggregates (Utsunomiya et al. 1980) has been investigated primarily in relation to platelet/vessel wall interactions (Oates et al. 1988). It also has some fibrinolytic activity (Saldeen 1983) which may add to its effects on blood flow in patients with severe sepsis and ARDS in whom activation of the coagulation cascade may contribute to vascular damage within the lungs and other organs (Carvalho et al. 1982; Saldeen 1983; Carvalho 1985). How important are these properties (which make PGI_2 a very different sort of vasodilator indeed!) remains to be seen because there is considerable controversy concerning the exact role of platelets ("culprits or innocent bystanders?") in the pulmonary damage associated with ARDS, let alone in the multiple organ failure syndrome itself (Heffner et al. 1987). The same concern surrounds the role of the neutrophil in the pathogenesis of ARDS since the spate of publications describing increasing numbers of neutropenic patients who develop severe ARDS despite having no neutrophils in their circulations or lungs (Ognibene et al. 1986; Rinaldo and Rogers 1986; Maunder et al. 1986). Certainly, both PGE_1 and PGI_2 have been shown to inhibit neutrophil activation (Goldstein et al. 1977; Issekutz and Movat 1982) and PGI_2 does reduce the adhesion of neutrophils to damaged endothelium (Jones and Hurley 1984). Yet if these actions are so important, one might have expected better results with the various steroid trials since these agents are particularly potent at inhibiting white cell function in vitro. Yet they have been so disappointing in the controlled clinical trials of septic shock and ARDS (Weigelt et al. 1985; Bone et al. 1987a,b; The Veterans Administration Systemic Sepsis Cooperative Study Group 1987).

Effects on Cytokine Release from the Activated Monocyte/Macrophage Cell System

These observations have led to the emergence of the activated monocyte–macrophage, e.g. the alveolar macrophage in the lung, the Kuppfer cell in the liver, as the fashionable cell system mediating in part the evolution of cell death and organ failure associated with sepsis (Henson and Johnston 1987; Nathan 1987; Matuschak and Rinaldo 1988). Among the many secretory products of the macrophage are those originating from arachidonic acid via the cyclooxygenase enzyme, specifically thromboxane A_2 (TXA_2), PGE_2 and PGI_2 (Nathan 1987). Some lipoxygenase compounds are also produced and the profile of eicosanoids synthesized by the cell appears to be related to its state of activation (Needleman and Tripp 1986). As the macrophage becomes activated, expressing the Ia antigen, it synthesizes mainly products of the lipoxygenase enzyme and TXA_2 whilst turning off the production of PGE_2 and PGI_2. It seems that these two latter prostaglandins are important modulators of the state of activation tending to inhibit the process. The exogenous administration of both PGE_2 and PGI_2 to activated mouse peritoneal macrophages leads to a reduction in the secretion of interleukin-1 (IL-1) and tumour necrosis factor (TNF) suggesting that these two prostaglandins do indeed inhibit activation (Kunkel et al. 1986a,b). PGE_1 has not been studied in this system but probably has the same effects. Again, as more emphasis is placed upon the role of various monokines (IL-1, TNF etc.) as mediators in septic shock and multiple organ failure (Larrick et al. 1987; Girardin et al. 1988; Michie et al. 1988; Stephens et al. 1988; Zeigler 1988), this action of prostacyclin may be seen as both important and beneficial in the prevention of tissue damage.

Cytoprotection with Prostaglandins

Another property of prostacyclin and prostaglandins of the "E" series is that of "cytoprotection" (Robert 1977). This rather inexact term, coined by Jacobson, has been used to describe the protection of a variety of cells from very different organ systems in animal models, single organ perfusion preparations and "in vitro" tissue culture models from the lethal effects of endotoxin, hypoxia and several other toxic molecules. This effect, analogous to the often quoted action of "lysosomal and membrane stabilization" attributed to steroids, is apparently independent of changes in blood flow but remains difficult to identify and measure in critically ill patients. This phenemenon has been extensively studied in relation to gastric mucosal ulceration and seems to be a very real effect of PGI_2, PGE_2 and several of its analogues. Moreover, several studies (Araki and Lefer 1980; Sikujara et al. 1983) have demonstrated that PGI_2 in particular will prevent hypoxia-associated damage of hepatocytes in an isolated perfused liver. PGI_2 also affords rodent hepatocytes protection against a wide variety of insults, such as paracetamol (Guarner et al. 1988), galactosamine (Noda 1986) and carbon tetrachloride (Stachura et al. 1981). Given the importance of maintaining hepatic synthetic function in the prevention of multiple organ failure (Cerra et al. 1979; Clowes et al. 1985; Matuschak and Rinaldo 1988), this property may have particular significance. Moreover, in the animal models of acute respiratory failure associated with either endotoxin (Demling et al. 1981; Brigham et al. 1988) or oleic acid (Slotman et al. 1982), PGI_2 and PGE_2 reduce both the severity of the endothelial cell injury and the release of damaging inflammatory mediators as assessed by their concentration in lung lymph. Similarly, whilst the PGI_2/TXA_2 axis has been implicated in the pathogenesis of acute renal failure (Lelcuk et al. 1985; Badr et al. 1986), there are numerous studies demonstrating the protective effects of PGI_2 and its analogues in various animal models of ischaemic acute renal failure (Kaufman et al. 1987; Tobimatsu et al. 1988).

The mechanism of prostaglandin-induced cytoprotection remains unclear but may be related to an increase in intracellular concentrations of cAMP. This may prevent the uncontrolled influx of calcium ions into susceptible cells, a process often thought to be the final common pathway of cell damage and death (Farber 1982). This proposed mechanism makes "cytoprotection" an extremely important property in the prevention or reduction of a reperfusion injury. It would make more sense to reperfuse ischaemic/hypoxic tissues with, and in the presence of, a cytoprotective agent; theoretically, further tissue injury following the re-establishment of blood flow would be more limited using a vasodilatory prostaglandin rather than with any other means of increasing blood flow. A greater effect might be achieved in combination with a calcium antagonist. Obviously, this hypothesis is difficult to prove in the ITU but adds to the rationale for using PGI_2 or PGE_1 not only on their own, but also in combination with other compounds, to improve tissue perfusion in the critically ill.

Effects on Pulmonary Function

In patients with severe acute respiratory failure (ARDS) of any cause, special consideration should be given to the preservation of both lung function and lung tissue. The entire process of mechanical ventilation with positive pressure depends upon the recruitment of healthy or near-normal lung tissue to maintain gas exchange. The Milan group has emphasized how this approach may lead to further pulmonary dysfunction as normal ventilation:perfusion units are hyperventilated (to maintain a normal arterial carbon dioxide tension) and subjected to high peak and mean airway pressures (a consequence of their normal compliance) (Pesenti 1987; Gattinoni et al. 1988). In the absence of some form of extracorporeal support, this may be unavoidable but the development of hypoxic pulmonary vasoconstriction in areas of severe pathology, whilst reducing the shunt, may lead to further pulmonary damage, as suggested earlier, through the process of ischaemia and infarction. Furthermore, the associated pulmonary hypertension has direct consequences for the right ventricle, the failure of which is a common occurrence in the natural history of ARDS (Thijs et al. 1988). A reduction in pulmonary artery pressure with an increase in cardiac output is an important aspect of the vasodilatation produced by PGI_2 and PGE_1 in patients with ARDS. Neither compound is a specific pulmonary vasodilator but we have observed a median reduction of 15% in pulmonary artery pressure with a median increase of 25% in cardiac output in our 27 septic patients with acute respiratory failure (Bihari et al. 1987). The effect of PGI_2 was more marked in those cases with the more severe pulmonary hypertension but very often was associated with a decrease in arterial oxygen tension and an increase in the calculated shunt fraction. This is of some physiological interest since some investigators have suggested that the severe arterial hypoxaemia of ARDS is related to a relative "failure" of pulmonary hypoxic vasoconstriction so that perfusion continues to relatively diseased alveolar ventilation units. Indeed, it has been proposed that this lack of vasoconstriction is mediated through the increased secretion of PGI_2 by pulmonary endothelial cells, presumably stimulated in part by local hypoxia. Recently, a Canadian group reported that indomethacin, (1 mg kg^{-1}) increases the arterial oxygen tension in patients with severe bacterial pneumonia requiring mechanical ventilation (Hanly et al. 1987). They suggested that the cyclooxygenase inhibitor had reduced the synthesis of PGI_2 in the pulmonary circulation and so had enhanced the hypoxic pulmonary vasoconstriction reflex; pulmonary venous admixture was then presumably reduced. Similar effects of NSAIDs have been observed in various animal models of an acute lung injury (Sprague et al. 1987). The implication of these studies was that non-steroidal anti-inflammatory drugs might be useful in patients with an acute lung injury to maintain arterial oxygenation. Philosophically, this line of reasoning is not appealing! Although pulmonary hypoxic vasoconstriction may be life-saving for the whole organism, the arterial oxygen tension is preserved only at the expense of further compromising blood flow to a damaged part of the lung. Again, it is important to emphasize that pulmonary arterial blood flow has an, often forgotten but important, "nutrient" role especially in sustaining the structure and function of alveolar type II cells. Also, any increase in bronchial arterial blood flow (leading to a rise in bonchopulmonary anastomotic flow) which usually accompanies and may compensate for reductions in pulmonary arterial flow is probably mediated by the release of PGI_2 (Deffebach et al. 1987). Thus, ignoring all the other protective effects which might occur through the release of PGI_2 by the damaged endothelium, maintenance of pulmonary and bronchial arterial flow to the injured regions of the lung will prevent further damage through frank infarction or a later reperfusion injury. The administration of PGI_2 may well reduce the arterial oxygen tension but this is relatively unimportant since we have shown that oxygen delivery to tissues goes up with the increase in cardiac output. The maintenance of the nutrient blood supply to damaged lung, endothelial cell protection through its antiplatelet/white cell effects or directly through the process of "cytoprotection", together with the reduction of pulmonary arterial pressure by pulmonary vasodilatation are all factors which may contribute to the successful outcome of a patient with sepsis and ARDS. Of course, as with any other therapy, there are special considerations which must be taken into account. Importantly, the hazards of reducing right coronary perfusion pressure in the face of increasing end diastolic and systolic ventricular pressures have been extensively investigated in animal models (Prewitt 1987) and such a manoeuvre may well induce further right ventricular dysfunction, a consequence of myocardial ischaemia.

Prostaglandins and Sepsis – "To Give and/or To Block?"

The preceding discussion depends upon a variety of different observations – some clinical and some taken from animal models or tissue culture systems – spiced with raw speculation. However, the evidence from controlled clinical trials for a beneficial effect of these prostaglandins is at best scanty, and at worst non-existent! In this, one is reminded yet again of the steroid debate, the controversy that surrounds the use of low-dose dopamine, mannitol and frusemide in preserving renal function and the difficulties inherent in the construction of clinical trials in critically ill patients in the ITU.

The well-known trial (Holcroft et al. 1986) using PGE_1 for the management of ARDS associated with sepsis and trauma demonstrated that this prostaglandin substantially reduced mortality. At 30 days after the end of the infusion, 15 (71%) of the 21 patients treated with the PGE_1 were alive compared with only 7 (35%) of the 20 placebo-treated patients. However, there was no statistically significant difference between the two groups in "overall survival". Nevertheless, of the six PGE_1 patients free of severe organ failure at time of entry, all survived to leave hospital. By contrast, of the 10 placebo patients initially free of severe organ failure, only four survived. Following on from this, a larger multi-centre trial in the USA has failed to confirm these observations although the results from this study have yet to be published. The results from a similar European study also could not demonstrate a difference in survival between 58 placebo (34 (59%) survivors) and 51 PGE_1 (28 (55%) survivors) treated patients (Upjohn Ltd, UK, personal communication). Again, it looks as if a promising new treatment will not be shown to improve outcome from ARDS in large multi-centre studies. But is this because the compound is ineffective or perhaps it is related to the problems of trial design (with only late cases of fully established ARDS being included) or an effect of the many centres taking part? It is interesting to note the high mortality rate apparent in Holcroft et al.'s placebo group compared with the European study and this suggests that case definition, aetiology, the stage of disease on entry and centre effects play an important role in outcome. It also emphasizes the importance of the inclusion of some attempt to score the chronic health status and severity of illness of patients on entry to such trials since it is impossible to interpret the vague statements, such as "free of severe organ failure" which appear in many of the written reports. Whilst it is easy to criticize, we have made no attempt, ourselves, so far to assess the effects of PGI_2 in this way, believing that in our ITU, the population of patients with sepsis is too small and heterogeneous to justify a controlled trial.

With the more recent studies of the beneficial effects of some non-steroidal anti-inflammatory drugs (NSAIDs), in particular ibuprofen, on outcome from septic shock and ARDS (Jacobs et al. 1982; Utsunomiya et al. 1982; Balk et al. 1986; Ogletree et al. 1986; Steinberg et al. 1987), there has come the suggestion that full prostaglandin therapy should be an attempt to block the synthesis of all eicosanoids (including platelet activating factor, TXA_2 and the leukotrienes) whilst treating the patient with the beneficial compounds PGI_2, PGE_2 (or some analogue) and/or PGE_1. A possible regimen might include: high dose steroids for 24 hours to inhibit the phospholipase A_2 enzyme and the breakdown of membrane phospholipid to arachidonic acid with the liberation of platelet-activating factor; ibuprofen or some other NSAID to inhibit the cyclooxygenase enzyme; and finally, PGI_2 or PGE_1, for the reasons already mentioned. In the future, a specific lipoxygenase inhibitor or a leukotriene antagonist might also be required to provide more protection from this group of mediators. Toxicity from such a regimen would require careful assessment especially since NSAIDs are such an important cause of acute renal failure, a disaster in this group of patients. It is still not clear that in sepsis, the mechanism of action of NSAIDs (again ibuprofen in particular) is through cyclooxygenase inhibition. Ibuprofen has been shown in some studies to alter the ratio of circulating concentrations of TXB_2 and 6-keto $PGF_{1\alpha}$ so that prostacyclin synthesis appears paradoxically to be promoted (Shinozawa et al. 1986). Cyclooxygenase-independent white cell inhibition may also be an important mechanism.

The Prevention of Multiple Organ Failure

Most physicians are not involved in the evaluation of new compounds and quite rightly, do not practice an experimental approach to therapeutics as outlined above. What then, is on general offer for the prevention and management of multiple organ failure in the ICU? This subject has been reviewed in depth elsewhere and only some general guidelines (with few references, reflecting an intensely personal bias) can be provided below. The interested reader should refer to our two previous publications on the subject (Kox and Bihari 1988; Cerra and Bihari 1989).

In short, the treatment of the primary underlying problem which has precipitated the crisis, the elimination of "delivery dependent oxygen consumption" and finally, metabolic support i.e. some sort of nutrition with careful attention to fluid balance are usually regarded as the three fundamental aspects of management. The prevention of nosocomial infection is a fourth aspect of care which is receiving an increasing amount of attention and is reviewed by Noone (Chapter 3). The physician's ethical platform for such care (and its withdrawal) has been well defined: the preservation of life; the alleviation of suffering; patient or patient surrogate (i.e. "the person who loves that patient the most") autonomy (with the implication of truth telling by the physician); informed consent or conversely, informed refusal; and finally, a sense of responsibility and justice within the physician for the community at large (Ruark et al. 1988).

Source Control

Certainly, no patient will get better unless the underlying problems, whatever they are – sepsis, heart failure, liver failure, persisting hypovolaemia related to surgical bleeding, fractured long bones, a perforated viscus, dead gut, acalculus cholecystitis etc. – are firstly reversible, and secondly addressed as a matter of urgency. "Find and drain the pus" is a surgical principle never to be forgotten in the management of these patients but unfortunately, it is more easily said (or written down) than done. The imaging techniques available, (plain radiography, ultrasound, CT, radiolabelled gallium and white cell scanning) suffer from variable false negative rates with a considerable cost in terms of expense and perhaps more importantly, in time wasted. Since surgical (rather than "radiological" percutaneous) drainage is the definitive treatment for localized sepsis, it often falls upon the attending physician to support a more aggressive surgical approach rather than pursuing the less-invasive but more time-consuming avenue of more sophisticated, non-contributory scans! No-one likes "a death on the table" but a death in the ICU from multiple organ failure related to resectable dead gut or localized infection is worse. If the physical signs suggest a problem in the abdomen together with deteriorating pulmonary, renal or liver function, then that abdomen must be explored. However, pulmonary sepsis is often present and must always be suspected in patients with ARDS running a prolonged undulant course in whom the abdomen appears to be essentially innocent (Coalson 1986)!

Elimination of "Delivery Dependency"

The elimination of delivery dependency (which I consider impossible in some cases without specific microcirculatory intervention) is essential in the critically ill septic patient. Careful attention to some basic aspects of cardiopulmonary function is all that is required in the majority of patients (Haupt et al. 1985; Demling 1986; Shoemaker 1987). Inadequate resuscitation (most commonly, unrecognized hypovolaemia) must be avoided or rapidly corrected. Importantly, ventilation (spontaneous or mechanical) and fluid therapy (crystalloid or colloid) must be manipulated to maintain cardiac output and systemic oxygen transport at levels greater than normal so as to meet the patient's metabolic requirements which are greater than normal (Shoemaker 1987). In principle, spontaneous breathing with continuous positive airways pressure (CPAP) is preferable to sedation, muscle paralysis and full mechanical ventilation. Nevertheless, the latter is at times life saving by correcting a severe respiratory acidosis, removing the work of breathing, reducing oxygen demands and off-loading a failing, dilated left ventricle. Again, it is emphasized that adequate volume replacement must be achieved rapidly and severe anaemia corrected. The optimal haemoglobin concentration (or haematocrit) for a patient with sepsis, respiratory failure and arterial hypoxaemia is unknown but is probably greater than the 9–10 g dl^{-1} that is commonly observed and often accepted in such cases. We aim for 12–14 g dl^{-1}, trading off increases in whole blood viscosity against increases in oxygen-carrying capacity. Even in the absence of hypotension, early intervention with inotropes (preferably dobutamine) to maintain a high systemic flow is important. Although a low-dose dopamine infusion (1–3 µg kg^{-1} min^{-1}) to increase renal, splanchnic and hepatic blood flow is often said to be of unproven value (if not entirely useless) (Lazarus, Chapter 24), it does little, if any, harm whilst it may have some beneficial effects (Polson et al. 1987). A similar attitude pertains to the use of frusemide and mannitol. Although there is little evidence that these agents can prevent acute renal failure in septic patients, or affect overall survival rates, the management of such cases is made much easier if the patient continues to pass urine. One approach to a rising serum creatinine and blood urea and a falling urine flow rate in the presence of an adequate blood pressure and more than adequate blood and extracellular volume, is a low-dose dopamine infusion, a bolus of mannitol (0.5–1.0 g kg^{-1}) with some regular frusemide in an attempt to make the patient polyuric. If the urine flow rate increases, a urine replacement regimen (the previous hour's urine output + 30 ml adjusted according to the patient's fluid balance and other fluid requirements) is often used to maintain hourly flow rates of more than 200 ml h^{-1}. Again, it is important to emphasize that this approach is only useful if the underlying problem has been successfully addressed and should be instituted early on rather than after a prolonged period of oligoanuria. Similarly, these measures are useless in the face of an inadequate renal perfusion pressure. Given the absence of autoregulation in the acutely failed animal kidney and the failure of the renal circulation to vasoconstrict in response to noradrenaline (Kelleher et al. 1984), the relatively early administration of a vasopressor (adrenaline or noradrenaline depending upon the measured systemic vascular resistance) to maintain renal perfusion is advocated.

Nutritional Support and Fluid Balance

Finally, some sort of nutrition is essential although we recognize that this statement is no more than a "gut" feeling reflecting the well-documented fact that malnutrition in surgical patients is a co-variable determining a fatal outcome

(Little et al. Chapter 29). Presumably, if it is to be given, then nutrition (which may be enteral or parenteral), like all other forms of support, should be started as early on in the course of the illness as possible. Thus, as soon as the patient has been resuscitated, with the optimization of oxygen delivery to tissues, attention should focus on daily fluid requirements and the nature of the fluids administered.

There has been considerable argument over the role of fluid overload in the development of ARDS together with the merits, or otherwise, of diuresing these patients while limiting their fluid intake (Lawson and Bihari 1988). There is evidence to suggest that patients who survive an episode of severe acute respiratory failure go into significant negative fluid balance and lose weight early on in the course of their illness whereas those patients who subsequently die continue to retain fluid and tend to increase their weight (Simmons et al. 1987). Of course, this does not mean that a forced diuresis alone will necessarily convert a non-survivor into a survivor. More likely, it reflects the severity of the generalized capillary leak so that the more severely ill patients require more fluid to maintain their intravascular volumes. In other cases, the iatrogenic factor – fluid overload with a normal pulmonary arterial occlusion pressure and a reduced plasma oncotic pressure – makes an important contribution to the syndrome of "adult respiratory distress" but can be treated relatively easily with diuretics. These considerations emphasize the importance of attention to daily fluid balance with the aim of keeping the patient in balance or slightly negative. It has been said that all critically ill patients with peripheral oedema who require respiratory support have substantial amounts of pulmonary oedema which may contribute to chest X-ray abnormalities and defects in gas exchange (R. Wright, personal communication). This may well be the case but it does not necessarily mean that the extra lung water can be mobilized using diuretics. Moreover, there is little evidence that peripheral oedema, *per se*, forms any sort of independent risk factor in ICU patients. Whilst it has often been suggested that peripheral oedema might be a marker for other vital organ oedema, contributing to defective oxygenation by increasing diffusion distance from capillary into cell, or by limiting capillary perfusion through increases in interstitial pressure (Shah et al. 1981), these possibilities remain hypothetical. On the other hand, by "drying out" the patient, one risks the development of prerenal oliguria which, when combined with all the other insults (bacteraemia or endotoxaemia, systemic mediator release, hypoxaemia, positive intrathoracic pressure, aminoglycosides and NSAIDs etc.) can very rapidly become established acute renal failure. It is our practice to assess carefully the fluid balance status of a patient when haemodynamic stability has been attained. We tend to rely on fluid balance charts, prehospital and subsequent measurements of weight, a careful physical examination and the usual cardiovascular pressures and laboratory data to get some idea of the contribution of fluid overload to the patient's problems. If a decision is taken to diurese a patient or to remove fluid by ultrafiltration, the response in terms of changes in physical signs, chest X-ray appearance, pulmonary compliance and gas exchange are carefully monitored. If no improvement in lung function can be detected over 48–72 hours (with a calculated negative fluid balance of 2.5–5.0 litres in that period), these attempts to "dry out" the patient are abandoned. In such cases, we accept that the lung injury is severe and there is no easily reversible factor in terms of pulmonary oedema that can be mobilized with diuretics. Very often, these are the patients who require prolonged respiratory support and the preservation of their renal function is essential for a successful outcome.

Having determined the volume of fluid to be given to a patient over a 24 hour period, the route of administration must be chosen. If the gut is functioning, enteral nutrition is preferred. This simplifies management enormously and may have a number of important (but unproven) effects. It may reduce the prevalence of serious stress ulceration associated with gastrointestinal haemorrhage and limit colonization of the gut by potentially pathogenic organisms. Feeding by the enteral route, by stimulating the release of secretin and cholecystokinin, promotes gall bladder emptying. This may help to avoid the development of acalculus cholecystitis and biliary sludge, of which the latter often contributes to intrahepatic cholestasis and abnormal liver function. Presumably, enteral nutrition stimulates splanchnic blood flow, thereby reducing the likelihood of ischaemic mucosal changes. Again, although these theoretical advantages are impressive, there are no controlled data supporting the assertion that enteral feeding is superior to the parenteral route. Moreover, a considerable amount of "feeding" time can be lost during which efforts are made to establish, very often unsuccessfully, nutrition by the enteral route. For this reason, nutritional support must not only occur early on in the course of the illness, but it must also be administered in a reliable, continuous fashion. Gastrointestinal function is extremely variable in the first 48 hours after resuscitation from septic shock and acute respiratory failure. An ileus is common and many of the drugs administered (muscle relaxants, sedatives etc.) tend to reduce motility. Moreover, the formation of "gut oedema" is a presumed but unknown quantity. Interestingly, for a given severity of illness (measured by APACHE II scores), abnormal gut function which precludes enteral feeding seems to be an independent variable predictive of a fatal outcome. Thus, while an attempt is made to establish nutritional support by the enteral route over the first 72 hours of illness, a reliable source of nutrient is ensured by the parenteral route.

In the absence of reliable measurements of oxygen consumption, CO_2 production and nitrogen balance, the assessment of the nutritional requirements of individual patients is difficult. As a rule of thumb, these critically ill patients require 30–40 non-protein kcal $kg^{-1} 24 h^{-1}$ and 0.2–0.4 g $kg^{-1} 24 h^{-1}$ of nitrogen. Thus, a 70 kg man should receive around 2100 non-protein kcal and 18–21 g of nitrogen a day. There is not a lot to choose between the various enteral feeding solutions although "Pulmocare" (Ross Laboratories) provides a high-calorie, high-fat, low-carbohydrate diet which may be useful in reducing CO_2 production. The source of the calories in parenteral nutrition solutions may be from carbohydrate alone (dextrose 20%–70%) or together in varying proportions with fat (usually "Intralipid" 10% or 20%, KabiVitrium). Whereas there is agreement that a mixed source of calories on a daily basis is preferable, (glucose intolerance is less likely; there is a reduction in CO_2 production; essential fatty acid deficiency is avoided), if more expensive, there is no consensus concerning the correct ratio of carbohydrate to lipid calories. Cerra has recommended that no more than 20%–30% of the daily calories should be given as fat since defective white cell function, reductions in pulmonary gas exchange and "flocculation" within the microcirculation (calcium-dependent agglutination of liposomes by C-reactive protein) can all accompany the hypertriglyceridaemia associated with excessive fat administration (Pingleton and Harmon 1987; Skeie et al. 1988). In our unit, oxygen consumption and CO_2 production are estimated and the resting energy expenditure of the patient is calculated. Attempts are then made to keep the patient in "calorie balance" by the provision of at least that number of calories. Daily Intralipid 20% is used as a fat source supplying up to 50% of the daily calorie requirements providing the patient's plasma does not become lipaemic and the blood triglyceride concentration remains less than 3.0 (the upper limit of normal being 1.5) mmol l^{-1}. Nitrogen is administered in the form of conventional amino acid solutions ("Synthamin", Travenol; "Vamin", KabiVitrium) since enriched branched-chain amino acid solutions are unavailable. Whilst there are no survival data supporting the use of branched-chain solutions, there is some evidence to suggest that in critically ill patients, they are associated with less-severe nitrogen depletion at any given level of nitrogen intake compared with the standard solutions.

Feeding has been described as "the icing on the intensive care cake" (Bihari), which perhaps undervalues its importance. Nevertheless, many surgeons put much too much faith in the effects of parenteral nutrition and this can sometimes guide them away from dealing definitively with the underlying problem which caused the acute lung injury and other organ failure in the first place. Adequate nutrition cannot drain pus, nor join together dehisced bowel anastomoses. It is only a form of support but in that context, it is vital. "Fix the underlying problem" should be the motto of the present day intensive care unit but sadly, all too often, the problems with which the physician is faced are irreversible. In these cases, the fundamental aspect of their intensive care is the recognition of the irreversibility of the disease process. It is then appropriate to change the goals of care away from "cure" towards "comfort" and the alleviation of suffering in the patient and family. We would do well to remember the early comments of Professor Dornhorst concerning physicians involved in the development of intensive care in the UK in the 1960s – "all too often, they are more intensive than caring!" Despite the science, are we any better today?

Summary

There is considerable evidence from animal and human studies of sepsis and acute lung injury that prostacyclin and PGE_1 may have a beneficial effect on tissue perfusion with a reduction in the severity of tissue damage associated with these disorders. As yet, there are no good data from controlled clinical trials that these agents improve survival and it is not clear whether in the future, such data will be forthcoming. Nevertheless, using various physiological endpoints, both prostaglandins seem to be beneficial in sepsis and when used in combination with the whole process of intensive therapy, may contribute to the survival of some cases. Although the assessment of combinations of agents designed to inhibit mediator release might be more useful (Sielaff et al. 1987), it remains to be seen whether the relatively insensitive controlled clinical trial, with survival as its endpoint, is the appropriate tool for assessing efficacy in the ITU. Perhaps, the "consensus" approach has something more to offer in this situation! At present, we are left with a number of basic clinical measures which are considered by the majority of interested physicians and clinical investigators to be "reasonable medical practice" and most importantly, unlikely to do any harm.

Acknowledgements. I would like to thank Drs Malcom Fisher, Ray Raper, Ross Wilson and all my medical and nursing colleagues at the Royal North Shore Hospital, Sydney, for their stimulating company and enthusiastic support for many of these ideas. It has certainly been a great honour to work in their midst and to learn how to practise intensive care medicine to the highest possible standard. Without them, few of these ideas would have come to fruition.

(The opinions expressed above are those of the author and do not necessarily reflect the protocols or standard clinical practice at the Royal North Shore Hospital.)

References

Araki H, Lefer A (1980) Cytoprotective actions of prostacyclin during hypoxia in the isolated perfused cat liver. Am J Physiol 238: H176–H181
Astiz M, Rackow E, Falk J, Kaufman B, Weil M (1987) Oxygen delivery and consumption in patients with hyperdynamic septic shock. Crit Care Med 15: 26–28
Badr K, Kelley V, Rennke H, Brenner B (1986) Role for thromboxane A_2 and leukotrienes in endotoxin-induced acute renal failure. Kidney Int 30: 474–480
Baker J, Deitch E, Berg R, Specian R (1988) Hemorrhagic shock induces bacterial translocation from the gut. J Trauma 28: 896–906
Balk R, Tryka A, Bone R, Mazurek G, Holst L, Townsend J (1986) The effect of ibuprofen on endotoxin-induced injury in sheep. J Crit Care 1: 230–240
Bartlett R, Mault J, Dechert R, Palmer J, Swartz R, Port F (1986) Continuous arteriovenous haemofiltration: Improved survival in surgical acute renal failure? Surgery 100: 400–408
Beutler B, Cerami A (1987) Cachectin: more than a tumour necrosis factor. N Engl J Med 316: 379–385
Bihari D (1987a) Mismatch of the oxygen supply and demand in septic shock. In: Vincent J-L, Thijs L (eds) Septic shock – a European view. Springer-Verlag, Berlin, pp 148–160
Bihari D (1987b) Indomethacin and arterial oxygenation in critically ill patients with severe bacterial pneumonia. Lancet I: 755 (letter)
Bihari D (1988a) Oxygen delivery and consumption in the critically ill; their relation to the development of multiple organ failure. In: Kox W, Bihari D (eds) Shock and the adult respiratory distress syndrome. Springer-Verlag, Berlin, pp 95–121
Bihari D (1988b) Effects of prostacyclin on oxygen delivery and uptake in critically ill patients. N Engl J Med 318: 855 (letter)
Bihari D, Gimson A, Williams R (1986) Cardiovascular, pulmonary and renal complications of fulminant hepatic failure. Semin Liver Dis 6: 119–128
Bihari D, Smithies M, Gimson A, Tinker J (1987) The effects of vasodilatation with prostacyclin on oxygen delivery and uptake in critically ill patients. N Engl J Med 317: 397–403
Bone R, Fisher C, Clemmer T, Slotman G, Metz C, Balk R, Methylprednisolone severe sepsis study group (1987a) A controlled clinical trial of high dose methylprednisolone in the treatment of severe sepsis and septic shock. N Engl J Med 317: 653–658
Bone R, Fisher C, Clemmer T, Slotman G, Metz C, Methylprednisolone severe sepsis study group (1987b) Early methylprednisolone treatment for the septic syndrome and the adult respiratory distress syndrome. Chest 92: 1032–1036
Brezis M, Rosen S, Silva P, Epstein F (1984) Renal ischaemia: a new perspective. Kidney Int 26: 375–383
Brezis M, Shina S, Kidroni G, Epstein F, Rosen S (1988) Calcium and hypoxic injury in the renal medulla of the perfused rat kidney. Kidney Int 34: 186–194
Brigham K, Meyrick B (1986) Endotoxin and lung injury. Am Rev Respir Dis 133: 913–927
Brigham K, Serafin W, Zadoff A, Blair I, Meyrick B, Oates J (1988) Prostaglandin E_2 attenuation of sheep lung responses to endotoxin. J Appl Physiol 64: 2568–2574
Bryan-Brown C (1988) Blood flow to organs: parameters for function and survival in critical illness. Crit Care Med 16: 170–178
Cain S (1984) Supply dependency of oxygen uptake in the adult respiratory distress syndrome – myth or reality? Am J Med Sci 288: 119–124
Cameron JS (1986) Acute renal failure in the intensive care unit today. Intensive Care Med 12: 64–70

Carrico C, Meakins J, Marshall J, Fry D, Maier R (1986) Multiple organ failure syndrome. Arch Surg 121: 196–208
Carvalho A (1985) Blood alterations during ARDS. In: Zapol W, Falke K (eds) Acute respiratory failure. Marcel Dekker, New York, pp 303–346
Carvalho A, Bellman S, Saullo V, Quinn D, Zapol W (1982) Altered factor VIII in acute respiratory failure. N Engl J Med 307: 1113–1119
Cerra F, Bihari D (eds) (1989) Multiple organ failure. New Horizons Volume 3, Society of Critical Care Medicine, Fullerton, California
Cerra F, Siegel J, Border J, Wiles J, McMenamy R (1979) The hepatic failure of sepsis – cellular versus substrate. Surgery 86: 409–422
Cerra F, West M, Keller G, Mazuski J, Simmons R (1988) Hypermetabolism and organ failure – the role of the activated macrophage as a metabolic regulator. In: Bond R, Adams H, Chaudry I (eds) Perspectives in shock research, progress in clinical and biological research, vol 264. Alan R. Liss, New York, pp 27–42
Clowes G, Hirsch E, George B, Bigatello L, Mazuski J, Villee C (1985) Survival from sepsis – the significance of altered protein metabolism regulated by proteolysis inducing factor, the circulating cleavage product of interleukin-1. Ann Surg 202: 446–458
Coalson J (1986) Pathology of sepsis, septic shock and multiple organ failure. In: Sibbald W, Sprung C (eds) Perspectives on sepsis and septic shock, New Horizons Volume 1, Society of Critical Care Medicine, Fullerton, California, pp 27–60
Deffebach M, Charan N, Lakshminarayan S, Butler J (1987) The bronchial circulation – a small but a vital attribute of the lung. Am Rev Respir Dis 135: 463–481
Demling R (1986) Colloid or crystalloid resuscitation in sepsis. In: Sibbald W, Sprung C (eds) Perspectives on sepsis and septic shock, New Horizons Volume 1, Society of Critical Care Medicine, Fullerton, California, pp 275–300
Demling R (1988) The role of mediators in human ARDS. J Crit Care 3: 56–72
Demling R, Smith M, Gunther R, Gee M, Flynn J (1981) The effect of a prostacyclin infusion on endotoxin-induced lung injury. Surgery 89: 257–263
Epstein F, Balaban R, Ross B (1982) Redox state of cytochrome aa_3 in isolated perfused rat kidney. Am J Physiol 243: F356–F363
Falke K, Steinhoff H (1985) Renal function during acute respiratory failure. In: Zapol W, Falke K (eds) Acute respiratory failure. Marcel Dekker, New York, pp 577–598
Farber J (1982) Membrane injury and calcium homeostasis in the pathogenesis of coagulative necrosis. Lab Invest 47: 114–123
Fitzgerald G, Dargie H, Watkins J, Brown M, Friedman L, Lewis P (1981) Cardiac effects of prostacyclin in man. In: Lewis P, O'Grady J (eds) Clinical Pharmacology of prostacyclin. Raven Press, New York, pp 145–152
Gardner T, Stewart J, Casale A, Downey J, Chambers D (1983) Reduction of myocardial ischaemic injury with oxygen derived free radical scavengers. Surgery 94: 423–427
Gattinoni L, Pesenti A, Marcolin R, Mascheroni D, Fumagalli R, Riboni A, Rossi F, Scarani F, Avalli L, Giuffrida A (1988) Extracorporeal support in acute respiratory failure. In: Kox W, Bihari D (eds) Shock and the adult respiratory distress syndrome. Springer-Verlag, Berlin, pp 167–176
George R, Tinker J (1983) The pathogenesis of shock. In: Tinker J, Rapin M (eds) The care of the critically ill patient. Springer-Verlag, Berlin, pp 168–188
Gillis C, Pitt B, Wiedemann H, Hammond G (1986) Depressed prostaglandin E_1 and 5-hydroxytryptamine removal in patients with adult respiratory distress syndrome. Am Rev Respir Dis 134: 739–744
Gimson A, Braude S, Mellon P, Canalese J, Williams R (1982) Earlier charcoal haemoperfusion in fulminant hepatic failure. Lancet II: 681–683
Girardin E, Grau G, Dayer J-M, Roux-Lombard P, the J5 Study Group and Lambert P-H (1988) Tumour necrosis factor and interleukin-1 in the serum of children with severe infectious purpura. N Engl J Med 319: 397–400
Goldstein I, Malmsten C, Samuelsson B, Weissmann G (1977) Prostaglandins, thromboxanes and polymorphonuclear leukocytes. Inflammation 2: 309–317
Goris R, te Boekhorst T, Nuytinck J, Gimbrere J (1985) Multiple organ failure: generalised autodestructive inflammation. Arch Surg 120: 1109–1115
Guarner F, Boughton-Smith N, Blackwell G, Moncada S (1988) Reduction by prostacyclin of acetaminophen-induced liver toxicity in the mouse. Hepatology 8: 248–253
Gutierrez G, Pohil R (1986) Oxygen consumption is linearly related to the oxygen supply in critically ill patients. J Crit Care 1: 45–53
Halliwell B (1987) Oxidants and human disease: some new concepts. FASEB J 1: 358–364

Hanly P, Roberts D, Dobson K, Light R (1987) Effect of indomethacin on arterial oxygenation in critically ill patients with severe bacterial pneumonia. Lancet I: 351–354

Haupt M, Gilbert E, Carlson R (1985) Fluid loading increases oxygen consumption in septic patients with lactic acidosis. Am Rev Respir Dis 131: 912–916

Heffner J, Sahn S, Repine J (1987) The role of platelets in the adult respiratory distress syndrome; culprits or bystanders. Am Rev Respir Dis 135: 482–492

Henson P, Johnston R (1987) Tissue injury in inflammation; oxidants, proteinases and cationic proteins. J Clin Invest 79: 669–674

Holcroft J, Vassar M, Weber C (1986) Prostaglandin E_1 and survival in patients with the adult respiratory distress syndrome. A prospective trial. Ann Surg 203: 371–378

Hyers T, Gee M, Andreadis N (1987) Cellular interactions in the multiple organ injury syndrome. Am Rev Respir Dis 135: 952–953

Issekutz A, Movat H (1982) The effect of vasodilatory prostaglandins on polymorphonuclear leukocyte infiltration and vascular injury. Am J Pathol 107: 300–309

Jacobs E, Soulsby M, Bone R, Wilson F, Hiller F (1982) Ibuprofen in canine endotoxin shock. J Clin Invest 70: 536–541

Jones G, Hurley J (1984) The effect of prostacyclin on the adhesion of leucocytes to injured vascular endothelium. J Pathol 142: 51–59

Kaufman R, Anner H, Kobzik L, Valeri C, Shepro D, Hechtman H (1987) Vasodilator prostaglandins prevent renal damage after ischemia. Ann Surg 204: 195–198

Kelleher S, Robinette J, Conger J (1984) Sympathetic nervous system in the loss of autoregulation in acute renal failure. Am J Physiol 246: F379–F386

Knaus W, Zimmerman J (1985) Prediction of outcome from intensive care. Clin Anaesthesiol 3: 811–829

Knaus W, Draper E, Wagner D, Zimmerman J (1985a) APACHE II: a severity of disease classification system. Crit Care Med 13: 818–829

Knaus W, Draper E, Wagner D, Zimmerman J (1985b) Prognosis in acute organ system failure. Ann Surg 6: 685–693

Knaus W, Draper E, Wagner D, Zimmerman J (1986) An evaluation of outcome from intensive care in major medical centers. Ann Intern Med 104: 410–418

Kolobow T, Moretti M, Fumagalli R, Mascheroni D, Prato P, Chen V, Joris M (1987) Severe impairment in lung function induced by high peak airway pressure during mechanical ventilation – an experimental study. Am Rev Respir Dis 135: 312–315

Kox W, Bihari D (eds) (1988) Shock and the adult respiratory distress syndrome. Springer-Verlag, Berlin

Kunkel S, Wiggins R, Chensue S, Larrick J (1986a) Regulation of macrophage tumour necrosis factor production by prostaglandin E_2. Biochem Biophys Res Commun 137: 404–410

Kunkel S, Chensue S, Phan S (1986b) Prostaglandins as endogenous mediators of interleukin 1 production. J Immunol 136: 186–192

Larrick J, Graham D, Toy K, Lin L, Senyk G, Fendly B (1987) Recombinant tumour necrosis factor causes activation of human granulocytes. Blood 69: 640–644

Lawson A, Bihari D (1988) The clinical presentation and diagnosis of the adult respiratory distress syndrome. In: Kox W, Bihari D (eds) Shock and the adult respiratory distress syndrome. Springer-Verlag, Berlin, pp 225–234

Lelcuk S, Alexander F, Kobzik L, Valeri C, Shepro D, Hechtman H (1985) Prostacyclin and thromboxane A_2 moderate postischaemic renal failure. Surgery 98: 207–212

Machlin L, Bendich A (1987) Free radical tissue damage: protective role of antioxidant nutrients. FASEB J 1: 441–445

Mason J, Torhorst J, Welsch J (1984) Role of the medullary perfusion defect in the pathogenesis of ischemic renal failure. Kidney Int 26: 283–293

Matuschak G, Rinaldo J (1988) Organ interactions in the adult respiratory distress syndrome during sepsis: role of the liver in host defense. Chest 94: 400–406

Maunder R, Hackman R, Riff E, Albert R, Springmeyer S (1986) Occurrence of the adult respiratory distress syndrome in neutropenic patients. Am Rev Respir Dis 133: 313–316

McCord J (1985) Oxygen derived free radicals in postischemic tissue injury. N Engl J Med 312: 159–163

McCoy R, Hill K, Ayon M, Stein J, Burk R (1988) Oxidant stress following renal ischemia: changes in the glutathione redox ratio. Kidney Int 33: 812–817

Michie H, Manogue K, Spriggs D, Ravhaug A, O'Dwyer S, Dinarello C, Cerami A, Wolff S, Wilmore D (1988) Detection of circulating tumour necrosis factor after endotoxin administration. N Engl J Med 318: 1482–1486

Miller S, Anderson R (1987) The kidney in acute respiratory failure. J Crit Care 2: 45–48
Morrison D, Ulevitch R (1978) The effects of bacterial endotoxins on host mediation systems. Am J Pathol 93: 527–617
Movat H, Cybulsky M, Colditz I, Chan M, Dinarello C (1987) Acute inflammation in gram negative infection: endotoxin, interleukin 1, tumour necrosis factor and neutrophils. Fed Proc 46: 97–104
Nathan C (1987) Secretory products of macrophages. J Clin Invest 79: 319–326
Needleman P, Tripp C (1986) The regulation and function of macrophage eicosanoid metabolism in tissue injury. Proceedings, sixth international conference on prostaglandins and related compounds, Florence, p 484
Noda Y, Hughes R, Williams R (1986) Effect of prostacyclin and a prostaglandin analogue BW 245C on galactosamine-induced hepatic necrosis. J Hepatol 2: 53–64
Oates J, FitzGerald G, Branch R, Jackson E, Knapp H, Roberts L (1988) Clinical implications of prostaglandin and thromboxane A_2 formation (in two parts). N Engl J Med 319: 689–699; 761–767
Ogletree M, Begley C, King G, Brigham K (1986) Influence of steroidal and non-steroidal anti-inflammatory agents on the accumulation of arachidonic acid metabolites in plasma and lung lymph after endotoxaemia in awake sheep: measurements of prostacyclin and thromboxane metabolites and 12-HETE. Am Rev Respir Dis 133: 55–61
Ognibene F, Martin S, Parker M, Schlesinger T, Roach P, Burch C, Shelhamer J, Parrillo J (1986) Adult respiratory distress syndrome in patients with severe neutropenia. N Engl J Med 315: 547–551
Paller M, Sikora J (1988) Renal work, glutathione and susceptibility to free radical mediated postischemic injury. Kidney Int 33: 843–849
Pesenti A, Gattinoni L, Coffano B (1987) Extracorporeal support in acute respiratory failure. In: Vincent J-L (ed) Update in intensive care and emergency medicine. Springer-Verlag, Berlin, pp 253–262
Pingleton S, (1988) Complications of acute renal failure. Am Rev Respir Dis 137: 1463–1493
Pingleton S, Harmon G (1987) Nutritional management in acute respiratory failure. JAMA 257: 3094–3099
Polson R, Park G, Lindop M, Farman J, Calne R, Williams R (1987) The prevention of renal impairment in patients undergoing orthotopic liver grafting by infusion of low dose dopamine. Anaesthesia 42: 15–19
Prewitt R (1987) Pathophysiology and treatment of pulmonary hypertension in acute respiratory failure. J Crit Care 2: 206–218
Rinaldo J, Rogers R (1986) Adult respiratory distress syndrome (editorial). N Engl J Med 315: 578–580
Robert A (1979) Cytoprotection by prostaglandins. Gastroenterology 77: 761–777
Ruark J, Raffin T, Stanford University Medical Centre Committee on Ethics (1988) Initiating and withdrawing life support: principles and practice in adult medicine. N Engl J Med 318: 25–30
Saldeen T (1983) Clotting, microembolism and inhibition of fibrinolysis in adult respiratory distress. Surg Clin North Am 63: 285–304
Schrier R, Arnold P, Putten V, Burke T (1987) Cellular calcium in ischemic acute renal failure: role of calcium entry blockers. Kidney Int 32: 313–321
Schumacker P, Cain S (1987) The concept of a critical oxygen delivery. Intensive Care Med 13: 223–229
Shah D, Newell J, Saba T (1981) Defects in peripheral oxygen utilisation following trauma and shock. Arch Surg 171: 1277–1281
Shinozawa Y, Hales C, Jung W, Burke J (1986) Ibuprofen prevents synthetic smoke induced pulmonary oedema. Am Rev Respir Dis 134: 1145–1148
Shoemaker W (1987) Relation of oxygen transport patterns to the pathophysiology and therapy of shock states. Intensive Care Medicine 13: 230–243
Shoemaker W, Appel P (1986) Effects of prostaglandin E_1 in adult respiratory distress syndrome. Surgery 99: 275–282
Sielaff T, Sugerman H, Tatum J, Kellum J, Blocher C (1987) Treatment of porcine pseudomonas ARDS with combination drug therapy. J Trauma 27: 1313–1322
Sikujara O, Monden M, Toyoshima K, Okamura J, Kosaki G (1983) Cytoprotective effect of prostaglandin I_2 (prostacyclin) on ischaemia induced hepatic cell injury. Transplantation 36: 238–243
Simmons R, Berdine G, Seidenfeld J, Prihoda T, Harris G, Smith J, Gilbert T, Mota E, Johanson W (1987) Fluid balance and the adult respiratory distress syndrome. Am Rev Respir Dis 135: 924–929
Simonds AK, Mansell MA (1986) Haemodialysis or haemofiltration in the intensive therapy unit? Intensive Crit Care Digest 5: 5–7

Simpson HK, Allison ME, Telfer AB (1987) Improving the prognosis in acute renal and respiratory failure. Renal Failure 10: 45–54
Skeie B, Askanazi J, Rothkopf M, Rosenbaum S, Kvetan V, Thomashow B (1988) Intravenous fat emulsions and lung function – a review. Crit Care Med 16: 183–194
Slotman G, Machiedo G, Casey K, Lyons M (1982) Histological and haemodynamic effects of prostacyclin and prostaglandin E_1 following oleic acid infusion. Surgery 92: 93–100
Sprague R, Stephenson A, Dahms T, Asner N, Lonigro A (1987) Effects of ibuprofen on the hypoxaemia of established ethclorvynol-induced unilateral acute lung injury in anaesthetised dogs. Chest 92: 1088–1093
Stachura J, Tarnawski A, Ivey K, Mach T, Bogdal J, Szczudrawa J, Klimczyk B (1981) Prostaglandin protection of carbon tetrachloride induced liver cell necrosis in the rat. Gastroenterology 81: 211–217
Steinberg S, Dehring D, Martin D, Gower W, Carey L, Cloutier C (1987) Amelioration of pulmonary pathophysiology of adult respiratory distress syndrome by sulindac, a cyclo-oxygenase inhibitor. J Trauma 27: 1323–1331
Stephens K, Ishizaka A, Larrick J, Raffin T (1988) Tumour necrosis factor causes increased pulmonary permeability and edema – comparison to septic acute lung injury. Am Rev Respir Dis 137: 1364–1370
Sweet SJ, Glenney CU, FitzGibbon JP, Friedmann P, Teres D (1981) Synergistic effect of acute renal failure and respiratory failure in a surgical intensive care unit. Am J Surg 141: 492–496
Thijs L, Groeneveld A, Schneider A (1988) Changing haemodynamic concepts in human septic shock. In: Kox W, Bihari D (eds) Shock and the adult respiratory distress syndrome. Springer-Verlag, Berlin, pp 79–94
Tobimatsu M, Ueda Y, Saito S, Tsumagari T, Konomi K (1988) Effects of a stable prostacyclin analog on experimental ischemic acute renal failure. Ann Surg 208: 65–70
Tokioka H, Kobayashi O, Ohta Y, Wakabayashi T, Kosaka F (1985) The acute effects of prostaglandin E_1 on the pulmonary circulation and oxygen delivery in patients with the adult respiratory distress syndrome. Intensive Care Med 11: 61–64
Utsunomiya T, Krausz M, Dunham B, Valeri C, Shepro D, Hechtman H (1980) Treatment of pulmonary embolism with prostacyclin. Surgery 88: 25–30
Utsunomiya T, Krausz M, Dunham B, Valeri C, Levine L, Shepro D, Hechtman H (1982) Modification of inflammatory response to aspiration with ibuprofen. Am J Physiol 243: H903–H910
Veterans Administration Systemic Sepsis Cooperative Study Group (1987) Effect of high-dose glucocorticoid therapy on mortality in patients with clinical signs of systemic sepsis. N Engl J Med 317: 659–665
Wardle N (1982) Acute renal failure in the 1980s: the importance of septic shock and endotoxaemia. Nephron 30: 193–200
Weigelt J, Norcross J, Borman K et al. (1985) Early steroid therapy for respiratory failure. Arch Surg 120: 536–540
Weinberg J (1984) Calcium as a mediator of renal tubular cell injury. Semin Nephrol 4: 174–191
Wendon J, Smithies M, Sheppard M, Bullen K, Tinker J, Bihari D (1989) Continuous high volume venous-venous haemofiltration in acute renal failure. Intensive Care Med (in press)
Westaby S (1986) Mechanisms of membrane damage and surfactant depletion in acute lung injury. Intensive Care Med 12: 2–5
Wheeler DC, Feehally J, Walls J (1986) High risk acute renal failure. Q J Med 61: 977–984
Zeigler E (1988) Tumour necrosis factor in humans. N Engl J Med 318: 1533–1535

Final Discussion

Dr Bihari opened the final discussion by describing the first clinical decision that had to be taken in assessing a patient with severe combined acute respiratory and renal failure. This decision taken together with the nursing staff and the relatives of the patient was whether or not to resuscitate the patient in the first place and attempt to keep that patient alive in the intensive care unit. This decision was often not explicit and was usually taken rapidly since it was deemed safer to resuscitate the patient and then re-assess the appropriateness of this action, rather than to let the patient die. This was not always the case, and on some occasions in consultation with the relatives, the lives of certain patients were not prolonged. Dr Bihari went on to describe the six principles of ethical practice of medical care in the intensive care setting as set down by the Stanford University Human Rights Committee. These included first the preservation of life and second the alleviation of suffering. The third principle was that of the autonomy of the patient or an elected surrogate; the fourth principle depended on the concept of "informed consent" or "informed refusal". The fifth relied upon a belief in "truth telling" by the physician. Finally, and at the bottom of the list, was the suggestion that the sixth principle might be a sense of justice in the allocation of resources and a sense of responsibility to the community. This subject was debated in depth. Dr Epstein emphasized that it was very important for an organization of intensive care physicians to take some sort of principled stand on the initiation and withdrawal of life support. He thought that there had been a great deal of loose talk about the physicians' responsibility to society for it seemed to him that their primary responsibility lay with their patients. Certainly, no one would suggest, claimed Dr Epstein, that a doctor's responsibility to his patient consisted of employing a treatment, expensive or inexpensive to society, when that treatment had been demonstrated to be ineffective. Dr Noone supported this view. He said that his personal involvement in the treatment of leukaemia had convinced him that the very aggressive approach of the oncologists had brought about an enormously improved survival in some groups of patients. He felt that it was not the role of the physician to act as a resource allocator; he should never be made to say to his patient "I am sorry, society cannot afford this; the marginal cost of curing you is too much for our community to bear". He doubted the ethics of doctors involved in resource management and was convinced that such administrative tasks took them away from their clinical duties and distorted their clinical view. Dr Bion thought that resource management put the ball into the doctors' court in so far as physicians working in intensive care had to demonstrate that what they did actually worked and improved the survival of certain patients. He did not agree that doctors should do their best for the patients regardless of cost and regardless of consequences to the rest of society. Dr Linton ageed and described this as "medical ostrich behaviour". He also agreed entirely with Dr Epstein in terms of the basic philosophical approach, but the fact that the cost of health care clearly exceeded that which society was prepared to pay for, had to be accepted. Doctors had to act as responsible managers and divert resources into those subjects from which patients could benefit.

Dr Myers then led the discussion towards a definition of the history of acute renal failure that was haemodynamically mediated. He felt it was important to consider the natural history so that one might identify the critical point at which intervention would be effective. He used the cardiac surgical patient as an example of haemodynamically mediated acute renal failure and described three stages in the natural history of the condition; first, there was the initiation stage during which the insult took place. This was a very short stage in isolation, perhaps covering a period of 40–60 minutes. Dr Myers thought it was only possible to intervene in such cases if one was forewarned. Planned intervention was possible during the initiation phase in such cases as pre-planned high risk surgery and in patients receiving radiocontrast media in the presence of certain risk factors for acute renal failure. In the case of high risk surgery it seemed that the prevalence of acute renal failure had fallen from 35% (and death in 20% of all such persons) to less than 5%. This was clearly the best form of prophylaxis, intervention before the event that was going to cause the renal failure. Mannitol and saline volume expansion seemed to have worked well and other compounds might also be useful. The second stage of haemodynamically mediated acute renal failure was the maintenance phase, during which the injury has become established in the wake of the insult. Dr Myers thought that renal protection before the application of the insult could produce a very abbreviated form of renal injury in 50% of cases. Thus, whilst the injury produced an immediate steep drop in GFR to $10 \, \text{ml} \, \text{min}^{-1}$, the patient promptly entered a recovery phase and within a period of about 7 days, could have a GFR approaching normal. Dr Myers emphasized that this relatively benign course should not be confused with patients who become more seriously ill. The serum creatinine is usually unhelpful because it is a poor guide to the GFR. Dr Myers emphasized that measurement of the creatinine clearance in the intensive care unit was an important daily measurement. The timed collection of urine over a period of 2-4 hours in the early morning, at least 8 hours after the last administration of frusemide, was an important daily investigation. He felt it was possible to distinguish between protected acute renal failure which was usually non-oliguric in a patient compared with prolonged, severe acute renal failure reflecting poor myocardial function.

Dr Linton agreed with Dr Myers' analysis of the particular situation pertaining to the post-cardiovascular surgery patient but thought that the acute renal failure associated with sepsis was somewhat different in its clinical presentation. Dr Linton emphasized that the septic sheep model of acute renal failure had demonstrated quite convincingly that sodium retention in the presence of massive volume loading occurred as the GFR fell. Dr Schrier was convinced that these sheep were prerenal, but Dr Linton pointed out that this was a rather circuitous argument since Dr Schrier believed that they were prerenal simply because they were retaining sodium. By the usual clinical criteria these sheep were actually full of salt and water. Dr Linton proposed that acute renal failure associated with sepsis should be split off from the other forms of renal failure that were thought to be haemodynamically mediated. All discussants agreed that acute renal failure in the intensive care unit was a sort of rag bag of different conditions and indeed the pathophysiology might well be different in so many, and various settings. Dr Neild thought that there was close agreement between Doctors Linton and Schrier. Dr Neild thought that Dr Schrier was probably describing a kidney that was not being adequately perfused; or if the kidney was being perfused it was not sensing that it was being perfused. This abnormality, Dr Neild went on to say, emphasized the ignorance that surrounded the relationship between cardiac output, systemic blood pressure, arteriovascular filling and renal perfusion. All discussants agreed that what was needed was an adequate method for the measurement of renal plasma flow at the bed side. A number of discussants again pointed out the similarity between the acute renal failure associated with sepsis as described by Dr Linton, and functional renal failure as seen in patients with acute and chronic liver disease. Dr Neild suggested that abnormalities in renal oxygen delivery might be the primary stimulus in all these conditions for the reduction in sodium excretion. Dr Epstein did not like that idea, chiefly because some animal experiments had demonstrated that renal hypoxia, short of making the kidney necrotic, caused a diuresis.

Dr Epstein returned to the hepatorenal syndrome. He thought its consideration was important since the assessment of volume status was critical in such cases. He thought it extremely relevant that the introduction of the Levene shunt, which in some way restores the dislocation of the general circulation, can reverse the azotaemia of the hepatorenal syndrome. Thus it appears that selective renal vasoconstriction somehow responds not to local therapy, but to the correction of the underfilling of the arteriovascular compartment. He also observed that if one transplants a kidney from a patient with hepatorenal syndrome into a normal environment, it may function almost immediately. Dr Myers asked the participants about fluid resuscitation in patients with sepsis. How much fluid was enough and should this be given as crystalloid or colloid? He also asked whether there was a level of tissue oedema, which could be detrimental in terms of oxygen transport from capillaries into cells? No one could answer these questions, although a general discussion of the use of crystalloid and colloid followed. In general it was felt that oedema was essentially a bad sign in so far as ankle oedema probably occurred in a setting in which pulmonary and cerebral oedema were also present. Dr Epstein emphasized that from the clinical point of view it was too much fluid volume which caused embarrassment of the respiratory system. This volume tended to be extremely variable, being related in some way to the underlying pathology. In the presence of sepsis, pneumonia, pulmonary aspiration etc., only a small volume could cause quite severe pulmonary oedema. Dr Bihari concluded this discussion by saying that in general most intensive care physicians use both crystalloid and colloid to resuscitate patients in an attempt to give them an adequate volume load, whilst preventing a dramatic fall in the oncotic pressure.

The discussion then moved on to consider the role of controlled clinical trials in the assessment of various prophylactic regimens available in the management of acute renal failure. Both Dr Epstein and Dr Linton thought that all medical therapy had to be assessed on the basis of controlled clinical trials, whilst Dr Bihari doubted that it was possible to obtain positive results for a useful treatment in many of the groups of severely ill patients that were looked after in intensive care. He was concerned that if these patients were randomized into a controlled trial, then a useful treatment might be discarded because such a trial would have great difficulty in demonstrating efficacy. This had been the case with steroids, prostaglandin E and other compounds used in the intensive care unit. However, the consensus view was that controlled clinical trials were essential in order to demonstrate the effectiveness of the various prophylactic regimens available.

Dr Myers summarized the conclusions of the workshop up to this point. He thought that the discussants had agreed that protection before an insult was very successful in preventing acute renal failure in discrete settings. Saline or mannitol seemed to do this particular job quite well and there was really no need to introduce more exotic substances at the moment, since there had been a dramatic reduction in the incidence of acute renal failure in these settings. It was in the intensive care unit during the maintenance phase of acute tubular necrosis that most investigators felt that a controlled trial of some new agent should be undertaken. Obviously it was necessary to decide on a reasonable level of fluid repletion and this was both clinically and physiologically difficult to assess. At this stage Dr Epstein proposed the inclusion of prevention of infection as an important priority in the management of patients with acute renal failure in the intensive care unit. He thought that physicians had to go back and look carefully at such things as hand washing, unnecessary instrumentations and the role of H_2 antagonists in the prevention of stress ulceration. He thought that nosocomial infections in the ICU could be reduced by 20% and this on its own could improve survival. Dr Bihari was still not clear at what stage any one of the discussants would randomize a patient with acute renal failure into a controlled clinical trial. He doubted whether this could be done on the basis of urinary electrolytes alone. He described the difficulties he had experienced whilst participating in a controlled clinical trial of PGE_1 in the management of patients with the adult respiratory distress syndrome and he re-emphasized his dislike of controlled clinical trials in the ICU with their ever-present risk of a Type-II statistical error. He finished by stating that one of the most important messages he had got from the workshop was that episodes of hypotension associated with haemodialysis were extremely bad for the failed ATN kidney. This message, which depended upon a lack of autoregulation in the failed ATN kidney, was something to be taken away.

All other participants agreed with this view. In the absence of data to the contrary, the Chairman of the Workshop emphasized that the Renal Physician and Intensive Care Physician had to treat the patient with acute renal failure as if renal autoregulation had disappeared. In this setting, any technique that reduced the number of episodes of hypotension during treatment would be advantageous in overall care. Dr Schrier emphasized that the decreases in blood pressure need not be great, and whilst the dialysis nurse might be satisfied to accept a systolic blood pressure falling from 130 mmHg to 105 mmHg, this could be associated with significant reductions in renal blood flow.

Finally, Dr Bihari raised the problem of uraemic control. He thought that renal replacement therapy was just one part of intensive care that was required in a patient who developed multiple organ failure associated with the systemic effects of sepsis. Whilst he agreed that data demonstrating that a tight control of uraemia improved survival were somewhat scarce, he felt it was complacent to sit back and let the blood urea rise to more than 25 mmol l^{-1} and the serum creatinine to more than 300 µmol l^{-1}. He did not find convincing, nor acceptable, the argument that few if any, controlled clinical trials had clearly demonstrated improved survival in patients treated more aggressively. Dr Bihari's view was that much of the therapy given in the intensive care unit had not been shown to be of proven value using this methodology of the controlled clinical trial, and it was best to think of intensive care as a "package" which could be offered to a patient who got into difficulties. As far as the costs of intensive care were concerned, Dr Bihari felt that since the majority of the cost lay in providing the salaries of the nursing staff, it was inappropriate to be overly concerned about the cost of individual drugs, the filter used during haemofiltration or dialysis, the volume of haemofiltration fluid infused, the cost of parenteral nutrition, antibiotics, prostacyclin etc. It was much more appropriate to be concerned about the standard of medical and nursing care offered to patients who were admitted to an intensive care area. Cost containment could not go on at the bed side and in his view, it was more appropriate to limit the number of patients receiving intensive care in the first place on the basis of some clinical judgement concerning their likelihood of survival. All discussants agreed that in order to preserve the autonomy of the patient, the patient himself, or an elected surrogate, would have to participate in this decision-making process of whether or not to pursue active treatment. This was the appropriate path to follow.

In conclusion, the Chairman of the Workshop and the delegates voiced their appreciation of Fisons plc for sponsoring the Workshop, and in particular the delegates thanked Mr Phillip White for his superb organization and administration.

Subject Index

Abdominal aortic surgery 168, 223
Acetylcholine 57, 201, 299
Achlorhydria 22
Acinebacter 30
Acinetobacter 24, 25, 31
Acute interstitial nephritis (AIN) 160–1
Acute intrinsic renal failure (AIRF) 196–8
Acute renal failure (ARF)
    aetiology 13–16, 280
    after surgery 4
    antibiotic-induced 3
    associated complications 16
    background causes 35
    causes of death 14–15
    changing patterns 14
    correlation between structure and function 183
    definition 41, 193
    diagnosis 36, 42, 182
    differential diagnosis 193–9
    drug-induced. *See* Drug-induced ARF
    endotoxin-induced 121–2
    epidemiology. *See* Epidemiology
    established 42
    factors involved in induction and maintenance of 78
    from medical causes 3
    glycerol-induced 84
    haemodynamically mediated 381
    hospital-acquired 18–19
    in multiple organ failure 4, 12, 18, 42, 360–4
    preventive methods 370–5
    in old age 41–4
    in the rat 103–14
    incidence of 13, 280
    ischaemic 103–14, 119–21
    isolated 3
    management in ITU 193–214
    mortality 4, 13–16, 19, 23, 27
    myoglobinuric 215–18
    nephrotoxic 14, 115
    non-oliguric 205–6
    NSAID-induced 123
    oliguric 205–6
    overall incidence 19–20
    pathogenesis 116, 120, 199–203, 226–30
    pathophysiology 27–8, 47, 118
    postcardiac surgical 174–7
    postischaemic, following aortic or cardiac surgery 167–80
    postpartum 14
    post-renal 42
    prediction of outcome 7–9
    prerenal 42
    present status 35–9
    prevention 5–6
    prognosis 4, 42
    prophylactic treatment. *See* Prophylactic treatment
    role of polypharmacy 41
    sepsis in. *See* Sepsis
    survival costs 19–20
    symposia 35
    syndromes 160
    treatment 43
    Type A 169, 174–8
    Type B 169, 174–8
    types characterized by low urine sodium 36
    undefined type 15
    unexpected causes 162–3
    vascular factors in induction and maintenance of 77
    see also under specific conditions
Acute tubular necrosis (ATN) 13, 21, 22, 35–8, 77, 83, 84, 143–4, 182–4, 187, 188, 194–6, 279, 283, 285, 287, 295, 298, 300, 336, 384
Adenosine 96
ADP 244, 246–8
Adrenaline 237
Adult respiratory distress syndrome (ARDS) 364, 366, 368–71, 373
Age effects 15–16
    see also Acute renal failure (ARF), in old age
Albumin 163
Aldosterone 133
Allergic interstitial nephritis (AIN) 198–9
Allopurinol 161
Alveolar-arterial oxygen tension gradient 274

Amikacin 29, 44
Amino acids 43–4, 163, 352, 375
Aminoglycosides 3, 16, 29, 33, 44, 157–9, 296, 363
Amphotericin 162
Anaesthetic agents 162
Analgesics 18
Angiotensin II 55, 129, 133, 135, 145, 147
Angiotensin-converting enzyme (ACE) 27
Angiotensin-converting enzyme (ACE) inhibitors 4, 195–6
Anoxic injury 93–5
Antibiotics 16, 17, 29–30, 33, 161, 248, 352
Anticoagulation, role of prostacyclin 337–45
Antidiuretic hormone (ADH) 60–1, 137
Antihypertensive agents 296–7
Anti-inflammatory therapy 364
Antithrombin III 207
Aortic surgery, postischaemic renal injury following 167–80
APACHE II score 8, 269–75, 271, 317, 374
Arachidonic acid 244, 246
  derivatives of 97
  metabolism in the kidney 116–17
Arterial oxygen tension 274
Arteriolar constriction 200
Arteriolar dilatation 200
Aspirin 253
ATN-like syndrome 162
ATP 105–7, 109–12, 114, 203
  depletion of cellular stores 95
  hydrolysis of 96
ATP-MgCl$_2$ 299
Atrial natriuresis 62, 66
Atrial natriuretic factor (ANF) 141, 207, 213, 297–8
Atrial natriuretic peptide 136, 141
Atrial pressures 59–73
  and renal sodium and water excretion 61–2
Azathioprine 237, 238
Azotaemia 194–9

Backleak theory 202
Behavioural alterations 267
Beta blockers 294–5
Beta-lactam antibiotics 248
Bleeding 243–54
  therapeutic strategies 251–2
Blood flow, maldistribution 361
Blood pressure during cardiopulmonary bypass 230
Blood trauma during extra-corporeal circulation 230
Blood urea nitrogen 193
Bradykinin 299
Brain
  biochemical changes in uraemia 258–9
  damage 221
  pathology in ARF 259–60
  subcellular studies 259

Calcium channel antagonists 364
Calcium channel arrest 201, 203
Calcium channel blockers 5, 201, 207, 295–6
Candida 238
Captopril 294, 296, 297
Cardiac denervation 66–72
Cardiac surgery 223
  ARF following 224–6
  postischaemic renal injury following 167–80
  postoperative cardiac output values for optimal renal function 229–30
  postoperative cardiac performance 227–8
  postoperative renal function 226–7
  study protocol 169
Cardiac transplantation 235–41
  cardio-respiratory support 237
  immunosuppression 237–8
  microbiology 238
  neurology 238–9
  nutrition in 238
  outcome 239
  patients studied 236
  postoperative laboratory data 239
  renal failure 236–7
Cardiopulmonary bypass 225, 227
  blood pressure during 230
  cerebral consequences of 233
  haemolysis and activation of complement system during 230
  management to prevent renal dysfunction 228–9
  systemic vascular resistance following 233
Cardiovascular surgery 382
Catabolism 7
Catecholamines 134, 201
CAVH 7, 319–26, 331, 336, 353
  comparison of spontaneous and pumped 323
  computer monitoring 324–5
  metabolic control in 321–3
  performance of 320–1
CAVHD 7, 322–9, 336
Cefotaxime 30
Cell swelling 201
Cellular ischaemia 203
Central nervous system 255
  in acute renal failure 257
  in chronic renal failure 258
  parathyroid hormone as uraemic toxin 260–1
Cephalosporins 33, 161, 249
Cerebral function 267
Charcoal haemoperfusion 155
Chlorhexidine 30
Chronic renal failure, haemostasis defect in 243–8
Cimetidine 194
Cirrhosis 131
  peritubular physical forces 132
Citrobacter 24, 25
CLINFO system 170

Subject Index

Clinical scoring 8
Clometacin 16
Cognitive function 267
Collagen 246
Colloid 311
Coma, role of 9
Combined acute respiratory and renal failure (CARRF) 380–1
Computerized tomography 159
Congestive heart failure 195
Continuous arterio-venous haemofiltration. *See* CAVH
Continuous arterio-venous haemofiltration combined with continuous haemodialysis. *See* CAVHD
Continuous positive airways pressure (CPAP) 12, 372
Continuous veno-venous haemofiltration. *See* CVVH
Contrast media, nephrotoxicity 166
Contrast nephropathy 159–60
  clinical features 159
  incidence and risk factors 160
Cortical blood flow 79
Cortical glomerular blood flow 47–57
Creatinine 193, 194, 206, 228, 229, 236, 244, 282, 296, 316
Crush injury 215–21
  resuscitation of patients with 220–1
Crush syndrome, therapeutic consideration 218–19
Cryoprecipitate 251
CUPID (continuous ultrafiltration and continuous bicarbonate haemodialysis) 312–18, 322
CVVH 332–4
Cyclosporin 39, 57, 267, 298
  in cardiac transplantation 235–41
  nephrotoxicity 129
Cyclosporin A nephrotoxicity 122–3
Cysteinyl leukotrienes 145, 146, 148, 152–3
Cytochrome aa_3 (cytochrome C oxidase) 92–3
Cytochrome b 95

Desferrioxamine 298–9
Desmopressin (dDAVP) 251, 254
Dextran 163, 165
Dialysis 205, 243, 311
  dementia 255, 262
  disequilibrium syndrome 255, 261–2
  encephalopathy 262–3
Diclofenac 16
Diltiazem 295, 296
Dimethylthiourea 298–9
Disseminated intravascular coagulation (DIC) 26–7, 86, 249–50
Diuresis 219
Diuretic poisoning 44
Diuretics 14, 161, 205, 290–4
Dobutamine 237

Dopamine 5, 14, 205, 213, 214, 233, 237, 294, 308
Drug-induced ARF 16–18, 123, 157–66
Drug treatment 289–300
Drugs reported to cause alteration of renal function 288

Effective arterial blood volume 195
Eicosanoids 115–29, 145, 148–53, 155
Electroencephalograms 257, 267
Electrolyte balance 204
Electrolyte metabolism 218
Enalapril 296, 297
Endothelial function 245
Endothelial injury 39, 85–6
Endothelium-derived constricting factors (EDCF) 81
Endothelium-derived relaxant factor (EDRF) 80
Endotoxins 25–6, 147–8, 183, 187, 188
Enterobacter 24, 25
Enterobacter cloacae 30
Environmental factors 267
Epidemiology 24–5
  in France 13–22
Epinephrine 244, 248
Epoprostenol 338
Epoxyeicosatetraenoic acids (EETs) 97
Erythropoietin (rHuEPO) 247–8, 251
Escherichia coli 24–6, 183
Extracellular fluid space 201
Extracellular fluid volume 279
  clinical evaluation 283–4
  establishment and maintenance of 286–7
Extracellular fluid volume compartment 72

Factor VIII 341
Factor X 337
Factor XII 26
Fasciotomy 219
Fluid balance 372–5
Fluid management 283–4
Free fatty acids 349
Frusemide 5, 213, 214
Frustose-1, 6-diphosphate 299
Furosemide 94, 205, 206, 289, 290

Gastrointestinal bleeding, prevention of 21
Gentamicin 29, 44, 157, 298
Glafenin 16, 21
Glasgow Coma Scale 269
Glomerular basement membrane (GBM) 78
Glomerular filtration rate (GFR) 27, 43, 44, 78, 79, 82–5, 109, 115, 121, 123, 132–5, 144–8, 151, 153, 162, 163, 167, 170–8, 184, 187, 189, 193–6, 199, 206, 212, 256, 282, 286, 382
Glomerular haemodynamics 80–2

Glomerular membrane permeability 200
Glomerulonephritis 15, 198
Glycerol 298
Glycoproteins 253
Gram-negative organisms 241
Gram-negative septicaemia 25–31, 188
  pathophysiology 26–7
Gram-positive infections 23–4
Guanidinosuccinic acid 244

Haemaccel 50
Haemodialysis 312, 319–26
  haemostasis defect during 250
Haemodynamic monitoring 204
Haemofiltration 311, 319–26
Haemolytic-uraemic syndrome (HUS) 250, 252
Haemostasis defect
  during haemodialysis 250
  in acute renal failure 248
  in chronic renal failure 243–8
Hageman Factor (Factor XII) 26
Heart and heart-lung transplantation. *See* Cardiac transplantation
Heparin 338, 339
Hepatic dysfunction and renal function 131–41
Hepatic sinusoid 155
Hepatorenal syndrome (HRS) 135, 143–55, 184, 195, 383
  haemodynamic changes in 144–5
  measures failing to reverse 153
  mediators 147–53
  pathogenesis of 146
  prostenoid excretion during 150–2
  vasoactive substances in 145
12-HETE 116
15-HETE 116
Humoral natriuretic factor 136–7
Hydrochlorothiazide 161
Hydrocortisone 29
Hyperalimentation 288–9
Hypermetabolism, pathogensis of 348
Hypoxic pulmonary vasoconstriction (HPV) 364

Iatrogenic disease 274
Imipenem 33
Indomethacin 146
Infrarenal aortic clamping 170–1
Injury, metabolic responses 348–9
Insulin 349, 350
Insulin-like growth factor 1 12
Intellectual dysfunction 255
Intellectual impairment 263
Interleukin-1 (IL-1) 148, 367
Interstitial nephritis 15, 17, 22
Intravascular coagulation 85–6
Intravascular fluid volume 283

establishment and maintenance of 286–7
Inulin 176

Juxtaglomerular apparatus (JGA) 79
Juxtamedullary glomerular blood flow 47–57

Kallikrein-kinin system 135
6-keto $PGF_{1\alpha}$ 120, 152, 185
6-keto $PGI_{1\alpha}$ 150
Kidney replacement therapy. *See* Renal replacement therapy
Kinin-kallikrein system 145
Klebsiella 24–6

Leukotrienes 118, 152–3
Liver disease 27, 131
Liver failure 143, 147, 155
Lung function 368–9
Lung tissue 368–9

Mannitol 5, 205, 206, 213, 214, 219, 233, 289, 290
Medulla, role in ARF 91–102
Medullary blood flow 79–80
Medullary hypoxia 95–6
Medullary injury 98–9
Medullary ischaemia 98
Medullary thick ascending limb (mTAL)
  ischaemic injury 95
  role of ATP depletion 95
  selective anoxic injury 93–4
Mercuric chloride 297, 298
Mesangial cell contraction 81–2
Metabolic changes associated with ARF 350–1
Metabolic responses to injury and sepsis 348–9
Methylprednisolone 238
Mineral abnormalities 218
Mitochondrial cytochromes 92–3
Multiple organ failure. *See under* Acute renal failure (ARF)
Multivariate analysis 8
Muscle destruction 221
Myocardial function 213
  effects of mechanical ventilation 233
Myocardial ischaemia 103, 369
Myoglobin 161
Myoglobinuric renal failure 215–18

Natriuretic factor 135–7, 201
Nephrotoxicity, avoidance or minimization of 287–8
Nephrotoxins 284, 298
Netilmicin 29, 44
Nifedipine 295
Nitrendipine 50
Nitrogen administration 43

Subject Index

Nitrogen balance 351–2
Nitroprusside 162–3
N-methylthiotetrazole (NMTT) 249
Non-esterified fatty acid (NEFA)
    concentration 349, 351
Non-steroidal anti-inflammatory drugs
    (NSAIDs) 16–18, 28, 44, 123–4, 161,
    248, 249, 364, 370
Noradrenaline 212
Norepinephrine 135, 298, 299
Nutrition 204–5, 311
    in cardiac transplantation 238
    management in ARF 351–3
Nutritional support 372–5
    in critically ill patients 347–57
    monitoring 12

Open heart surgery 223–33
Ouabain 94
6-oxo-PGF$_{1\alpha}$ 129
Oxygen and calcium paradox 361
Oxygen supply 91–2

^{31}P NMR
    in detection of renal ischaemia 105–7
    in timing of onset of renal ischaemia in the
        rat 108–12
Papaverine 299
Para-aminohippurate (PAH) 169, 176, 180
Parathyroid hormone (PTH) 246, 260–1
Parathyroidectomy 260
Parenteral nutrition 163, 351
PEEP 12
Penicillin G 248
Penicillins 161
Phenols 244
Plasma renin activity 147, 173
Plasma renin concentration (PRC) 133
Plasma volume expansion 62–5
Platelet activating factor (PAF) 137–8
Platelet aggregation, ristocetin-mediated 253
Platelet defects 244
Platelet function 245
Platelet membrane 253
Polysaccharides 163
Postischaemic renal injury. *See* under Renal
    injury
Postrenal azotaemia 194
Potassium balance 219
Prednisolone 238
Prerenal azotaemia 36, 194–6, 204, 283
Prerenal failure 15, 82–3
Prophylactic treatment 279–309
    approach to patient at increased risk
        285–300
    drugs 289–300
    role of controlled clinical trials 383
    selection of patients 280–5

susceptible patients or patients at increased
    risk 284–5
Propranolol 294
Prostacyclin 144, 254, 318
    effects on cytokine release from activated
        monocyte/macrophage cell system 366
    effects on platelet and white cell function
        366
    effects on pulmonary function 368–9
    in anticoagulation and extracorporeal
        circuits 337–45
    in preventing multiple organ failure
        associated with sepsis 364–9
    vasodilatation with 365
Prostaglandins 97, 116, 117, 129, 134–5, 144,
    148–50, 196, 201, 206, 245–6, 297, 364,
    366, 383
    and sepsis 369–70
    cytoprotection with 367–8
    in acute renal failure 119–23
    renal actions of 118–19
    sites of synthesis and actions in the kidney
        118
    see also Prostacyclin
Prostanoids 146, 148
    excretion during development of HRS
        150–2
Proteus 24
Pseudomonas 31, 238
Pseudomonas aeruginosa 24, 25, 29, 30
Psychological testing 258
Pulmonary function 368–9
Pulmonary infection 22

Radiocontrast material 159
Reflectance coefficient 180
Renal blood flow (RBF) 77, 118, 122, 134,
    135, 144, 145, 162, 163, 196, 212, 229,
    308
    changes in response to injury 82–5
    control of 79–80
Renal failure 143
    see also Acute renal failure (ARF); Severe
        combined acute respiratory and renal
        failure (SCARRF)
Renal function
    and hepatic dysfunction 131–41
    drugs reported to cause alteration of 288
    initial evaluation of 281
    measurement of 281–3, 285–6
Renal hypoperfusion and glomerular filtration
    rate 28
Renal injury, postischaemic 167–80
Renal ischaemia 82–5
    detection by ^{31}P NMR 105–7
    timing onset of 108–12
Renal perfusion
    regional variations leading to established
        renal failure 83
    response to compromised 82–3

Renal plasma flow rates (RPF) 169, 170, 176
Renal protective dose 165
Renal replacement therapy 331-6
  advantages and disadvantages of techniques 334
  survey of medical, surgical or multidisciplinary ICUs 331-2
Renal vascular disorders 199
Renin-angiotensin system 118, 129, 144, 201, 256
  during induction of renal failure 82-4
Renin-angiotension-aldosterone axis 133
Renin-secretion ratio (RSR) 169, 173
Respiratory failure. *See* Severe combined acute respiratory and renal failure (SCARRF)
Rhabdomyolysis 160, 218, 221
  non-traumatic 161
Ristocetin 244
Ristocetin-mediated platelet aggregation 253

Sandoz IV 57
Scoring systems 269
Secretin 201, 299
Sepsis 5-7, 22, 181-9, 213, 241, 382
  animal model 184
  as major cause of death 23
  generalized 183-5
  management of 28-31
  metabolic responses 348-9
  microbiologist's view 23-33
  multiple organ failure associated with 360-4
  prophylaxis 30-1
  prostacyclin in prevention of multiple organ failure associated with 364-9
  prostaglandins in 369-70
  role of 9
  treatment of 6
Sepsis syndrome 241
Serratia 24, 25, 30, 31
Serum beta-2 microglobulin (B2MG) 313-14
Severe combined acute respiratory and renal failure (SCARRF) 359-85
Severity of illness, measurement of 269-75
Sodium balance 59-73, 83
Sodium excretion 196
Sodium retention 183
  in cirrhosis 132-8
Somatomedin C 12
Spironolactone 141
Staphylococcus aureus 24

Staphylococcus typhi 26
Steroids 364, 383
Stress syndromes 267
Sucralfate 6
Sulphinpyrazone 253
Suphonamides 161
Suprarenal aortic clamping 172-4
Sympathetic nervous system 134, 147

Temporary ischaemia 47-57
  methods 48-9
  results 49-50
Thrombin 244, 246
Thrombocytopenia 248
Thrombotic-thrombocytopenic purpura (TTP) 250, 252
Thromboxanes 116, 119-23, 129, 145, 148-52, 185, 201, 206, 297, 370
Thyroxine 298, 308
Total parenteral nutrition (TPN) 43, 353
Transport inhibitors 96-7
Trauma, multiple organ failure associated with 360-4
Trauma Score 269
Trimethoprim-sulphamethoxazole 194
Tubular obstruction 85, 202
Tumour necrosis factor (TNF) 148, 367

Ultrasound studies 282
Univariate analysis 9
Uraemic encephalopathy 255-67
  differential diagnosis 256-7
  incidence 256
Urea 244, 316
Ureidopenicillins 248
Urinary diagnostic indices 182

Vascular events 199-202
Vascular nephropathy 13, 15
Vasoconstriction mediators 201
Vasopressin 201
Verapamil 295
Volume receptor hypothesis 62
von Willebrand factor 245

Water balance 59-73
White wall syndrome 267